NUTRITION FOR LIVING

THIRD EDITION

Janet L. Christian

Janet L. Greger

University of Wisconsin-Madison

The Benjamin/Cummings Publishing Company, Inc.

Redwood City, California · Menlo Park, California · Reading, Massachusetts

New York · Don Mills, Ontario · Wokingham, U.K. · Amsterdam · Bonn

Sydney · Singapore · Tokyo · Madrid · San Juan

Sponsoring Editor: Pat Coryell
Development Editor: Lisa Donohoe
Associate Marketing Manager: Stacy Treco
Production Supervisors: Janet Vail, John Walker
Copy Editor: Melissa Andrews
Text and Cover Designer: Mark Ong
Illustrators: Joan Carol, Marilyn Hill, Rolin Graphics
Photo Researcher: Darcy Lanham
Composition and Film: York Graphic Services

Library of Congress Cataloging-in-Publication Data

Christian, Janet L.
  Nutrition for living/Janet L. Christian, Janet L. Greger.
    p. cm.
  Includes index.
  ISBN 0-8053-1002-9
  1. Nutrition. I. Greger, Janet L. II. Title.
QP141.C548 1991
613.2—dc20   90-25792
                                                      CIP

ABCDEFGHIJ-DO-9543210

Ordering Information
31002 Christian/Greger Text
31007 Assessment Pad
31013 Package (Text and Assessment Pad)

The Benjamin/Cummings Publishing Company, Inc.
390 Bridge Parkway
Redwood City, California 94065

To my husband Jack, who kept everything else together while I put words together; and to our son Jeff, now at his own creative endeavors.

Janet L. Christian

To all my students over the years; and, of course, to my parents and sister.

Janet L. Greger

Preface

This book is intended for students with little or no science background, enrolled in college introductory nutrition courses. Our goal in writing it is to present the science of nutrition in a lively and personal way. We want to help people focus on their own eating practices and evaluate their habits in keeping with guidelines that support good health. While intent on saying what nutrition can accomplish, we are equally straightforward about its limitations.

The basic organization of earlier editions of *Nutrition for Living* has been maintained; we have not changed the topics or the order in which they are covered. The scope of this book, though, has been broadened considerably to include topics that reflect the ever-changing study of nutrition.

Each chapter incorporates new scientific findings and nutrition recommendations that were released up to the time of the book's publication. For example, the 1989 *Recommended Dietary Allowances* are incorporated throughout the text, and the 1990 report *Nutrition During Pregnancy* substantially affected the content of Chapter 16. Even impending changes in nutrition labeling are mentioned in appropriate chapters, and the proposed Reference Daily Intakes (RDIs) and Daily Reference Values (DRVs) are provided in Appendix J.

Some chapters contain so much new material that they were almost completely rewritten; this is true for "Why You Eat What You Do," "Effects of Food Production and Processing on Nutrients," "Beyond Nutrients: What Else Is in Your Food?" and the entire life-cycle section. In response to current interests, we also developed certain topical themes more fully. Throughout this edition, you will find more information about vegetarian eating and about how nutrition and exercise together enhance good health.

Discussions in this text begin with nutrition and the human body, work through the individual nutrients and food safety, and end with a section dealing with life-cycle nutrition issues. Part One sets the stage for these topics by describing our understanding of how nutrition is important to health, by explaining and illustrating how we can assess our personal nutritional status, and by reviewing the basic anatomy and physiology of the gastrointestinal system.

Part Two presents the macronutrients, the building materials needed in large quantities by the body for energy production. The chapter "Energy

Sources and Uses" falls early in this section, following an opening chapter on water. This early position of the energy chapter provides useful background for the next chapters and also allows the flexibility to discuss weight control issues. The next three chapters—"Carbohydrates," "Lipids," and "Proteins"—make up most of the unit and discuss nutrient functions, distribution in the body, dietary sources, recommended levels of intake, health effects of deficiencies and excesses, evaluation of one's own nutritional status, and just enough about chemical structures to make all of that understandable.

Part Three on eating behaviors provides a change of pace and an opportunity to apply the technical material learned in Part Two to everyday life. The first chapter, "Why You Eat What You Do," spotlights the factors that influence our daily food choices. A favorite topic of students—body weight—is thoroughly discussed in the next chapter. Anorexia nervosa and bulimia are covered in a separate short chapter on eating disorders.

Part Four returns to the nutrients, with a comprehensive, up-to-date discussion of vitamins and minerals in the same detail as the macronutrient chapters. Part Five, *Food Safety: A Concern of the 90s,* speaks to the worries many people have that our food supply is exposing us to more hazards and providing us with fewer nutrients than it did before. We'll look at the effects of food processing on nutrients and consider whether we are likely to be at risk from food-borne microorganisms, environmental toxicants, naturally occurring toxicants, and additives.

The final unit, *Nutrition Through Your Life,* examines how nutritional needs change as we grow older. Each phase of life—from infancy through adulthood—requires special consideration regarding nutrition. Topics covered include breast-feeding versus bottle-feeding of infants, obesity in children, nutrition and behavior, and the importance of both nutrition and exercise in maintaining long-term health. Finally, we will see that our education in nutrition must be a continuing process.

We created this book to be flexible enough to meet the restrictions of almost any course calendar and the preferences of most instructors. It will continue to serve as a useful reference after the course is over. Although it is logical to cover the nutrient chapters before those on the life cycle, the other topics can be read in almost any sequence. For example, Chapter 9 ("Why You Eat What You Do") could be discussed at any time, and the weight control chapter, Chapter 10, could be covered elsewhere in the course. Similarly, the food science chapters in Part Five could easily be relocated as a unit or used independently.

Features of This Book

In the Third Edition, we enhanced the features that teachers and students have valued in the earlier editions. A new Critical Thinking feature will challenge your students further and be the basis for lively classroom discussion.

Critical Thinking Case Studies.   The important new attractions of the Third Edition are the Critical Thinking Case Studies. These concern nutrition topics that are controversial, timely, and have no easy answers: "Is Bottled Water Better?" "Fiber, Fiber Everywhere—So What?" and "Food Safety of Poultry: Whose Job?" These sections help students gain experience in making operational decisions (whether to eat a certain type of food, for example), even when current scientific knowledge is unable to support a clear-cut right answer.

To help students make decisions about such issues, each Critical Thinking exercise consists of four parts (1) *The Situation* provides a context for the facts. (2) The accuracy of the presented facts is examined in *Is the information accurate and relevant?* (3) Other important factors regarding the issue are discussed in *What else needs to be considered?* (4) *What do you think?* presents a series of viable options. The student is challenged to choose what action is most suitable for him or her.

Slice of Life.   By popular demand, Slice of Life returns to the Third Edition. These case study examples—both ordinary and extraordinary—bring to life the relevance of the information just presented. This feature helps students see how nutritional principles apply to themselves and the foods they typically eat.

Margin Glossary.   Important terms appear in red boldface type and are defined in the margins of the text, where the word first appears.

Assessment Exercises.   The twelve self-assessment sections encourage your students to see how their nutrient intake compares with recommended intakes. Some assessments are taken directly from the second edition of *Nutrition for Living,* while others are completely new or modified from past assessments. For example, a new assessment in the energy chapter uses formulas published in the 1989 RDAs to estimate daily energy needs, and a new assessment in the carbohydrate chapter invites students to estimate their dietary fiber intake, a topic of great current interest.

For the convenience of both teachers and students, an Assessment Pad is packaged free with this text at the option of the professor. This pad contains 4 copies of each assessment.

Nutrition for Living.   The Nutrition for Living sections offer advice about how to achieve better nutrition habits. They include suggestions regarding food planning, selection, and preparation methods that are consistent with current nutrition goals.

Supplementary Materials

A complete package of supplementary materials accompanies this text.

- The student **Study Guide,** written by Dr. Susan Nitzke of the University of Wisconsin-Madison. This helpful guide follows the organization of the textbook. Each chapter provides an overview of the equivalent text chapter, a suggested study plan, learning objectives, a detailed chapter outline, a section on helpful memory aids, self-testing exercises, and application exercises. The memory aids section includes suggestions for constructing one or more concept maps, which are diagrams that show important concepts and the relationship between them. This unique exercise will help the students organize their knowledge in such a way that they are more likely to retain it. Every chapter of the study guide ends with a sample concept map, a list of answers to the testing exercises, and sample answers to the application exercises.

• The **Instructor's Guide,** by Dr. Susan Nitzke. This guide includes chapter learning objectives, a brief outline of each chapter in the text, suggestions for how to use the new critical thinking case studies in the classroom, a list of additional classroom resources, and a testbank of multiple choice and short answer questions. Testbank questions are correlated with the learning objectives and are classified according to level of difficulty.

• **Computerized Testing Software.** All test questions in the Instructor's Guide are also available on The Benjamin/Cummings Microcomputer Testing Software, available for the IBM PC, AT, and XT, the Apple II family, and the Macintosh computers. This software is available for qualified adopters of *Nutrition for Living* by contacting the publisher or your local representative.

• **Color Transparencies.** A set of 50 transparency acetates of key illustrations and tables in the text will be available to qualified adopters of the text.

Acknowledgments

Each edition of this text has provided proof-positive that a book requires the cooperation of many people; we do, indeed, have a large number to thank.

At Benjamin/Cummings, we have appreciated the strong commitment to this project from the outset; it was extremely helpful to meet early on with the entire staff assigned to the book, plus General Manager Sally Elliott, to plan this edition. The members of the editorial team—Connie Spatz, Pat Coryell, and Lisa Donohoe—each have added their unique perspectives and insights to help in shaping this edition. Connie handled the important transition between editions and got the wheels in motion for this one before moving along to greater responsibilities. Pat, new to Benjamin/Cummings, arrived brimming with ideas, but also respected our convictions. Lisa brought her very successful experience from other projects to this one, and raised our consciousness about consumer interests . . . and parenting twins!

We thank designer Mark Ong for the clean and engaging appearance of the book and for carrying on the tradition of our text covers with this edition's luscious-looking pineapple. And thanks to Darcy Lanham whose colorful "photo finds" highlight the messages on these pages. Finally, we appreciate Janet Vail's and John Walker's effective orchestration and steady tempo through the complicated production process; their efforts brought all the disconnected notes, phrases, and themes together into a harmonious book.

Here at home, we thank our friend and colleague Susan Nitzke, the author of the Instructor's Guide and student Study Guide that accompany this text. In these ancillaries, she has utilized not only her extensive nutrition knowledge but also her expertise about how people learn. In addition, her stamp is on the text: As a leader in the use of critical thinking in nutrition education, she has been a valued resource as we developed the new Critical Thinking Case Studies; in fact, she has been a helpful soundingboard throughout our writing of the text.

Finally, we appreciate the many careful reviewers and consultants who scrutinized and commented on various portions of this book, contributing to its refinement; and we are indebted to all those instructors who shared their experiences with using previous editions. Their classrooms are reflected in the pages of this edition.

We warmly thank you all.

Reviewers and Consultants

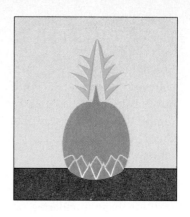

Paul Addis, University of Minnesota
Andrea Arguitt, Oklahoma State University
Rebecca A. Benedict, St. Olaf College
Nancy Betts, University of Nebraska
Laurel Jean Branen, Washington State University
Wen Chiu, Shoreline Community College
Maxine Cochran, William Penn College
Dorothy Coltrin, De Anza College
Marie Cross, University of Kansas
Lael Cutler, Northeastern University
Marjorie Dibble, Syracuse University
Susan Dougherty, Monroe Community College
Joan Downham, Normandale Community College
Bessie Fick, Auburn University
B. L. Frye, University of Texas
Sylvia Gartung, Michigan State University
Nancy Green, Florida State University
Yolanda Gutierrez, University of San Francisco
Ed Hart, Bridgewater State College
Wendy Hunt, American River College
Amy Ireson, College of San Mateo
Charlotte Juntunen, University of Minnesota, Duluth
Joan Karkeck, University of Washington
Janet King, University of California, Berkeley
Sondra King, Northern Illinois University
Judith Listman, Purdue University
Bo Lonnerdal, University of California, Davis
Sharleen Matter, University of Louisville
Sally McGill, Canada College
Glen McNeil, Arizona State University

Barbara Mitchell, University of Houston
Elizabeth Mills, Central Michigan University
Susan Nitzke, University of Wisconsin-Madison
Earl Nolenberger, Shippensburg University
Mary Ann Page, Dixie College
Ellen Parham, Northern Illinois University
Ellyn Satter, Jackson Clinic, Madison
Barbara Schneeman, University of California, Davis
Charles Seiger, Atlantic Community College
Jean Skinner, University of Tennessee
Anne Smith, University of Utah
Katherine Staples, North Dakota State University
Bernice Stewart, Prince George's Community College
Jon Story, Purdue University
Susan Strahs, California State University, Long Beach
Kathryn Sucher, San Jose State University
Barry Swanson, Washington State University
Steve Taylor, University of Wisconsin-Madison
Mary Ann Thompson, Waubonsee Community College
Linda Vaughan, Arizona State University
Jane Voichick, University of Wisconsin
Kathy Watson, Arizona Western College
Margaret West, Chicago State University
Billie Wood, Daytona Beach Community College
Kathy Yadrick, University of Southern Mississippi
Margaret Younathan, Louisiana State University

Brief Contents

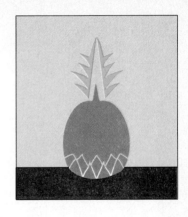

Detailed Contents

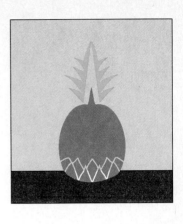

Topic Capsules

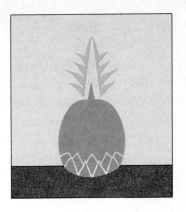

Each of the following Topic Capsules pertains to a subject that is treated, as appropriate, in several chapters in the book. Each capsule is an outline of all major points made on the topic through the book. Page numbers are show to the right.

Nutrition for the Athlete

The term *athlete,* as used in this text, applies to a person who trains for several hours daily to improve strength, agility, and/or stamina. Although the athlete needs exactly the same *kinds* of nutrients as the non-athlete, the *amounts* needed of certain nutrients may differ.

The athlete requires substantially more water to replace losses from perspiration.　97

Net loss of body water has a negative effect on physical performance.　98–99

Water lost during endurance activity should be replaced at the rate of 2 cups per pound of water-weight lost, or "replaced ahead."
98–99

Several hours are required from the time a person drinks fluid until the negative effect of dehydration on strength is relieved.　98

The athlete requires more kcalories.

Energy needs vary according to the type of activity, duration of activity, and the person's body weight.　115–118

The body simultaneously metabolizes fat and carbohydrate during exercise; proportions depend on the aerobic/anaerobic nature of the activity, its duration, state of training, typical diet composition, and scarcity of fat and/or carbohydrate.　135–138

Some experts believe that high carbohydrate intake is of greater benefit to the endurance athlete than larger amounts of the other energy nutrients because it promotes glycogen storage (carbohydrate loading) and longer endurance.　161–162

The athlete does not need large increases in protein. Although the exact protein needs of the athlete are not known with certainty, many experts believe that intakes between the athlete's RDA and twice the RDA are adequate and safe. Another guideline suggests getting 10–15% of kcalories from protein when weight is being maintained. Most North Americans consume this amount easily.　256–264

Although the need for some B vitamins increases slightly with high energy intakes, food sources can supply them; supplements are not needed.　403

Needs for most minerals are not significantly greater for the athlete, although there are a few concerns.

Iron status may warrant concern for some athletes; female athletes are more likely to become anemic.　448

Mineral losses in sweat do not usually need replacement unless water losses are substantial.
444–445

Nutritional supplements are not needed by most athletes, although they are heavily promoted by supplement manufacturers.   **601–603**

Athletic performance can be influenced by what is consumed a few hours beforehand.

A large pre-event meal should not be eaten sooner than three hours before intense activity, although a small meal is not likely to interfere with performance.   **79**

Ingestion of caffeine before exercising has been thought to prolong endurance, but more recently research puts this in doubt.   **521**

Extreme and/or rapid weight loss has negative effects for anybody, but there are some special concerns for athletes.

In women, low body fatness may lead to cessation of menstruation and, if sustained, eventually increased risk of osteoporosis.   **310, 436**

In wrestlers who use extreme measures to "make weight," performance may be negatively affected as a result of physiological stresses, and subsequent resting metabolic rate may be reduced.   **334, 602**

Vegetarian Diets

Vegetarian diets consist primarily or exclusively of foods of plant origin; they exclude some or all foods of animal origin. There are many vegetarian eating styles.   **232–236**

Lacto-ovo vegetarian diets, which include milk and eggs, are relatively easy to make nutritionally adequate. The Basic Food Guide can help with food choices.   **49, 233**

Vegan diets, which exclude all foods of animal origin, are more challenging to make adequate.   **233–236**

Vegan diets may require vitamin supplementation or deliberate intake of food containing vitamin B-12, vitamin D, and/or riboflavin.   **417–418**

Vegan diets require emphasis on foods that are good sources of the minerals calcium, iron, and zinc due to lower levels present in plant foods and generally lower bioavailability.   **429–430**

The Basic Food Guide can be used to help select an adequate vegan diet for most healthy adults.   **234**

Pregnant and lactating vegan women have higher needs for nutrients and must therefore select their diets carefully. In addition to the above nutritional concerns, they should also take care to get adequate quantity and quality of protein. Special Basic Food Guidelines have been developed for pregnant vegans.   **236, 548**

It is difficult for young children to be adequately nourished on a vegan diet; their needs for growth can better be met by a lacto-ovo vegetarian diet.   **236**

U.S. subgroups that are vegetarian tend to have different health characteristics than omnivores (people who eat food from *all* sources).   **170–171**

Vegetarians tend to weigh less than a matched group of omnivores.   **338**

Vegetarians are less likely to experience constipation than omnivores.   **168**

Vegetarians tend to have less heart disease and cancer than the general population; however, other lifestyle factors may be involved.   **169, 212**

Food Labeling

Federal regulations control what information is given on domestic food labels and how it is presented. To make information on labels more consistent with current interests, Congress passed a nutrition labeling bill in late 1990; but at the time this book went to press, final regulations had not been established. Therefore, this textbook edition features labeling practices of late 1990 and describes proposed changes. New regulations may take effect during the life of this edition.   **16**

The ingredient list on a food label tells what is in the product.

Foods for which there is a standard of identity in the Code of Federal Regulation do not require an ingredient list. (In the future, this is likely to change.)   **146, 528**

Ingredients must be listed in order of occurrence by weight, from the heaviest to the lightest.   **146**

A nutrition label (headed "NUTRITION INFORMATION") provides quantitative information about nutrients in one serving of the product.
14–16

A nutrition label is mandatory only if nutrients have been added or if a nutritional claim is made about the product. (In the future, nutrition labels are likely to be required on many more types of products.)   **16**

The top section of a nutrition label identifies serving size; number of servings in the whole container; kcalories per serving; grams of protein, carbohydrate, and fat per serving; and milligrams of sodium per serving. (In the future, the substances quantified here are likely to change.)   **14–17**

The lower section of a nutrition label identifies what percentage of the U.S. RDA is present per serving of food for these nutrients: protein, vitamin A, vitamin C, thiamin, riboflavin, niacin, calcium, iron, and sodium; certain others may be given as well. (In the future, the U.S. RDA is likely to be replaced by Reference Daily Intakes.)   **14–16 Apx. J**

You can calculate approximate amounts of micronutrients in labeled food products. **40, 41**

Atherosclerosis and Coronary Heart Disease

Atherosclerosis is a condition in which certain materials gradually accumulate in the lining of blood vessels, narrowing and hardening them. It often results in serious health problems such as stroke or cerebrovascular accident (CVA), heart attack or myocardial infarction (MI), or coronary heart disease (CHD). These conditions occur with greater frequency in association with certain *risk factors*.   **197–203**

Some uncontrollable factors increase risk, such as being male, aging, and having a family history of atherosclerosis.   **200**

Certain clinical findings help identify risk. These factors include high blood pressure; obesity (and even the distribution of excess body fat); abnormal blood lipids (high total blood cholesterol, high

LDL cholesterol, or low HDL cholesterol); abnormal electrocardiogram; and diabetes.
195–197, 200–203, 309

Certain living habits put a person at increased risk, such as smoking, excess energy intake, excess fat consumption, and physical inactivity.   **200**

Some risk factors can be reduced.

Several interventions may be useful for lowering high blood pressure: achieving and maintaining body weight within a desirable range; regulating intake of certain electrolytes; and taking medication, if indicated and as prescribed.   **443–444**

Several interventions have been suggested for lowering high total blood cholesterol. (Not all experts agree with these recommendations or on whether the general public should be advised to change their diets as a preventive measure.)   **203–211**

Achieve and maintain body weight within a desirable range.   **204**

Limit total dietary fat to 30% of kcalorie intake, limit intake of saturated fat and cholesterol, and consume some food sources of polyunsaturated and monounsaturated vegetable oil. **204–208**

Consume some fish each week.   **205–207**

Increase intake of soluble fiber.   **169**

Reducing risk factors may help reduce risk to some degree.   **209–211**

Cancer

Cancer, the second largest cause of death in the U.S., is a disease or group of diseases characterized by uncontrolled growth of body cells; it can take decades to develop.   **211–212**

The occurrence of cancer is thought to be influenced by genetic and environmental factors, including several nutrition-related factors.   **211–214**

A high-fat diet has been statistically associated with a higher incidence of some types of cancer in some studies but not in others.   **212–214**

Overfatness puts a person at greater risk of certain types of cancer.   **213–214**

Lower intake of foods containing vitamins A and C correlates with higher incidence of cancer.
392, 413, 525

A low-fiber diet is associated with higher incidence of cancer of the colon.   **168–169**

More studies are needed regarding the effect of selenium on cancer incidence.   **455**

Certain naturally occurring toxicants encourage cancer growth.

Toxins produced by molds   **527**

Alcohol   **639**

Substances in coffee need more study   **521, 524**

Certain food additives have been tested for association with cancer.

Ethylene dibromide (EDB)   **517–518**

Food colorings   **532**

Nitrates and nitrites   **524–525**

Polycyclic aromatic compounds   **525–526**

Saccharin   **531–532**

Some foods contain substances that may have a protective effect against cancer.   **214, 215, 392, 413, 503, 525**

Dietary guidelines have been published for reduction of risk of cancer development. (Not all experts agree with these recommendations.)   **214–216**

Eat a variety of foods.

Maintain a desirable weight.

Reduce intake of dietary fat to 30% of kcalories.

Increase the consumption of whole grain products.

Increase the consumption of fruits and vegetables, especially A and C and members of the cabbage family.

Be moderate in consumption of salt-cured, smoked, and charcoal-broiled foods.

Be moderate in consumption of alcoholic beverages.

Although the evidence suggests that what we eat during our lifetime influences the probability of developing certain kinds of cancer, ". . . it is not now possible, and may never be possible, to specify a diet that would protect everyone against all forms of cancer" (Committee on Diet, Nutrition, and Cancer, 1982).

Alcohol Consumption

The term *alcohol*, when used in this book, refers to ethyl alcohol as found in beer, wine, hard liquor, and other alcoholic beverages. Alcohol is a drug that has the nutrient characteristic of providing energy.   **636**

Alcoholic beverages are of low nutrient density, since they contain only low levels of a few nutrients while furnishing a significant number of kcalories.   **Basic Food Guide, Apx. E**

Ingestion of alcohol has short-range nutrition effects.

Alcohol is rapidly absorbed and used for energy or converted to fat.   **131**

Alcohol influences appetite and the body's handling of other foods variably, depending on the amount of alcohol consumed.   **603, 636–637**

Alcohol consumption promotes water loss.   **99**

Strategies can be used to moderate these effects.   **637–638**

Chronic ingestion of alcohol during pregnancy may result in fetal alcohol syndrome (FAS).   **551–552**

Chronic ingestion of alcohol has long-range association with several diseases.

Various liver diseases, anemia, cardiovascular problems, nervous system disorders, immunological problems, and cancers are more common among people who drink regularly in large amounts.   **638–639**

Certain vitamin deficiencies are more common among people who drink regularly in large amounts. These effects may be accentuated among teenage drinkers.   **402, 603, 638**

Moderate alcohol consumption appears to raise a certain fraction of high density lipoprotein (HDL), but it may not be the fraction that protects against heart disease.   **639**

Alcohol dependency develops in some people who consume alcohol.   **639–640**

Osteoporosis

Osteoporosis is a disease in which bone mass is gradually lost, weakening the skeleton. (Bone mass typically *increases* until some time in the fourth decade of life, after which it gradually begins to *decrease*.) Loss of bone mass is referred to as osteoporosis only if the decrease is severe enough to meet certain medical criteria.   **433, 436–437**

Much remains to be learned about what causes this multifactorial disease; however, a number of factors are statistically related to the development of osteoporosis. 436–437

Risk of osteoporosis increases with age. 436

Hormones appear to be a factor; four times more women than men have osteoporosis, and bone loss becomes more rapid after the menopause. 433–436

People who initially have less bone mass generally are at greater risk. 436

Too little or too much weight-bearing exercise increases risk. 436

Low calcium intake is not consistently related to increased risk of osteoporosis. 436

A variety of methods have been tried to slow down the loss of bone mass; each method may provide some benefit, but excesses of any method will have negative consequences. 436–437

Estrogen (female hormone) therapy has been shown to be effective for maintaining bone mass in postmenopausal women. 436

Weight-bearing exercise regimens may help maintain bone mass; but when women exercise to such an extreme that menstruation ceases, they may be more prone to osteoporosis. 436, 599

Increased calcium intake may help prevent bone loss.

Recent studies show that postmenopausal women who increase their calcium intake and take modest doses of estrogen maintain bone mass better than women who do neither or who only take calcium supplements. 436

Adequate calcium intake during the years when bone mass is still being accumulated may be more helpful in preventing osteoporosis than increased intake during the middle or older adult years. 437

Vitamin D, because of its influence on calcium metabolism, may play a role in helping prevent or treat osteoporosis; however, since many people have adequate vitamin D status, and since vitamin D is the most toxic of vitamins, caution should be used in regard to vitamin D supplementation. 396–398

Fluoride may play a role on prevention and/or treatment of osteoporosis; however, treatment with fluoride is experimental and the potential for toxicity is great. 453

International Nutrition Concerns

Food production capacity is dependent on availability of basic production resources and advanced technology. Nutrition problems in developing countries are complex, with agricultural conditions, transportation, size of population, national politics and economics, and religious and ethnic factors all influencing per capita availability of food. 270–283

The average number of kcalories available per person per day differs considerably from developing to developed countries. 278

The typical proportions of kcalories that come from the energy nutrients differ considerably from developing to developed countries.

Carbohydrate often accounts for well over 50% of kcalories in developing countries but less than that in developed countries. 170

Fat may sometimes be below the recommended intake levels in developing countries, whereas it is often too high in many developed countries. 217

Protein intakes are sometimes too low in the developing countries, and usually occur in conjunction with inadequate energy intake; whereas in the developed countries, protein intakes are usually generous. 251–253

The major nutritional problems in developing countries are protein energy malnutrition (PEM) (p. 251), and deficiencies of iron (p. 446), vitamin A (p. 390), and iodine (p. 449). Also seen are multiple vitamin deficiencies (p. 400), and deficiencies of zinc (p. 427–428, 451) and selenium (p. 454). **as shown**

Breast feeding is encouraged in the developing countries because it usually provides nutritional, immunological, and sanitary advantages, and because infants and young children are the most drastically affected by inadequate nutrition. However, seriously malnourished mothers may produce an inadequate supply of milk. 557, 562

Foods in developing countries often contain substances that decrease the bioavailability of nutrients (p. 427–428), and/or may be toxic, particularly to malnourished individuals (p. 501). **as shown**

YOU ARE WHAT YOU EAT

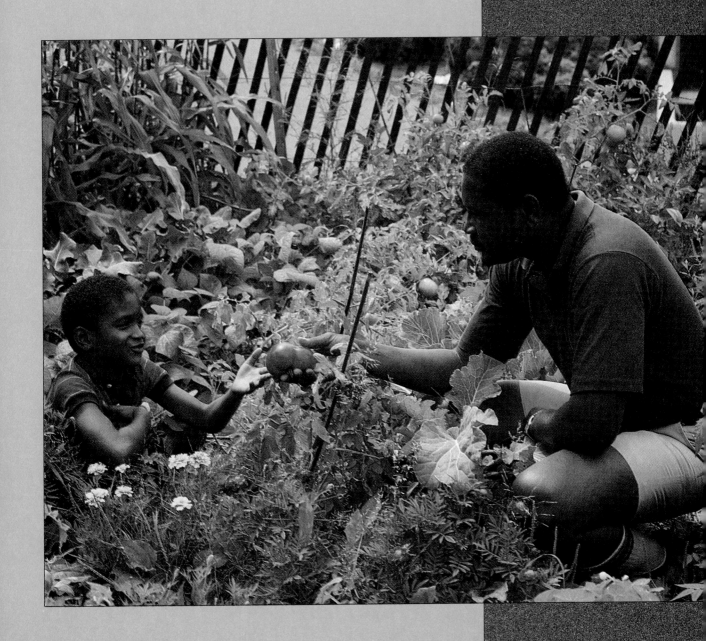

1

How Food Affects You

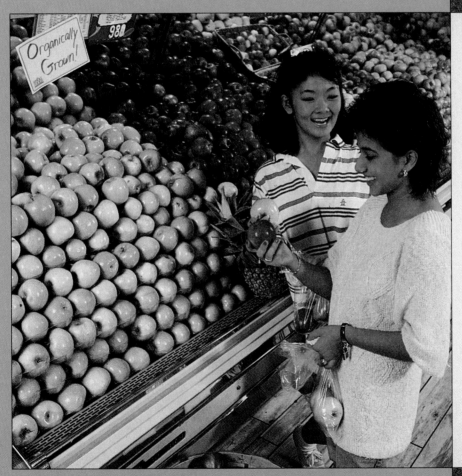

In This Chapter

- The Human Body Is Made of Elements That Must Be Obtained Mainly From Nutrients
- Nutrients Are Used for Three Basic Purposes
- Inadequate and Excessive Intakes of Nutrients Are Both Unhealthy
- The Effects of Nutrition Occur over Various Time Periods
- Different Types of Studies Document the Effects of Nutrition
- Good Nutrition Studies Require Careful Work

nutrition—the interactions between a living organism and
its food

T his is likely to be your first organized study of the science of nutrition.

Nevertheless, you have encountered a great deal of nutrition information already. Throughout your life, you have been gathering your own unique assortment of ideas and feelings about food and nutrition—simply by being a consumer, by participating in family, ethnic, and regional traditions, and by being exposed to advertising and information in the media. You have undoubtedly become convinced from such an ongoing blizzard of ideas (whether they are right or wrong) that food and nutrition are important to health and well-being.

We agree.

Nutrition has a broad scope: it includes all the interactions between a living organism and its food. Therefore, it involves physiological and biochemical processes, but is also affected by a myriad of psychological, social, economic, and technological factors.

Nutrition is so important that anthropologists who study the food habits of groups of people say that a society's patterns of choosing, obtaining, preparing, and serving its characteristic foods have a major influence in shaping its culture. Certainly, our food-related activities help to define us and our relationships to each other.

We will deal with such matters in various places throughout the book. But here, to begin, we are focusing on the importance of food for another reason—the nutrients it contains.

nutrient—a specific substance
that must be taken into the
body preformed and in sufficient quantity to meet the
body's needs

A **nutrient** is a substance in food that is used by the body for normal growth, reproduction, and maintenance of health. Nutrients are the basic materials from which the body is constructed and by which it is fueled and regulated.

Unfortunately, people in modern society do not instinctively eat foods that contain the nutrients they need. Human beings who have a more-than-adequate food supply must make choices from a spectrum of possibilities. We in North America have an especially wide selection, and each one of us has the responsibility for selecting foods that will provide adequate nourishment.

Deciding which foods are the most beneficial to eat is a challenge. If you have relied on the print and electronic media for nutrition information, you have probably found some contradictory views. How can you know which are true? (Figure 1.1.) For example, you may read different points of view on whether nutrition affects your moods or your ability to think. Or you may hear different suggestions about how the athlete should eat to enhance his or her performance. How can you sort out which information is valid and applicable to you?

We intend to speak to such concerns as the book proceeds. The way the information in this book may differ from some of what you read in the popular press is that we base our material on careful scientific investigation. Because research is time-consuming and expensive, there are still many gaps in the knowledge base; we will point out the limits of what is known.

We must also point out the limits of what nutrition can accomplish. Right

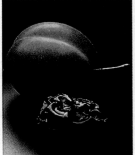

Some news about fiber you'll find easy to swallow.

You've heard a lot of news lately about fiber. How it's good for your health. How a high-fiber, low-fat diet may reduce the risk of some kinds of cancer.

Unfortunately, most high fiber foods just aren't very appetizing.

There is, however, a sweet way to get fiber. A bowl of prunes. Prunes have more dietary fiber, ounce-for-ounce, than almost any other food. A serving of six prunes has more fiber than two bowls of bran flakes.

The difference is, prunes are a spoonful of natural sweetness. Which means they're fiber you can actually enjoy.

And there's more. Prunes also give you potassium, vitamin A, no fat, no cholesterol, and almost no sodium.

So if you'd like to get more fiber in your diet, remember: Good nutrition doesn't have to put your taste buds to sleep.

Prunes. The high fiber fruit.

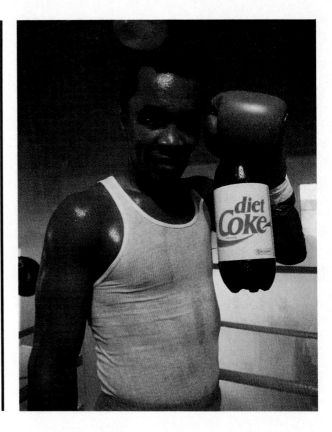

Figure 1.1 Nutrition ideas come from varied sources. What any individual knows about nutrition has been accumulated from different sources and is of variable quality. Some sources of information are much better than others, and the information in this book, which is based on scientific research, will help you sort out nutrition facts from wishful thinking or misleading pitches.

at the start, we acknowledge that nutrition, although it is needed for achieving and maintaining health, cannot by itself guarantee well-being. Other factors that influence health are the amount of exercise and sleep people get, whether they are genetically susceptible to disease, whether they smoke, whether they protect themselves from excessive environmental and psychological stresses, and whether they get good medical help when they need it. Important as these other aspects of living are, though, we will give them much less attention, since they are not the focus of this text.

This chapter explains more fully why nutrition is important. It describes what types of nutrients are needed by the body and what general roles they play. It points out the dangers of either deficiencies or excesses of nutrients, gives standards for recommended amounts of intake, and comments on how long it takes for nutrient effects to be noticed. The chapter concludes with a discussion of the kinds of studies that can provide valid information about nutrition.

The Human Body Is Made of Elements That Must Be Obtained Mainly from Nutrients

The basic components of which all things on the earth are constructed are the 105 elements, the most fundamental chemical substances known. When

Table 1.1 Classes of Essential Nutrients and Their Elemental Components

Water	Carbohydrates	Lipids	Proteins	Vitamins	Minerals
Oxygen	Oxygen	Oxygen	Oxygen	Oxygen	22 separate mineral elements
Hydrogen	Hydrogen	Hydrogen	Hydrogen	Hydrogen	
	Carbon	Carbon	Carbon	Carbon	
			Nitrogen	Nitrogen[a]	
			Sulfur[a]	Sulfur[a]	
				Cobalt[a]	

[a]Found in some but not all members of the class.

the human body is analyzed, 27 of these substances are usually identified, although many more are likely to be found in minute amounts if extremely sensitive testing methods are used.

Oxygen accounts for 65% of the body's weight, carbon for 18%, hydrogen for 10%, and nitrogen for 3%. The remaining 4% of the body's weight is contributed by all the other elements together.

Some elements can be used by the body only when they are consumed in chemically combined form (compounds). For example, hydrogen does nothing useful for the body if it is available in uncombined form as a gas, but the body readily makes use of various compounds that contain it. If hydrogen is combined with oxygen, carbon, and other elements into specific structures such as water, carbohydrates, fats, proteins, and vitamins, the body can incorporate the hydrogen. Therefore, the body's need is not for the hydrogen per se, but rather for certain compounds that contain it.

There are close to 50 specific substances that humans must take in preformed and in sufficient quantities to meet the body's needs; these essential materials are the nutrients. The nutrients are distinguished from thousands of nonessential substances that are found in food in that the nonessentials either can be produced within the body to meet its needs or are not needed by it.

The nutrients are grouped into six classes: *water, carbohydrates, lipids* (commonly called *fats*), *proteins, vitamins,* and *minerals.* Table 1.1 shows which elements they contain.

The classes of nutrients needed in the largest amounts are water, carbohydrates, lipids, and proteins; for this reason they are called *macronutrients.* Vitamins and minerals, which are needed in very small amounts, are *micronutrients.*

Nutrients Are Used for Three Basic Purposes

Nutrients have three functions in the body: (1) They constitute body structures, (2) they provide energy, and (3) they serve as regulators of body processes. This does not mean that a given nutrient can play only one role;

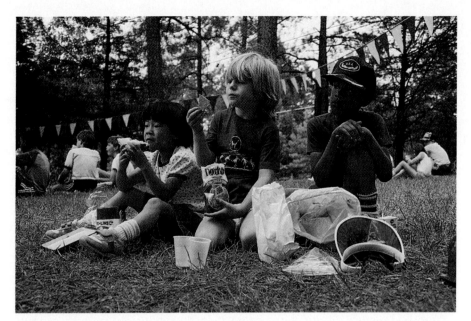

Figure 1.2 **You are what you eat . . . within limits.** The limits of your body's physical potential are determined by your genetic makeup; the degree to which you achieve that potential is substantially influenced by nutrition.

protein, for example, can be used in all three ways. At any given time, the proportions of body protein serving each function will depend on the body's total needs.

Structure

The cliche "You are what you eat" succinctly expresses the truth: your body consists of materials that were created from nutrients that you—or your mother when she was pregnant with you—consumed and biochemically reconstructed into your unique body substances.

This is not to say that you can completely determine what you become by what you eat. The limits of your body's physical potential are determined by your genetic makeup; the degree to which you achieve that potential is substantially influenced by nutrition (Figure 1.2).

For example, if your genes (the materials that determine hereditary characteristics) contain instructions for developing unusually long bones, you have a chance of being taller than others whose genes do not carry that information. But if you receive far less than the level of nutrients you should have as you grow, your chances for basketball stardom may be limited.

Similarly, if a baby is very seriously deprived of adequate nutrients during periods of rapid brain growth both before and after birth, brain size may be smaller than normal. For the body to be able to generate the full extent of well-organized tissues, organs, and systems for which it has the potential, it must have the appropriate level of raw materials.

The nutrient classes that contribute in a major way to body structure are water, proteins, lipids, and minerals.

Energy

Another vital function of nutrients is to provide energy. Without energy production, life ceases.

kilocalorie (kcalorie, kcal)—the amount of heat needed to raise the temperature of 1 kilogram of water 1 degree Celsius; a measure of energy

Energy is measured in a unit of heat called the **kilocalorie,** which will be abbreviated in this book as **kcalorie** or **kcal.** (The term *calorie* is in popular use, although this use is not technically correct, since a calorie is only 1/1000 as large as a kcalorie.) Most adults use between 1500 and 3000 kcalories in a day.

Carbohydrates, lipids, and proteins are nutrients that provide energy. These nutrients are available both from food and from your own body stores of these substances, as we will explain more thoroughly in Chapter 5 (on energy).

The energy nutrients do not provide equal numbers of kcalories. Carbohydrates and proteins each have the potential to produce 4 kcalories per gram, and fat produces 9. Alcohol, not usually classified as a nutrient, furnishes 7 kcalories per gram.

Your body generally functions better if energy is derived from more than one source. As we will discuss in Chapter 5, fat is utilized better if some carbohydrate is available simultaneously. This does not mean that it is best to take in equal amounts of carbohydrates, lipids, and proteins. Some distance athletes think that ingesting an increased proportion of carbohydrate (for example, getting 70% of their kcalories from carbohydrate) gives them greater endurance (Fig. 1.3). This will be discussed more thoroughly in Chapter 6.

Figure 1.3 Endurance and nutrition. Some distance athletes think that ingesting an increased proportion of carbohydrate gives them greater endurance.

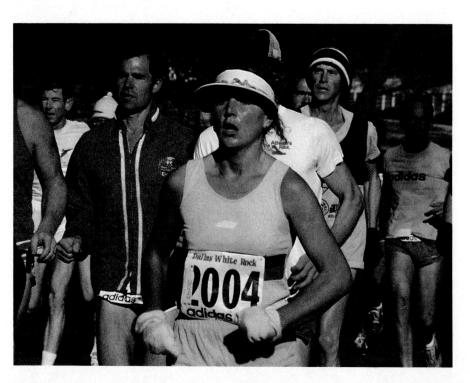

Regulation

The third important function that nutrients perform is regulation of body processes. The biochemical reactions that take place in a living system, which are cumulatively called **metabolism,** do not occur in random fashion; they are intricately controlled. Water, proteins, vitamins, and minerals are the chief regulators.

For example, many of the vitamins and minerals participate in the series of reactions that are needed to generate energy, although they themselves are not energy sources. If some of these nutrients are missing or inadequate, one of the effects will be that the body will not be as efficient a producer of energy and will therefore have poor work capacity and limited growth.

Certain essential minerals such as sodium and potassium also help regulate how water is distributed in the body; protein also performs this function.

Phosphorus and chloride influence the acidity or alkalinity (the opposite of acidity) of various body substances. This function is critical because a balance between acidity and alkalinity must be maintained in most of the body; departure from this balance in the blood can result in death. Normally, however, these mechanisms work so well that even though we take in foods and produce body substances of widely varying acidity and alkalinity, the balance in the blood is maintained.

metabolism—the biochemical reactions that take place in a living organism

Inadequate and Excessive Intakes of Nutrients Are Both Unhealthy

There is a beneficial range of intake for any nutrient; to go either below or above that range is usually undesirable, as shown in Figure 1.4. Both undernutrition and overnutrition are forms of **malnutrition.**

malnutrition—poor nutritional status resulting from intakes either above or below the beneficial range

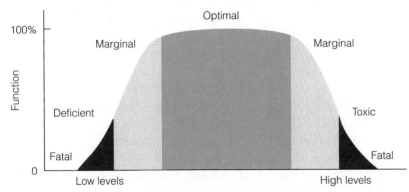

Figure 1.4 Effect of level of intake of a nutrient. Either too little or too much of a nutrient can interfere with growth and health. (Adapted from Mertz, W. 1983. The significance of trace elements for health. *Nutrition Today* 18(no.5):27. Reproduced with permission of *Nutrition Today* Magazine, P.O. Box 1829, Annapolis, MD 21404.)

Consequences of Inadequate Intake of Nutrients

If all or some of the nutrients are totally missing, the body will stop growing, fail to thrive, be more susceptible to infection, be incapable of reproduction, and eventually die. On the other hand, if all of the nutrients are present but are generally available in less-than-adequate amounts, the obvious consequences will be less severe: stunted growth is a likely result in children (Schelp et al., 1986) along with increased susceptibility to infection. The effect in adults is likely to be low body weight, poor work capacity, and increased susceptibility to infection.

If just one nutrient is restricted to low levels while the others are adequate, a more specific effect is likely to be apparent. For example, if your body did not get enough vitamin A over a period of years, you might begin to have reduced visual acuity at night (night blindness). Worse than that, eye damage (so serious as to eventually cause permanent blindness) could result in some situations. Although it would be unusual to see this severe a vitamin A deficiency in people in the developed countries, in the developing countries thousands of children become blind each year from this cause.

The chapters that deal with the nutrients will point out the consequences of severe, prolonged inadequate intake for each nutrient.

Consequences of Excessive Intake of Nutrients

Just as getting too little of a nutrient has damaging effects, a consistent and substantial overdose of a nutrient will have negative consequences as well. For example, if vitamin A is consumed in much higher-than-recommended amounts for a period of many months, toxicity symptoms including headache, nausea, and vomiting can occur. These high doses can result in elevated pressure of the fluid surrounding the central nervous system, sometimes causing the condition to be mistaken for a brain tumor. [See Chapter 12 (on vitamins).]

The dangers of excess nutrient intake have become more apparent in recent years. Because concentrated nutrients can be formulated inexpensively in the laboratory as pills, powders, or liquids, overdosing is possible if people use such products inappropriately (Figure 1.5). Although nutrient toxicities have resulted once in a great while from a person eating too much *food* that is high in a particular nutrient, nutrient overdoses are caused much more often by the indiscriminate use of nutritional *supplements.*

An example of the danger of supplement overdose involves vitamin B-6, a nutrient formerly thought to be safe at high levels of intake. Now we know that when vitamin B-6 is consumed for long periods of time in amounts that are hundreds or more times the recommended intake, nerve problems that make both large and small muscle control difficult can occur. Reports describe people who were no longer able to walk unassisted and office workers whose typing abilities were impaired.

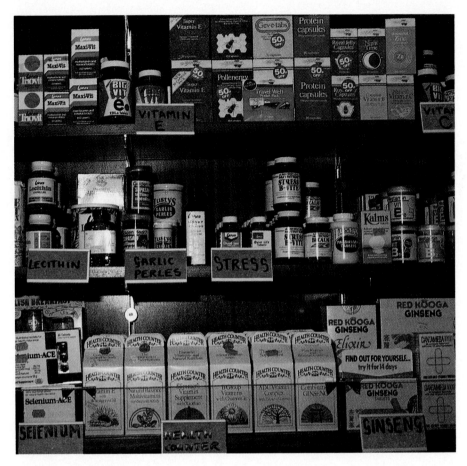

Figure 1.5 Nutritional supplements: boon or bane? Although concentrated nutritional supplements are useful in some circumstances, they also carry the potential for harm.

This is not to say that using vitamin supplements is always dangerous: there are situations in which they are very beneficial if used properly, as in infancy. In Chapter 12, we provide information on situations in which supplementation may be appropriate.

Nutrition Recommendations Suggest Healthy Levels of Intake

In the last half century, scientists around the world have conducted thousands of studies to ascertain what levels of nutrients should be consumed to meet nutritional needs. To make sense of this large body of research, various countries have assigned some of their top scientists to evaluate these findings and to make recommendations regarding nutrient intakes for their populations. Recommended levels of intake vary somewhat from one country to another; this occurs both because judgment of the scientific community plays a major role in establishing the recommended levels of intake and because differences in the types of foods available in various regions of the world can affect the extent to which nutrients can be utilized.

How can you know how much of the nutrients to consume daily? Two types of U.S. standards will be discussed in this section. Although these standards cannot be regarded as absolutes, they provide considerable guidance for achieving adequate and safe levels of intake.

Recommended Dietary Allowances (RDAs)

Recommended Dietary Allowances (RDAs)—daily nutrient intake recommendations established by the National Academy of Sciences

In the United States, the National Academy of Sciences (NAS) periodically appoints a committee to review recent research on nutrient needs. At the end of the evaluation, the committee prepares a report that is then thoroughly reviewed by other scientists. Following the reviewers' input, the NAS issues a new set of **Recommended Dietary Allowances (RDAs).** RDAs state the levels of nutrients that the scientists believe to be appropriate for daily intake by practically all healthy Americans, based on the most current evidence available. A table that summarizes the 1989 RDAs is inside the back cover and in Appendix A.

In Canada, a process similar to the development of the RDAs is undertaken by the Department of National Health and Welfare when they prepare their *Nutrition Recommendations.* The 1990 edition is in Appendix B.

gram (g)—metric unit of measure convenient for expressing macronutrient needs; 28 grams = approximately 1 ounce

Note that nutrients are measured in metric units; conversion factors for metric values and U.S. measures are shown in Appendix C. The macronutrients are expressed as **gram (g)** amounts; there are about 28 grams in an ounce. Most micronutrients are quantified in **milligrams (mg);** a milligram is a thousandth of a gram. The recommended intakes for some vitamins and minerals are so small that they are given in **micrograms (μg);** a microgram is a millionth of a gram.

milligram (mg), microgram (μg)—respectively, one-thousandth and one-millionth of a gram; used for expressing micronutrient needs

Research has shown that a person's actual level of need for any given nutrient can be influenced by sex, body size, growth, and reproductive status. Therefore, separate recommendations are made for various subgroups, defined by sex, age, pregnancy, and lactation.

There is also variability among individuals within any given subgroup. When the NAS establishes a recommended nutrient level, it usually makes it high enough to include the needs of practically all (98%) healthy people in that group. In addition, the recommendations are generous enough to allow for some loss of the nutrient as it makes its way through the body. For example, the RDA allows for losses such as those that occur during absorption or conversion from one chemical form to another, when some of the nutrient's activity may be decreased.

In addition to the nutrients for which RDAs have been established, recent editions of the RDA have included a number of Estimated Safe and Adequate Daily Dietary Intakes (ESADDI) of Selected Vitamins and Minerals. These are nutrients for which less data exist. The values are expressed in ranges, as shown in the summary table in Appendix A of this textbook.

The one set of values in the RDA that the NAS does not set high enough to meet the needs of almost all of the people in the category relates to energy intake as measured in kcalories. Recommendations for the number of kcalories have been established at an average level of need for each age group in order to discourage overconsumption. They are located in Table 5.2 in Chapter 5 (on energy).

The RDAs do not take into account the effects of illness or injury that raise the body's need for nutrients. People who are recovering from infection, surgery, and wounds (including burns) may need higher levels of nutrients; so may people who are taking certain medications. The RDAs apply to healthy people only.

A new edition of the RDAs was prepared for publication in 1985, but for the first time the NAS chose not to print the report the committee submitted. NAS President Frank Press gave as the reason "an impasse that resulted from . . . scientific differences of opinion" (Press, 1985). The debate that ensued calls into question the long-term future of the RDAs. Nonetheless, to get beyond the impasse of 1985, a subcommittee was eventually appointed to reconsider the report; with revision by the subcommittee, the tenth edition was finally released late in 1989.

Although many recommendations from the 1980 RDA were carried forward into the 1989 version of the RDA report, some changes were made. In general, the changes consisted of reductions of recommended levels, though there were notable exceptions. The recommendations for the minerals calcium and phosphorus were raised for people from ages 19–24; vitamin K and selenium were moved from the ESADDI table to the RDA table, reflecting an increase in confidence about what levels are most beneficial. Even at best, nutrient requirements have been established from data that are less than complete.

Guidelines to Prevent Toxicity of Vitamins and Minerals

Members of the general public and health care practitioners often wish that recommendations also could be made regarding what *upper limits* of micronutrient intake will protect against toxicity. We know that *some amount* in excess of the RDA can be consumed without risk, but *how much?*

It is difficult to answer this question, because this type of research often has not been done. Definitive research on toxicity in humans may be unethical to conduct and would surely be expensive. It would compete with more pressing nutritional issues for funding, so it seems unlikely that much of this type of research will be done in the near future. We therefore need to consider other sources of available information on which to base our thinking about toxicity of vitamins and minerals.

Much of the existing data come from instances in which people have overdosed themselves on micronutrients and, without realizing the source of the problems that followed, went to a health care professional who uncovered the cause. From such **case reports** (as well as from animal studies), we know that *certain nutrients are much more toxic than others*; for example,

case report or **case study**—a thorough evaluation of a carefully documented instance of one patient's illness.

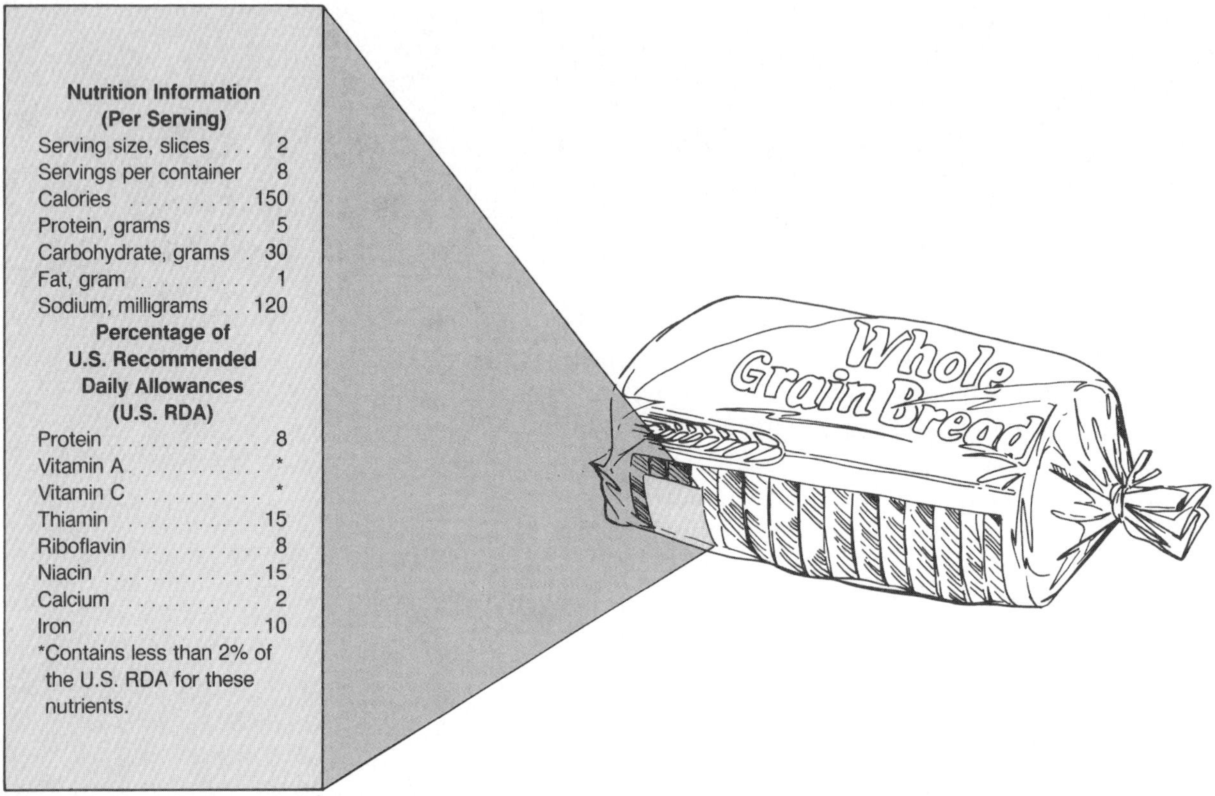

**Nutrition Information
(Per Serving)**

Serving size, slices . . . 2
Servings per container 8
Calories 150
Protein, grams 5
Carbohydrate, grams . 30
Fat, gram 1
Sodium, milligrams . . . 120

**Percentage of
U.S. Recommended
Daily Allowances
(U.S. RDA)**

Protein 8
Vitamin A . . . . *
Vitamin C . . . . *
Thiamin 15
Riboflavin 8
Niacin 15
Calcium 2
Iron 10
*Contains less than 2% of
the U.S. RDA for these
nutrients.

Figure 1.6 The U.S. RDA.
The U.S. RDA is a standard
that was developed for use
on food product labels to provide information about nutrient content and to allow comparisons between products.
This standard will be replaced
by Reference Daily Intakes
(RDIs) sometime in the early
1990s.

vitamins A and D have long been recognized for their ability to produce
adverse reactions at lower levels of excess than other vitamins. We have also
learned that toxicity symptoms may appear in some people, but not in others, at a given level of intake. Even the nature of the symptoms may vary
with the age and health of the people involved. For all these reasons, it
would be difficult to set individual upper limits and impossible to set a
general limit such as X-number-of-times-the-RDA for safe upper limits of
intake for all nutrients.

Despite all of these caveats about why "it can't be done," there are ways
of protecting against toxicity. In 1987, the American Medical Association's
Council on Scientific Affairs advised that people should not take supplements that exceed 150% of recommended levels; in 1989, the National Research Council recommended that people avoid taking dietary supplements
in excess of 100% of the RDA in any one day. The key point is that for the
normally healthy person, *there is no nutritional advantage to taking in more than
the RDA; more is not better.* But a modest supplement as described above,
added to the levels of micronutrients in the foods you eat, will not be so
excessive as to cause toxicity.

The best way to be confident that you will not experience toxicity is to eat
a varied diet (you will become acquainted with a plan for good overall nutrition called the Basic Food Guide in the next chapter), and forget about taking

Table 1.2 The U.S. Recommended Daily Allowance (U.S. RDA) as a Derivative of the Recommended Dietary Allowance (RDA)

Nutrient	RDA for Adult Man (1968)	RDA for Adult Woman (1968)	U.S. RDA for 4-Year-Olds through Adults
Nutrients that *must* appear on the label			
protein (higher quality) (g)[a]	—	—	45
protein (lower quality) (g)[a]	**65**	55	65
vitamin A (IU)[b]	**5000**	4000	5000
vitamin C (ascorbic acid) (mg)	**60**	55	60
thiamin (vitamin B-1) (mg)	1.4	1.0	1.5
riboflavin (vitamin B-2) (mg)	**1.7**	1.5	1.7
niacin (mg)	18	13	20
calcium (g)	0.8	0.8	1.0
iron (mg)	10	**18**	18
Nutrients that *may* appear on the label			
vitamin D (IU)[b]	—	—	400
vitamin E (IU)[b]	**30**	25	30
vitamin B-6 (mg)	**2.0**	2.0	2.0
folic acid (folacin) (mg)	**0.4**	0.4	0.4
vitamin B-12 (μg)	**6**	6	6
phosphorus (g)	0.8	0.8	1.0
iodine (μg)	120	100	150
magnesium (mg)	350	300	400
zinc (mg)	—	—	15
copper (mg)	—	—	2
biotin (mg)	—	—	0.3
pantothenic acid (mg)	—	—	10

The U.S. RDA was developed to be the standard for nutrition labeling. Based on the 1968 RDA (which was in use at that time), the U.S. RDA usually incorporates the highest RDA for each nutrient. (Note: there are differences between the 1968 RDA and the 1989 RDA.)

[a] Proteins found in food vary in their usefulness to humans. If a particular protein is very good for meeting people's needs, it is called a "high-quality protein," and the 45-gram standard is used. If the protein is of lower quality, the 65-gram standard is used.

[b] IU = International Units

supplements; as we mentioned earlier, concentrated nutritional supplements are generally the cause of nutrient toxicity when it occurs.

The U.S. Recommended Daily Allowances (U.S. RDA)

For a number of years, many food products have had nutrition information on their labels that refers to the "**U.S. RDA**" (Figure 1.6). *The U.S. RDA is different from the Recommended Dietary Allowances*, although it was derived from them. The U.S. RDA provides a standard that was designed for use in nutrition labeling, and the term applies to healthy people of various ages.

Table 1.2 shows the U.S. RDA. This standard was developed so that people would be able to see at a glance what relative levels of nutrients a serving

U.S. Recommended Daily Allowance (U.S. RDA)—standard used in nutrition labeling for a number of years; gives relative levels of nutrients in a serving of food; expressed as a percentage of a standard that includes the needs of almost all healthy people

of food contains, expressed as a percentage of the standard. The U.S. RDA standards were set to include the highest recommended level of intake for most nutrients on the RDA table for anybody from four years old through adulthood, except pregnant and lactating women.

Therefore, if a nutrition label states that a serving of canned corn provides 6% of the U.S. RDA for riboflavin, it means that four-year-olds through adults, except pregnant and lactating women, will get *at least* 6% of their RDA for riboflavin from a serving. The nutrition label must specify what serving size was analyzed.

U.S. RDAs can also be used to compare nutrient values between products. For example, labels show that a one-cup serving of canned peas provides approximately 10% of the U.S. RDA of protein, whereas an equal portion of canned carrots provides about 2%. On the other hand, the carrots have 600% of the U.S. RDA for vitamin A, and the peas have 15%.

Nutrition labeling is required on foods that have had nutrients added to them or whose labeling or advertising makes a claim about nutrition. For a number of years, many processors have voluntarily provided this information for other products as well.

In 1989 and 1990, extensive efforts were under way to bring about changes in nutrition labeling. Considerable interest was expressed in having nutrition labeling mandated for more types of foods. Government agencies, the food industry, and the general public suggested various improvements in content and format. These groups generally agreed that the information on labels should be easier to understand and more relevant to current nutrition and health concerns. Figure 1.7 shows the original label design and three alternative formats that have been suggested. As we go to press, an important proposal to update the standard used in nutrition labeling (currently the U.S. RDA) is also going through the process for change; the new standard is called the **Reference Daily Intakes (RDI)** (Appendix J). This standard differs from the U.S. RDA in two ways. It is based on the 1989 RDA and reflects a "weighted" average of the RDAs for various age groups so that the RDI represents the recommended intake of an average person in the population. It is possible that this new standard and a new label format will begin to appear on food products during the life of this book's third edition.

Reference Daily Intakes (RDI)— new standard proposed for nutrition labeling to replace U.S. RDAs; expressed as a percentage of a standard that reflects recommended intakes of an average person in the population

The Effects of Nutrition Occur Over Various Time Periods

There is tremendous variety in how long it takes for a nutrient—or the absence of a nutrient—to have an obvious effect on the body. The quickest effects can occur within minutes; at the other extreme, some effects take decades to develop.

ORIGINAL DESIGN

NUTRITIONAL INFORMATION
SERVING SIZE ....12 OZ.
SERVING PER BOX 1

PER SERVING
CALORIES 320
PROTEIN ....19 g
CARBOHYDRATES .... 39 g
FAT.. 10 g
SODIUM...................................... 700 mg

**PERCENTAGE OF U.S.
RECOMMENDED DAILY ALLOWANCES
PER SERVING**
PROTEIN.. 40%
VITAMIN A 5%
VITAMIN C 100%
VITAMIN B1.......................................30%
VITAMIN B2.......................................25%
NIACIN 20%
CALCIUM 5%
IRON..15%

* contains less than 2%

SUGGESTION A

Nutritional Information Per Serving

Serving Size ....12 OZ.
Servings per Container 1

Calories 320
Protein...19 g
Total Fat ....10 g
Saturated Fat ....4 g
Cholesterol ....10 mg
Sodium..700 mg

Fiber...1 g
Sugar...3 g

Percent of Daily Value

Protein...40%
Vitamin A 5%
Vitamin C...100%
Calcium..5%
Iron...15%

SUGGESTION B

NUTRIENTS PER 12 OZ. SERVING

320 Calories

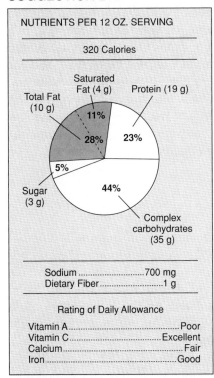

Sodium ....700 mg
Dietary Fiber...........................1 g

Rating of Daily Allowance

Vitamin A..Poor
Vitamin C...Excellent
Calcium...Fair
Iron..Good

SUGGESTION C

NUTRITION INFORMATION PER SERVING

Serving Size .... 12 ounces
Servings per Container.......... 1

Calories 320
Protein .... 19 grams
Carbohydrate
    Starch................................. 35 grams
    Sugar................................... 3 grams
    Total dietary fiber.............. 1 gram
Fat
    Total fat .... 10 grams
    Saturated fat..................... 4 grams
    Cholesterol .... 10 mg
Sodium.................................... 700 mg

PERCENTAGE OF DAILY VALUE

	0	25	50	75	100
Calories					
Protein					
Vitamin A					
Vitamin C					
Calcium					
Iron					

Figure 1.7 Proposed changes in nutrition labeling on food products. Consumers want information that addresses current nutrition and health concerns and is easy to understand. The original design and some suggested alternatives are shown here; all represent the same food product. By the time you use this book, one of these label styles—or, possibly, yet another—may be in use.

Short-Range Effects of Nutrition

Some effects of nutrition begin to take place within minutes or hours after a food or beverage is consumed. The way your body responds to your drinking something sugary, such as a carbonated beverage or lemonade, is an example of an almost immediate effect. If you consume the drink on an empty stomach, some of the sugar will appear in the bloodstream within minutes, and from there the sugar will move into your cells. You may even note that you feel more energetic as a result. But probably within an hour, depending on how much sugar you consumed and how active you were during the hour, you may feel hungry and tired.

Another example of rapid cause and effect is the way your body responds when it is deprived of water. A person who does not have access to drinking water will become thirsty and progressively more dehydrated—a condition that leads to headache, dizziness, confusion, and eventually unconsciousness and death, all within a few days. But if water becomes available soon enough, drinking it can quickly and dramatically reverse the symptoms of deprivation.

Intermediate-Range Effects of Nutrition

Some nutritional effects take weeks or months to manifest themselves. Generally, vitamin deficiencies and excesses fit into this category of effects that take an intermediate amount of time to become evident. For example, if you quit eating foods or drinking beverages that are sources of vitamin C, in a couple of months you may notice that your gums bleed slightly when you brush your teeth. The connection between low levels of vitamin C and the bleeding gums can be demonstrated by watching the gum condition improve in the days after vitamin C is put back into the diet.

Surplus kcalories show another intermediate-range effect: if a person regularly takes in excess amounts of the energy nutrients, in weeks or months those accumulated kcalories will become apparent as extra body fat.

Long-Range Effects of Nutrition

Some noticeable effects of nutrition take longer than months to appear. Links have been established, for example, between nutrition and the development of health problems such as heart disease and cancer, which take years—even decades—to become apparent. Because so much time intervenes and so many circumstances—called **risk factors**—apparently come into play in the development of these conditions, it is a great challenge to identify exactly how nutrition affects them.

When there are many risk factors that influence the development of a disease, it is referred to as **multifactorial.** Among the other factors that may

risk factor—a circumstance statistically associated with a particular disease

multifactorial—having many contributing factors or causes

be involved are inborn predisposition (genetically controlled likelihood of developing the disease), stress, detrimental substances in the environment, and level of exercise.

If nutrition is only partly responsible for a condition, then nutrition can play only a limited role in prevention. For example, if you have a strong genetic tendency to develop hypertension (high blood pressure), even if you take all the right dietary steps to try to prevent yourself from developing it, you probably will eventually develop hypertension anyway. In the meantime, however, you may at least delay its onset through your choice of diet. Similarly, if you do develop one of these conditions, diet can furnish only part of the treatment or control for it. Figure 1.8 illustrates the extent to which nutrient intervention is thought to be able to change the rate or course of certain diseases once they are in progress.

On the other hand, if you are *not* genetically predisposed to a certain disease, there is probably little need to concern yourself about risk factors for that disease; you're not likely to get it anyway. To extend the example above, if you have not inherited the tendency for your blood pressure to rise when you consume salt, you can use it with impunity and not worry about hypertension.

The only problem with this approach is that scientists currently don't know how to test for genetic predisposition for most diseases. It would be ideal if researchers could find easy-to-evaluate *biological markers* (such as a substance in blood or urine) that could serve as a reliable predictor of disease risk. By the turn of the century, some scientists expect to be able to "read" an individual's genetic code. This has exciting implications for predicting and treating inheritable diseases (McBean, 1990).

Unless and until such methods are accessible to most of the population, however, the public health establishment will encourage all people to try to reduce risk factors by modifying lifestyle factors, including diet. The possible benefits from reducing risk factors for heart disease and cancer are substantial, considering that deaths from these causes represent about two-thirds of all deaths in the United States (Surgeon General, 1988).

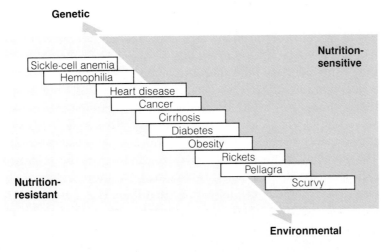

Figure 1.8 The influence of nutrition on some health conditions. Health conditions vary in the extent to which nutrition can influence them. You can estimate the relative effectiveness of nutrition in modifying these diseases if they already exist by noting how much of the bar is in color. (Adapted from Olson, R.E. 1978. Clinical nutrition—where human ecology and internal medicine meet. *Nutrition Today* 13(no.4):18–28. Reproduced with permission of *Nutrition Today* Magazine, P.O. Box 1829, Annapolis, MD 21404.)

Different Types of Studies Document the Effects of Nutrition

Generally speaking, research is conducted in one of two ways (National Research Council, 1989). In one method, investigators strictly *observe* situations that arise without intervening in them. The second general method involves *intervention:* scientists deliberately change conditions and measure the results. The latter is effective for proving cause and effect, whereas the former is usually not.

There are many scientific types of studies conducted in these two general ways. In this section, we will discuss several of the types of studies most commonly used for nutrition research, such as those used as the basis for the information in this book. We will also discuss which of these types of experiments are considered valid so that you can start to evaluate for yourself various claims about the effects of nutrition. The first, the epidemiological study, is of the observational type. The others are interventional.

Epidemiological Studies

epidemiological studies—
assessments of the health status of a large, defined group of people

Epidemiology is the study of disease as it occurs within populations. In **epidemiological studies** (also known as *ecological* or *correlation studies*), scientists assess the health status of a large, defined group of people, such as the population of a particular country or region. At the same time, the researchers observe the dietary patterns and other lifestyle features of the population. The people are not asked to change their diets in any way: the scientists simply record what is normally consumed. Then the researchers observe other populations that have different diets, recording their health status as well. They note which health factors and diets exist together.

For example, physicians practicing in Africa noticed that natives who ate high-fiber diets rarely developed appendicitis, bowel cancer, or heart disease but frequently contracted infectious diseases. On the other hand, Europeans living there had a different experience: they developed appendicitis, bowel cancer, and heart disease more frequently than the natives did but had much lower rates of infectious diseases. Their diets were different too: they contained less fiber than those of the Africans.

It is tempting to conclude that the level of fiber in the diets was responsible for the type of health problems these two groups of people experienced. However, *the coexistence of two conditions* (for example, a high-fiber diet and the incidence of infectious diseases) *does not prove that either causes the other.* The possibilities are that the two conditions may be present together by coincidence, that both may be caused by a third factor, or that one may cause the other; **one cannot *assume* that there is a cause and effect relationship between two coexisting conditions.** We cannot make this principle emphatic enough, since it is a common *mistake* for people to believe that *statistical correlation* means *causation.*

Even if there is a cause and effect relationship, other factors are also usually involved in the disease process. In this example, in addition to the different levels of fiber, the diets of the two groups also varied in levels of fat, protein, and other substances. Moreover, the activity levels and overall lifestyles of the two groups differed markedly.

The observations that come from epidemiological studies such as these nonetheless have great value, because they can raise important questions for further research. Scientists may form a hypothesis (theory) to try to explain what nutrition factors led to certain health consequences, which can then be tested by using other kinds of research methods. For example, many hypotheses regarding the relationship between fiber intake and health have been sparked by the epidemiological study just mentioned. We will discuss some of that research in later chapters.

Animal Studies

Laboratory animals can be fed controlled levels of nutrients or other food substances to determine causes and effects. This is a kind of information most epidemiological studies cannot provide. For animal studies, researchers design a set of diets in which the levels of the nutrient(s) or other food substances being studied are varied from one phase of the experiment to another or from one animal to another, while all other nutrient intakes are kept constant throughout. The researchers want to find out whether changes in the amount of the test substance(s) cause changes in the animals' body chemistry or in substances excreted in urine or feces (solid waste).

Animal metabolic studies have several advantages over human metabolic studies. The normal life span of a small laboratory animal such as a mouse, rat, or rabbit is just a fraction of a human's; therefore, an animal study that encompasses the whole life cycle can be done in a few years.

The fact that the animals are caged is another advantage because there is no possibility that they will consume other than the designated diet. In addition, it might be possible to feed the animals more extreme levels of nutrients than would be ethical to feed humans; seeing these effects may help scientists to forecast what might happen in people. Finally, since animals are usually sacrificed (killed) at the end of a study, a great deal of detailed information can be gained from postmortem examinations and chemical analyses of tissues and organs.

If the objective of an animal metabolic study is to yield information that could eventually contribute to knowledge of human nutrition, it is important to select a type of animal for the study that uses the test nutrient(s) in a way similar to the way people do. For example, vitamin C is an essential nutrient for humans, but rats do not need it in their diets because their own bodies produce it. Therefore, the guinea pig, which does require vitamin C, is a better choice for vitamin C research.

Animal studies yield a wealth of detailed information about the nutritional needs of *laboratory animals*. How much *human* nutrition information they provide depends on how carefully the study was designed and on appropriate interpretation of the results.

Human (Clinical) Studies

In human (clinical) studies, as in experiments with laboratory animals, careful chemical analyses are done. A major difference, however, is that in human studies the substances analyzed are unlikely to go beyond blood, urine, and feces. On the other hand, physical measurements such as blood pressure may be collected as well.

The scope of human metabolic or clinical studies may vary considerably. A study may involve as few as 8–12 subjects for a month or two, or it may involve up to thousands of subjects for years, depending on the objectives of the study. The *Slice of Life* on page 23 describes what it is like to be a subject in one type of small-scale metabolic study.

In the larger studies, fewer types of data are collected, and the collections are often at widely spaced intervals. The participants in smaller, shorter human studies are monitored daily for various biochemical changes, and often their food intake is rigidly controlled; therefore, subjects must be able and willing to tolerate food restriction for several weeks. Compliance is usually encouraged by paying the subjects for their cooperation.

Studies of this sort are sometimes used to establish levels of nutrient requirement by finding out how much of a nutrient the subject must get to stay "in balance"—that is, to have an intake of the nutrient equal to the need for the nutrient.

When researchers who conduct metabolic or clinical studies publish their results, they are careful to explain under what circumstances the findings were obtained. It is possible that the results might not have been the same if a different test diet or other conditions had been used.

Sometimes it is important to keep those involved in nutrition research from knowing who is receiving the test substance or during which phase of the study it is being administered. To accomplish this, a **placebo** (a food or pill made to look, taste, and smell like the test substance but without its effect) is given when the experimental treatment is not. Such studies are called **blind studies.**

In *single-blind studies,* only the subjects are kept unaware of whether the test substance is being administered. This is done for studies in which the subjects' expectations might influence test results. For example, if a study is being done to test the effect of caffeine on blood pressure, subjects should not know whether they received the caffeine or not, since blood pressure can be modified by psychological factors. The subjects' expectations may cause their blood pressure to rise or fall, which would confound the effects of the caffeine.

In *double-blind studies,* neither the subjects nor the researchers working directly with the subjects know who is receiving the test substance; this

placebo—a food or pill superficially identical to a substance being tested, but without its effect

blind studies—studies in which the subjects or the subjects and the researchers do not know who is receiving the test substance; the first type of study is a single-blind study, and the second is a double-blind study

eliminates the likelihood of bias on the part of the researchers as well. For example, if a test were being done on whether vitamin E supplements ease respiratory problems, and the person on the listening end of the stethoscope knew which subjects had received the vitamin, she might "hear" the person's breathing a little differently depending on her expectation. (Of course, somebody in charge of the study has to know who got what—but the information is not revealed until the study is over.)

Slice of Life

Being a Subject in a Clinical Study

As the alarm rings, Tom awakens with the realization that this is going to be an unusual day: it is *day one* of a clinical study regarding the mineral zinc, for which he has agreed to be a subject. He recalls the recent chain of events that led to his signing up: seeing the ad for subjects on a campus bulletin board, interviewing with the major professor and the graduate students who compose the research team, and being examined by the project's physician.

He shuts off the alarm and stretches, thinking about the ways in which his life will be different for the 51 days of the study. He will still live in his apartment, but he will get everything he eats and drinks from the kitchen of the research unit: 51 identical-looking and -tasting breakfasts, 51 identical lunches, and 51 identical dinners. Even the water he drinks must be from the study, since it must be distilled to get rid of the naturally occurring traces of minerals that would interfere with the study results.

He steps into the bathroom, realizing that even this activity will be different during the study. He will have to collect all body wastes in the containers given to the subjects.

During the weeks of study, Tom learns a great deal about himself, including his real relationship to food. At first he doesn't mind the repetitious menus and being restricted from eating other foods, but after about two weeks he realizes that he has the "blahs." He's tired of eating the same three meals a day—every day of the week—in the same place, and he'd like to leave town for a weekend. But the research team is depending on him to complete the study, and he wants to earn the full payment. Besides, he has come to enjoy the company of the other subjects and the "TLC" he gets from the researchers.

Finally, with just days to go, everybody is "counting down" the last meals and anticipating the party that will be held at the end of the study . . . with different food! And in the weeks to come, a gradual return to normalcy.

Tom's story demonstrates how totally accountable a subject in a clinical study needs to be regarding intake and output and provides an indication of the attention to detail that is characteristic of a properly planned and conducted study. Protocols for buying, preparing, portioning, and serving food are no less precise; the subsequent laboratory analysis, statistical handling, and writing of the papers for publication must be done with equal care.

Such efforts stand in sharp contrast to untested (or inadequately tested) nutrition claims. ▲

Molecular Biological Studies

molecular biology—area of science in which cellular metabolism is studied

Molecular biology involves the study of basic biological processes at the cellular and subcellular levels. Scientists in this rapidly growing field might, for example, study the differences between the ways normal human cells and cancerous cells metabolize nutrients, or they might even learn the ways nutrients gain entry into cells or cross membranes within cells.

These studies, which are conducted in a test tube or other laboratory systems, are referred to as *in vitro* studies (contrasted with *in vivo* studies, which involve studying effects within the living body). The new techniques of molecular biology allow greater precision than is attainable in in vivo studies and also make possible studies for which the technology has never before existed.

Molecular biology has much to offer to the nutritional sciences. However, this type of research will not replace the other types of studies; rather, it will help scientists complete the picture of how nutrition affects us.

Good Nutrition Studies Require Careful Work

Selecting the appropriate type of research method is not by itself enough to guarantee the validity of a study. Other factors are also characteristic of good work. The considerations discussed below will help you understand why scientists may be cautious in their comments about a newly published study.

Time Demands of Thorough Studies

Considerable time and effort are required to design, fund, operate, analyze, and publish valid nutrition studies. With all the steps involved, a "short" study may take anywhere from two to five years from the time a researcher conceives the idea for an experiment until the findings have been published. Studies in which the test period runs for several years take much longer in total.

Qualifications of Researchers and Nutrition Spokespersons

Ideally, researchers working in human nutrition should have earned *advanced degrees in human nutrition, medicine, or biochemistry from universities of good reputation.* Unfortunately, some "PhD" diplomas in nutrition are available by mail-order from unscrupulous groups for a price and do not denote authentic scientific training. Sometimes individuals with a PhD in literature, music, or some unrelated field claim to be nutrition experts also. This means the consumer can't automatically trust a person who claims to hold a degree.

Researchers must not only be qualified; it is also critical that people who communicate nutrition information to the general public have the appropriate background. These people include public health nutritionists, dietitians (preferably Registered Dietitians), and professionals in Cooperative Extension programs in every state.

As with research, there are some unqualified nutrition spokespersons, usually with meaningless certificates from "diploma mills," who are involved in individual counseling and/or product sales. Generally speaking, it is wise to be wary about nutrition information from nontraditional sources. People who sell nutrition products may be tempted to go beyond what is known by scientists about the effects of a substance: some overzealous or uninformed salespeople may present as facts ideas that are inadequately tested or are even wrong. It is as true about nutrition as it is with anything that what sounds too good to be true probably is. At times, skepticism may protect your health and, at the same time, save you from misspending your money (American Dietetic Association, 1988).

Reputation of Journals

A careful scientist will also be particular about having his or her research published in respected journals. Journals that are *refereed* are more likely to contain accurate information, because articles submitted to them are carefully critiqued by other experts in the field before they can be published. A list of refereed publications that carry nutrition research and review articles is given in Appendix D. Journals that do not use a rigorous review process are more likely to contain errors in study procedures and/or conclusions.

Reproducibility of Results

Even after publication the work is not immediately accepted. Only after thorough discussion by fellow scientists, and replication (repeating) of the same study elsewhere with similar results, does the new information become a part of mainstream thinking within the nutrition community. Of course, the time, expertise, equipment, and effort involved in conducting research costs money. Depending on where they do their work, scientists may have to secure funds from a variety of sources to pay for their projects. Researchers at a public university, for example, may receive some support from their institution; but they also may have to compete for grants from government agencies, industry, and/or private foundations in order to hire help, buy equipment and supplies, or even secure part of their own salaries. For this reason, it may take years for the scientific community to prove or disprove new theories and recommendations about nutrition.

Looking at the research picture as a whole, it is desirable that there be a balance of public and private funding sources, because the funding agency determines which projects they will support. Private funds have supported much worthwhile research that would otherwise have required tax dollars (or perhaps might not have been done at all). However, sufficient public funding is also critical for maintaining research programs that respond to broad general public interests.

Inadequacy of Anecdotal Reports

anecdotal report—a superficial description of an isolated case

One type of "evidence" that is not reliable is the **anecdotal report.** An anecdotal report is someone's personal testimony (in superficial terms) supporting a nutritional claim. For example, somebody might say, "I had a red, itchy rash on one leg for a couple of weeks, but after I took these nutritional supplements for a few days, it cleared up. This is wonderful stuff." Such personal experience can be interesting and is often dramatic, but it cannot prove anything about the relationship between the condition and nutrition.

Anecdotal "evidence" is sometimes given by celebrities who are deservedly respected for work in their own fields but who have little understanding of the science of nutrition. When these individuals promote various dietary products and services, you have no guarantee that the product is either safe or effective.

Anecdotal reports are different from case studies or case reports, which are often used in the medical literature to illustrate a particular condition and its treatment. In a case study, extensive scientific evidence is given regarding a particular patient's initial condition and the consequences of efforts to modify it. Well-documented though it may be, even the case report is not by itself sufficient evidence of a nutrition cause and effect relationship because it does not employ enough subjects or have adequate controls.

We put all this emphasis on the characteristics of good research to help you understand the difference between valid work and that which looks interesting and persuasive at first glance but which lacks scientific rigor. A study of this kind does not prove what it claims.

This chapter's *Critical Thinking* (following page) gives you the opportunity to consider what is likely to be right and wrong in a sample study.

Why is all of this important to know? We hope that it will help you to understand the difference in quality and reliability between science-based information and wishful thinking. It can also help you appreciate that since judgment is needed to interpret scientific data and to relate the results of studies to each other, there can be legitimate disagreement among scientists about the practical implications of study findings. The lively debates currently taking place on many nutrition issues attest that nutrition is a dynamic and healthy field of inquiry.

You can be confident that the information in this book is based on scientific experiment. For issues that are still under investigation and are therefore still open to debate, we will present the various points of view currently being aired, so you can make a tentative decision that will serve you until more conclusive evidence is available.

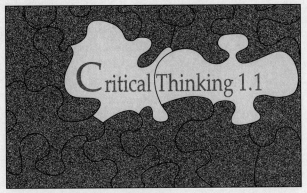

Is This Study Valid?

The situation

You are scanning the array of vitamin preparations in the nutritional supplement section of your grocery store, and you notice a stack of brochures entitled, "Vitamin X—An Aid to Physical Performance." You pick up a copy and drop it in your shopping cart.

At home, you sit down to read the brochure. It states that an independent testing lab studied the effects of "vitamin X" on healthy young men who ran the same two-mile course every day for three weeks. There were two groups of 10 men; the experimental group received the vitamin at the U.S. RDA level in a single dose every day, and the control group received a placebo. The study was double blind.

Every day, after each man had completed his run, he was asked for a *Rating of Perceived Exertion (RPE)* on a scale from 6 to 20, with 6 representing no effort and 20 for maximal effort. When the results were analyzed, 8 of 10 of the men who had received the vitamin supplement perceived their effort to be 3 points less at the end of a three-week study than it had been at the beginning, indicating that it felt easier to run the course.

Is the information accurate and relevant?

■ You can only assume that the data supplied by researchers was accurately reported; all re-

search depends on this trust. (When an occasional scientist is found to have fabricated or falsified data, it makes big news in the scientific community, and the person's career is summarily over.)

■ Rating of Perceived Exertion (RPE) is a self-awareness tool developed by sports psychologists and exercise physiologists (Morgan, 1981). When these subjective ratings are used in research, physiological measurements also usually are taken to provide objective data (Wilmore et al., 1986). In this brochure, however, only RPEs were reported.

What else needs to be considered?

An individual's RPE at a given moment is affected by complex physiological and psychological factors (Morgan, 1981). Certainly, such factors mutually *affect* physical performance, but RPE does not *measure* performance. There *are* tests that effectively measure performance; a simple one could have been to time the subjects' two-mile runs every day, after instructing them to run as fast as they could and still complete the course. Perhaps this was done, but if so, the brochure neglected to mention it.

Another important consideration: to evaluate the effect of any variable (in this case, "vitamin X") on physical performance, you need to separate the effect of the variable from other factors in the study. Here, you need to control for the fact that running daily will improve running performance over time and that it will improve it to the greatest extent in previously untrained individuals. Therefore, the two groups of men need to be carefully matched so that their initial *training states* are similar. It would be valuable to have two additional matched groups of men who did not run throughout the study; one group would take the vitamin, the other would not.

Focusing next on the nutrient, the brochure says only that the experimental group received a daily supplement containing the U.S. RDA for "nutrient X," but you do not know their intake of this substance from foods and beverages. Depend-

Continues

ing on their diets, it is possible that some of the men *not taking the supplement* could have consumed as much or more "nutrient X" as the men *receiving the supplement;* another possibility is that some of those not receiving the supplement and not getting much of it in their diets may have had a marginal deficiency of the nutrient. The levels of other nutrients could also have been important, since nutrients can substantially affect one another. None of these considerations were addressed.

The report of results was also lacking in information: how did the control group fare? We are told nothing about their results; they may have done worse, better, or the same as the experimental group.

On the back of the brochure is a statement that the complete study is available on request. The brochure was published by a manufacturer of nutritional supplements.

What do you think?

How useful is the information in the brochure?

- ■ Option 1   Trust the information as presented. Give the benefit of the doubt that all appropriate tests were done—but not reported in this brief brochure—and that the data support the stated outcome of better performance.
- ■ Option 2   Trust the information that seems well documented (which do you think is valid?) but not the rest.
- ■ Option 3   Reserve judgment. Send for the complete study and evaluate it on the basis of all available information.
- ■ Option 4   Be skeptical of this study, but consult trustworthy sources such as this nutrition text; or ask your instructor or a Registered Dietitian (RD) at a sports medicine clinic or hospital whether this nutrient is known to enhance physical performance.
- ■ Option 5   Disregard the study totally. No amount of additional information could validate this study.

What additional options or combinations of options do you see? Which do you think is correct?

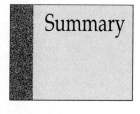

Summary

► **Nutrition** is the sum of all the interactions between an organism and the food it consumes. Foods contain **nutrients** and other substances, and each of us is responsible for selecting foods that will provide us with adequate nourishment. We are bombarded with information about what we should or should not eat, and learning to evaluate this information is an important goal.

► The human body is composed of elements that must be obtained primarily from nutrients. Some of these elements can be used by the body only if they are chemically combined with others. In our diets we require about 50 such essential substances, the **nutrients,** which can be grouped into six classes: **water, carbohydrates, lipids, proteins, vitamins,** and **minerals.** The first four classes are **macronutrients;** vitamins and minerals are **micronutrients.**

► Nutrients are used for three basic purposes. (1) They constitute body structures (such as bones and blood). (2) They provide energy, which is measured in **kilocalories.** (3) They help to regulate the body's biochemical reactions, collectively called **metabolism.**

► Both inadequate and excessive intakes of nutrients are unhealthy, and both result in **malnutrition.** The effects of malnutrition can be general or specific, depending on which nutrients and what level of deficiency or excess are involved.

▶ Standards of recommended intake called the **Recommended Dietary Allowances (RDAs)** have been established by the National Academy of Sciences. Since many factors influence nutrition needs, the recommendations vary for people of different sexes, ages, and reproductive statuses. The **U.S. Recommended Daily Allowances (U.S. RDAs) and Reference Daily Intakes (RDIs)** are derived from the RDAs and have been designed for use in food labeling. They give the relative levels of nutrients in a serving of food, expressed as a percentage of a standard that includes the needs of almost all healthy people.

▶ The effects of nutrition occur in various time frames, taking anywhere from a few minutes to many years to become apparent. Some of the long-range effects of nutrition are now thought to be among the factors involved in certain diseases of **multifactorial** origin for which there are multiple **risk factors.**

▶ **Epidemiological studies** address the health status of large groups of people, whereas **animal** and **human** (or clinical) **studies** usually involve more detailed assessments of the effects that occur when controlled levels of nutrients are given. Single- and double-**blind studies** and the use of **placebos** help to remove some of the possible sources of bias created by human expectations and other psychological factors. Experiments using animals must be designed and interpreted with care if they are to yield any meaningful information about human nutrition. Research in **molecular biology** can clarify the effects of nutrition at the cellular level. Personal testimony does *not* provide valid support for nutrition claims.

▶ Validated scientific studies are most likely to be conducted by qualified researchers, published in refereed journals, and replicated by other scientists before the conclusions become generally accepted. Good studies take years to complete, and since their interpretation requires judgment, there can be legitimate disagreement among experts about what the findings mean. These debates often spark future research that may eventually lead to clear answers.

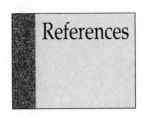

American Dietetic Association. 1988. Position of the American Dietetic Association: Identifying food and nutrition misinformation. *Journal of the American Dietetic Association* 88:1589–1591.

Council on Scientific Affairs. American Medical Association. 1987. Vitamin preparations as dietary supplements and as therapeutic agents. *Journal of the American Medical Association* 257:1929–1936.

McBean, L.D. 1990. Genetics and nutrition. *Dairy Council Digest* 61(no. 1):1–5.

Morgan, W.P. 1981. The 1980 C.H. McCloy research lecture: Psychophysiology of self-awareness during vigorous physical activity. *Research Quarterly for Exercise and Sport* 52:385–427.

National Research Council. 1989. *Diet and health.* Washington, DC: National Academy Press.

Press, F. 1985. Letter from Frank Press, NAS. *Journal of Nutrition Education* 17:191–192.

RDA Subcommittee. 1989. *Recommended dietary allowances.* Washington DC: National Academy Press.

Schelp, F.P., P. Pongpaew, N. Vudhivai, and S. Sornmani. 1986. Relationship of "weight for height" to "height for age"—a longitudinal study. *Nutrition Research* 6:369–373.

Scientific Review Committee. 1990. *Nutrition Recommendations.* Ottawa, Canada: Health and Welfare Canada.

Surgeon General. 1988. *The Surgeon General's report on nutrition and health.* Washington, DC: U.S. Department of Health and Human Services.

Wilmore, J.H., F.B. Roby, P.R. Stanforth, M.J. Buono, S.H. Constable, Y. Tsao, and B.J. Lowdon. 1986. Ratings of perceived exertion, heart rate, and power output in predicting maximal oxygen uptake during submaximal cycle ergometry. *The Physician and Sports Medicine* 14:133–143.

2

How Do You Rate Nutritionally?

In This Chapter

- Long-Term Extremes in Intake Are Unhealthy
- Body-based Measures of Nutritional Status Have Limitations for Ordinary Use
- Diet Analysis is Ordinarily Useful for Estimating Nutritional Status

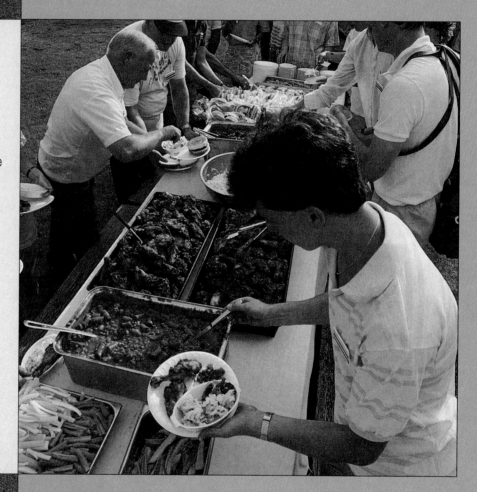

ow can you tell whether you are getting the right amounts of the essential nutrients to meet your needs? What kind of clues can alert you to inadequate or excessive intakes or reassure you that your consumption is on target?

There are many suggestions in the popular press about what conditions are caused by malnutrition. Are they accurate? For example, when you are continually tired, does this mean you have iron-deficiency anemia? If you have cracks at the corners of your mouth, are you vitamin deficient? If your skin has taken on a yellowish cast, could it be from eating too many carrots? Such questions will be answered in this chapter as various **nutritional assessment techniques** are discussed.

nutritional assessment techniques—methods of rating nutritional status

Before discussing those techniques, however, we will describe what happens in the body when a person consumes a nutrient at levels that deviate from the amount the person actually needs. This information is important background for understanding nutritional assessment.

Long-Term Extremes in Intake Are Unhealthy

Nobody gets exactly the amounts of nutrients that are needed each day. All of us typically deviate somewhat from optimal levels. Usually, a person alternates between brief periods of moderate underconsumption and overconsumption of nutrients. This is normal and is not known to damage health.

For example, if cheese sandwiches and milk have been the mainstay of your lunches recently, your intake of calcium may have been above what you need, since cheese and milk contain generous amounts of that mineral. If you change your menu to peanut butter sandwiches and orange juice for a few days, your intake of calcium may be less than optimal, but your intake of vitamin C may be higher.

Such short-term deviations can be handled easily by a healthy person, since the body stores at least some of the surplus nutrients it receives, and makes use of them later when intake is not as high. Even the nutrients that are the least storable or stable in the body, such as vitamin C and the B vitamins, won't be completely depleted as a result of just a couple of days of low intake.

Sometimes a person consistently *under*consumes a particular nutrient or group of nutrients for weeks or months at a time. The body's initial response is to mobilize the stored nutrient and circulate it via the bloodstream to where it is needed, as it does in the case of a temporary shortage. But when the inadequate intake continues, there is eventually a decrease in the level of the nutrient and sometimes other related compounds in the body's tissues, blood, and urine. There is no consistent order in which these events will occur; it varies from one nutrient to another.

When the blood levels have been very low for a time, some of the body's functions and structures begin to change, and the person starts to look and feel unhealthy. Death can result from severe, prolonged deficiency of energy, vitamins, and/or minerals.

In the United States, death directly from undernutrition is quite rare. Marginal undernutrition is more common, but it is very difficult to determine the extent of its effects on health and longevity.

Severe undernutrition *is* a common cause of death in the developing countries. There, tens of thousands of children die each day from hunger and related causes.

Now consider what happens when a person consistently *over*consumes a nutrient for a long period of time. Each nutrient has a slightly different ceiling, or saturation point, for storage in the body. Generally, only small amounts of nutrients that are soluble in water can be stored; large excesses of water-soluble substances or their metabolites (products of metabolism) are usually filtered out by the kidneys into the urine.

Originally it was thought that all water-soluble excesses were excreted and would cause no problems; more recent evidence, however, indicates that there are circumstances in which large excesses of water-soluble nutrients can have undesired effects on the body. For example, vitamin B-6 in repeated, large doses may cause nervous system malfunction in some people.

Some substances, notably the fat-soluble vitamins A and D, can accumulate to much higher levels than the water-soluble nutrients can. If overconsumed for long periods, vitamins A and D can eventually increase in tissues to a toxic (damaging) level that causes a person to look and feel sick. Some serious permanent effects have occurred from such overdosing.

Moderately excessive intake of some nutrients may be detrimental as well. For example, excess sodium intake can result in the development of hypertension in people who are genetically sensitive to salt. Excessive intake of the energy nutrients will cause overweight and may contribute to the development of heart disease or cancer in people genetically predisposed to those conditions.

To summarize the effects of long-term malnutrition: deficiencies or excesses influence the levels of nutrients and their metabolites in tissues, blood, and/or urine before they affect a person's appearance or sense of well-being. The entire process may take anywhere from months to several years, depending on the specific nutrient(s) involved.

Even with what is known about the effects of malnutrition, it is not easy to get an exact and comprehensive evaluation of what nutrients are present in the body at a given time. Two general types of methods are used to assess nutritional status. With the first type, the body itself is evaluated to determine what level of a given nutrient or its metabolites is present. With the second type, the diet is examined: the amounts of nutrients consumed are compared to a standard for adequate intake. Since you can use the dietary techniques by yourself without professional help or special equipment, these are the methods we will emphasize throughout the book.

Body-based Measures of Nutritional Status Have Limitations for Ordinary Use

In the following sections, body-based means of measuring nutritional status are discussed; those that yield more specific data are mentioned first and those that furnish less precise information later.

Biochemical Tests

Biochemical tests involve chemical analysis of substances from the body. Blood and urine are the materials most often analyzed.

biochemical tests—chemical analyses of body substances such as blood or urine

Blood Tests   Blood tests are techniques for professional use only. The skin and an underlying blood vessel are pierced to collect a blood sample, which is analyzed to determine whether certain nutrients and their metabolites are within normal ranges. For example, physicians often have several analyses conducted on blood samples that indicate whether an individual is anemic. The anemia may be due to iron deficiency. Even though some of these techniques show what levels of nutritional substances are circulating, they do not necessarily indicate how much is present elsewhere in the body.

Abnormal levels of nutrients in the blood do not always mean that something is wrong with the person's diet: an illness could be the real culprit, causing the nutrients to be handled in an abnormal way. For example, a high level of blood sugar (glucose) could mean that a person has recently consumed a large amount of sugar, or it might mean that the individual's body is incapable of handling even a moderate sugar intake in a normal way, due to a disease such as diabetes mellitus.

Because blood tests are also very helpful for diagnosing and monitoring disease conditions, they have become a fairly routine part of general health checkups and hospitalizations, as well as nutritional status surveys. It is surprising how many people (adults as well as children!) resist these procedures, but the wealth of information they yield to aid in a person's health care makes them extremely valuable.

Urine Tests   Chemical analysis of urine also involves laboratory procedures that require skill. Like blood tests, urine tests can reveal whether the levels of some nutrients and/or their metabolites are within normal ranges, giving clues to nutritional status or the presence of disease. This technique is commonly used in general health checkups, hospitalizations, and nutritional status surveys.

Anthropometric Tests

Anthropometric tests involve taking various external measurements and comparing them with population standards; such assessments provide in-

anthropometric tests—external measurements of the body such as height, weight, and skinfold thickness

formation about overall nutritional status and are less specific than the biochemical tests. The most commonly used anthropometric tests are described here.

Height and Weight Measurements of height and weight have some value for nutritional assessment. Remember that although growth is influenced by your intake, genetics sets the limit on how tall you potentially can become. Nutrition helps determine how far you grow toward that limit.

In children, measures of both height and weight can provide a rough evaluation of general nutritional status, particularly of energy intake and output. In adults, weight changes usually testify either to *fluctuation in body water, body fat, muscle mass,* or even *bone mass* (Frisancho, 1988).

Height/weight tables are the standards to which an individual's measurements are compared. They appear in Chapter 10 (on body weight), where their limitations are also discussed.

skinfold calipers—device to measure thickness of skin and underlying fat

Skinfold Thickness Judgments about past energy intake and expenditure can also be made when an experienced professional measures the thickness of the skin and underlying fat layer at various body sites using special **skinfold calipers** (Figure 2.1). If many more kcalories have been eaten than expended over a period of time, the fat layer will be thicker than before. Conversely, if a person used more energy than was consumed during past weeks or months, the fat layer will be measurably thinner.

Tables based on large numbers of people have been developed to show typical fat thicknesses at various body sites. Any individual's measurements can be compared to the tables to determine body fatness relative to the reference group.

Such measurements are useful for assessing changes in fatness. Chapter

Figure 2.1 Using skinfold calipers to measure body fatness. One way of determining how much body fat a person has is to measure the fat that has accumulated under the skin in various locations on the body. This figure illustrates just two of many possible locations at which the skinfold can be measured.

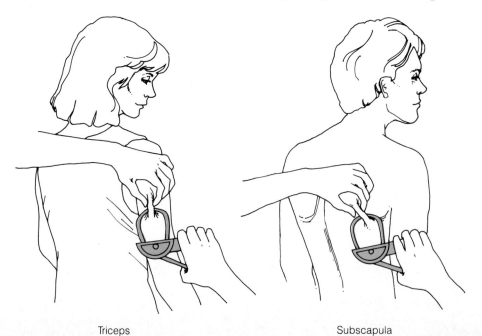

Triceps   Subscapula

10 describes why it is difficult to make accurate determinations of absolute levels or percentages of body fat by using this method.

Appearance and Sense of Well-Being

Of the methods of nutritional assessment, appearance and sense of well-being are the least specific. Nonetheless, they indicate that a problem exists, and they may provide useful clues to further testing.

Appearance   Changes in appearance are sometimes used as a rough means of assessing nutrition status. Table 2.1 shows some typical outward signs that often accompany severe, long-term malnutrition.

   Since looking for these changes requires no special equipment, you might think that this would be a good method of assessment to use for yourself. However, because even trained health professionals do not always identify malnutrition or its cause correctly when using it, this method is not reliable by itself.

Table 2.1 A Few Signs of Nutritional Problems . . . or Something Else?[a]

Noticeable Sign	Possible Nutrient Involvement(s)	Possible Other Explanation(s)
Dry, scaling skin	Deficiency of vitamin A, zinc, protein, or essential fatty acid	Chapping from cold or wind
		Sunburn
	Excess of vitamin A	Chemical irritation, e.g., detergents
Increased yellow pigmentation of skin	Excess of carotene, a compound in carrots and other vegetables and fruits that becomes vitamin A (otherwise harmless condition)	Liver disease (serious health problem)
Swollen, bleeding gums	Deficiency of vitamin C	Poor dental hygiene
		Particular medication
Swelling of feet and ankles due to fluid retention (edema)	Deficiency of thiamin or protein	Pregnancy
		Hot weather
		Standing for long periods
		Some medications
		Cardiovascular problems
		Kidney disease
Cracks in lips and at corners of mouth (cheilosis)	Deficiency of riboflavin, multiple B vitamins, or protein	Cold, windy weather
		Repeated wetting or rubbing of lips
		Viral infections
Obesity	Excessive kcalorie intake in relation to energy output	Possible hormone imbalance in rare cases

[a]References: McLaren, D.S. 1988. Clinical manifestations of nutritional disorders. In *Modern Nutrition in Health and Disease*, eds. M.E. Shils and V.R. Young. Philadelphia: Lea & Febiger; and Heymsfield, S.B. and P.J. Williams. 1988. Nutritional assessment by clinical and biochemical methods. In *Modern Nutrition in Health and Disease*, as above. Some data drawn from Weinsier, R.L. and C.E. Butterworth, 1981. Handbook of Clinical Nutrition. St. Louis: The C.V. Mosby Company.

There is another reason that assessing appearance is not very useful: few people in the United States, especially in the young adult population, experience malnutrition severe enough to result in obvious external changes. If you have one of the signs, it has more likely resulted from some cause other than nutrition. Notice the alternative explanations for some external symptoms in Table 2.1.

North Americans who might be undernourished enough to show such signs are the elderly and the chronically (persistently) ill, including alcoholics. Developing countries offer many more examples of obvious undernutrition than our area of the world does.

One type of obvious overnutrition that is commonly seen in North America is obesity. Cases of overnutrition of specific nutrients, on the other hand, are more unusual but do occur.

Sense of Well-Being Sometimes, but not always, a person is aware of changes in the way he or she feels or functions. Like changes in appearance, these self-reports are of limited value because they are very subjective and could be the result of circumstances other than nutrition-related ones. For example, tiredness could result from prolonged inadequate iron or kcalorie intake, or from nonnutritional factors such as too little sleep, mental depression, or other illness. Increased frequency of minor health problems (e.g., colds, digestive upsets) may also relate to poor nutritional status. On the other hand, some people are surprised when they are diagnosed as having severe health or nutritional problems on the basis of blood tests; they may claim that they felt fine, or they may have ignored not feeling well.

No matter what the cause may be, you should report such observations to your doctor so that professional evaluation can be done, a diagnosis made, and appropriate care initiated.

Tests of Limited or Very Questionable Value

Several types of tests do *not* provide useful information about an individual's nutritional status. Moreover, these tests can be very expensive.

Hair analysis has very limited valid use. It can sometimes help in identifying mineral poisoning (arsenic poisoning, for example) and in comparing the status of various population groups in regard to certain minerals. But that's all.

In recent years, some enterprising pseudoscientists have marketed the service of analyzing hair samples to see what nutrients they contain and reporting their findings as evidence of nutritional status. This is not a reliable means of nutritional assessment.

Why? Biochemistry experts say that although it certainly is possible to analyze the amounts of various minerals present in hair—and some scientists do this for various experimental purposes—there are currently few standards as to what values are normal. Furthermore, the composition of hair is not likely to reflect the current composition of other body tissues. In addition, products that come in contact with hair can change its chemical composition: shampoos, bleaches, dyes, solutions used for permanents, and even the water supply can remove or add chemicals. All of this means that hair analysis currently has little value for nutritional assessment or for diagnosis and treatment of diseases (Klevay, 1987).

In addition, there is evidence that laboratories that market hair analysis to the general public may not do consistent work. The *Slice of Life* below makes the point.

Some tests have even less validity. The *cytotoxic test*, in which a blood sample is mixed with food extracts and then the activity of the white blood cells is observed under a microscope, supposedly identifies allergies—but the "test" is useless. *Applied kinesiology* is said to be a way of assessing muscle weakness that can be corrected by nutritional supplementation—but the method has no scientific basis (Jarvis, 1989).

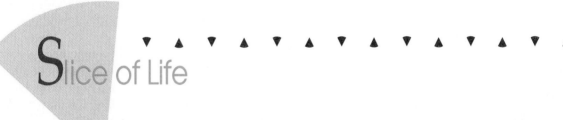

Slice of Life

The Unreliability of Hair Analysis

Stephen Barrett, a physician who helped found the National Council Against Health Fraud, put to the test some laboratories that chemically analyze hair samples.

He took hair samples from two healthy 17-year-old girls and sent cuttings from each of them to 13 labs for mineral analysis. The reports he received back from them varied widely: several laboratories reported values for most minerals that were at least ten times those stated by others. One lab reported 2200 times more of a certain mineral than another!

Six labs included supplement advice in their reports, and the types and amounts suggested varied widely from lab to lab for each girl. Some reports noted "trends or tendencies" to diseases; among the conditions suggested for these two girls were goiter, uremia (toxic metabolites in the blood), and "depression of central nervous system" (Barrett, 1985).

Since the girls were known to be healthy, the most charitable statement that can be made about the lab reports is that many of them seem to have been in error. Of course, people who receive reports from such laboratories are likely to take them seriously, since they trusted the service enough to seek it out. Unfortunately, what they may actually be receiving for their money is needless worry about their health. When advice is given to purchase nutritional supplements to correct the supposed "nutritional deficits," people spend even more money on products that are probably unnecessary or may even be dangerous. ▲

Diet Analysis Is Ordinarily Useful for Estimating Nutritional Status

A thorough nutritional assessment includes techniques that focus not only on the body, as just discussed, but also on dietary evaluation. This involves analyzing a person's intake and comparing it to a predetermined standard for adequacy. Because of its convenience, we will emphasize diet analysis in this text for people who have no apparent health problems.

Describing Your Diet

To analyze your diet, you first need to describe your intake. Three methods are discussed in this section. These methods are only valid if you are very careful to remember and record everything you eat and drink. This can be a challenge, especially when it comes to details like the mayonnaise on a sandwich or the butter in which an egg is fried. Another task is to estimate correctly the *amounts* you consumed. Correctly estimating serving sizes takes practice. Measuring several food items can help you become a better judge.

Twenty-Four-Hour Recall   A 24-hour recall consists of remembering everything you consumed for an entire day (usually the preceding day). Be sure to include all eating situations—whether you would classify them as meals, snacks, or "just having something to drink because I was thirsty." Many people get 10–20% of their intake for the day at times other than during meals (Food and Nutrition Board, 1986).

   Now ask yourself whether your list is representative of your eating; it may or may not be. After all, people's diets vary considerably from day to day. For example, you probably don't eat the same way on weekends as on weekdays; you may have eaten unusual items or amounts that day; or you may eat differently during one season than another (Medlin and Skinner, 1988). The more typical the diet you analyze, the more useful the information can be to you.

Food Records   A way to avoid forgetting what you consume is to record what you take in as a day goes along. This technique may tempt you to change your eating habits to reflect what you think you *ought* to eat instead of the way you usually *do* eat. When you keep a food record, try to eat as you usually do, and record exactly what you ate. Carry your record with you throughout the day.

   However, one day's worth of data—whether collected by the recall method or with a food record—is not very useful by itself, because energy intake often varies by 25% from day to day, and nutrients may vary up to 50% (Dwyer, 1988). You can get a more accurate picture of what you eat by keeping records for many consecutive days and averaging the results. Experts in diet analysis have suggested various minimal time periods for achieving reasonable accuracy, such as three or four days or a week. Although it seems that any length of time has its limitations, longer recording periods generally provide a more accurate picture of typical nutrient intake.

The next *Slice of Life* highlights some pitfalls of using these techniques. Despite the fact that food records are not perfect—no method is—we will encourage you to keep records many times throughout this textbook. When possible, record several days of food intake for a more accurate result.

Slice of Life

What Did You Eat? Guess Again!

It's not as easy to do a 24-hour recall or a food record as you might think. The point came home to Jane when she tried it herself.

Jane started jotting down what she had eaten the day before. *Let's see . . . I had a bagel with cream cheese just before I left for my 9:55 Econ class . . . a bowl of chili and a carton of yogurt when I met Ted at the cafeteria for lunch . . . didn't eat again until I got home after work. . . .*

As she looked over the list she had made, she realized that she had forgotten to list the beverages she had drunk, both with her meals and in between. When she tried to recall them, she remembered that she had taken a vitamin pill with orange juice when she first got up; she added it to her list. *Oh, yes, somebody made popcorn at work . . . and I'd better write down the oil it's popped in, too.*

Estimating amounts was another challenge. *How much popcorn did I eat? Maybe five handfuls, but how much is in a handful? And how much chili do you get at the cafeteria?* She couldn't exactly recall the size of the bowls.

Jane decided that she would do a food record the next day and try to improve her accuracy regarding amounts by actually measuring the things she ate at home.

She was on the right track with this idea. Training your eye by looking at a known quantity of food can improve subsequent estimates. At Ohio University at Athens, it was found that students who were given a 10-minute training session using food models made better estimates than untrained students made (Yuhas et al., 1989). In an earlier study at Penn State University, Helen Guthrie, PhD, RD (Registered Dietitian), also found that people tend to be poor judges of the amounts they consume. She offered a free breakfast or lunch to 147 young adults and asked them to write down what and how much they had taken from the buffet table. Among the most common errors were overestimating use of butter and forgetting to mention salad dressing, and four out of ten were more than 50% off in judging the amount of milk they poured on their cereal (Guthrie, 1985). In the Ohio University study, solids (meatloaf and fish) were better estimated than liquids (soup and milk), which were better estimated than amorphous items (spaghetti and applesauce).

Studies such as these show that in order to prepare yourself for estimating food quantities, it might be worth taking the time to measure your typical portion sizes to "develop an eye" for food quantities. ▲

food frequency questionnaire—
tool for ascertaining intakes
of foods or groups of foods in
specific time period; used for
estimating intake of one or
more nutrients

Food Frequency Questionnaires　Another approach that is sometimes used for collecting food intake data is the **food frequency questionnaire,** which takes a more general approach. It involves considering a list of common foods or categories of food and indicating how many times a day (or some other time period) you are likely to consume them. This method can be used for overall nutritional assessment or for estimating your intake of specific nutrients. You will have an opportunity to use food frequency data in Chapter 7 while doing an assessment of your fat intake.

The results of food frequency questionnaires are likely to have somewhat larger margins of error than the results of food records (Krall and Dwyer, 1987). Even so, their popularity may be increasing owing to the ease with which they can be administered and analyzed; and since data can be collected in one interview, compliance is not a problem. For these reasons, it is anticipated that efforts will be made to improve the validity and accuracy of this technique (Medlin and Skinner, 1988).

Analyzing Your Diet

Once you have described your diet, you can use several approaches to analyze it. The Assessments that follow can help you with diet analysis by comparing the use of food composition tables, food group plans, and various other dietary guidelines.

Food Composition Data　Thousands of foods have been analyzed by government, university, and industry laboratories to discover what levels of nutrients they contain. This is a costly and slow process because of the substantial time, skill, and special equipment that are involved.

The U.S. Department of Agriculture (USDA) has been the leader in the United States in analyzing food and assembling and publishing information about food composition. USDA's *Agricultural Handbook 8*, which is now under revision, will eventually contain more than 4000 items. Other authors have also pulled together food composition data from USDA and other sources. In Appendix E, you will find approximately 1500 items from one such compilation. Do not be surprised if you consult several food composition tables and find that the values for a particular food do not agree exactly (Hollman and Katan, 1988); different laboratory methods by which data can be derived are likely to yield somewhat different results.

Assessment 2.1 presents the steps to follow in performing a diet analysis with information from a food composition table, shows an example of an analysis, and suggests a form to follow.

Food composition information also is often available from the labels of specific food products; currently, 61% of packaged foods carry nutrition labeling (Stark, 1990). The nutrition label format in use in 1990 (see Figure 1.6) expresses the amounts of some nutrients in absolute terms (protein, fat, carbohydrate, and sodium); these values can be used directly in doing

Assessment 2.1. However, the amounts of other nutrients are shown as *percentages* of the U.S. RDA (vitamin A, vitamin C, thiamin, riboflavin, niacin, calcium, and iron). To use the latter type of information in Assessment 2.1, you need to convert the percentages into absolute values: multiply the nutrient values of the U.S. RDA in Table 1.2 by the percentages of the U.S. RDA indicated on the label. (When RDIs replace U.S. RDAs on labels, you can convert those percentages into absolute values by the same method, using the RDIs listed in Appendix J.)

Using the method outlined in Assessment 2.1 will give you a means of determining your approximate nutritional status for a number of nutrients. This method lends itself very well to computerization. Nutrient data bases and diet analysis software are being used increasingly in research, health care, and nutrition education, thereby saving much time that would otherwise have been spent in hand calculation.

Some notes of caution need to be sounded about computerized diet analysis. One is that there is considerable variation in the quality of the data in available software. In some computerized data banks, for example, foods for which some nutrient values have not been entered are included in the data set. When intake values are compiled for the day, nutrients for which some values were missing will be artificially low. This is particularly apt to occur in regard to analyses of dietary fiber, copper, selenium, and vitamin B_6. Another consideration when shopping for diet analysis software is that different programs produce very different kinds of output. If you are ever in the position of choosing such software, be sure you are getting the features you want.

Another type of diet evaluation is faster to use than analyzing food composition data, although it sacrifices much detail; this method uses the food group plans. Such plans are convenient both for evaluating past intakes and for planning future consumption.

Food Group Plans The food group plans pay less attention to what specific foods were eaten, and more to the general type of products that were consumed. This is a workable approach because related foods often have similar nutrient values. For example, the grains rice, wheat, and oats are significant sources of carbohydrate, thiamin, and niacin (although the amounts of the nutrients are not identical from one grain to another). Given this similarity in the composition of the foods, a person who eats several servings of various grains per day can be confident of having an appreciable intake of those nutrients (Table 2.2).

Given the nutrient characteristics of each group, it is then possible to construct an eating plan that contains close to RDA levels of nutrients by recommending how many servings from each group should be eaten daily. Using this type of plan, you can evaluate whether a person's consumption has been generally satisfactory without directly calculating how many milligrams of thiamin or niacin or any other nutrient were in it.

Many food group plans have been developed over the last four decades to

Analyzing a Day's Intake Using Food Composition Data

Assessment 2.1

1. Look up the items in your diet on a food composition table (for example, Appendices E and F), and record the amounts of nutrients in them. You will have to adjust the nutrient values for different serving sizes. (If you drank ½ cup of milk but the table gives the values for 1 cup, you will need to divide all values in half before you record them.)

2. If you want to use food composition information from food product labels, you need to convert values given as percentages of the U.S. RDA or RDI to absolute values (see text).

3. After entering all the items, calculate the sum for each nutrient.

4. Enter the RDA (see inside back cover) for your sex, age, and reproductive status on the line below the sums. Note: there is no RDA for total fat, unsaturated fat, and carbohydrate.

5. Compare the sums to your RDAs. How far apart are they? Calculate what percentage of your RDA you obtained for each nutrient by dividing the sum for a given nutrient by your RDA for it. Multiply your answer by 100 to get the percentage (move the decimal point two spaces to the

Food or Beverage	Approximate Measure	Food Energy kcal	Protein g	Total Fat g	Unsaturated Fat g	Carbohydrate g
Egg bagel	1	180	7	1	1	35
Jelly	1 T.	49	tr	tr	tr	13
Orange pop	12 oz.	170	0	0	0	42
McDonald's cheeseburgers	2	636	30	32	14	58
French fries	regular	220	3	12	8	26
McDonald's cookies	small box	308	4	10	6	49
Cola drink	12 oz.	151	0	0	0	39
Pork chop—lean only	2½ oz.	172	21	9	6	0
Baked potato	1 avg.	145	3	tr	tr	34
Frozen peas	½ c.	63	4	tr	tr	11
Butter	2 t.	68	0	8	2	tr
Iceberg lettuce	2 c.	14	2	0	0	2
French dressing	2 T.	134	tr	18	10	1
2% milk	½ c.	61	4	2	1	6
Graham crackers	2 squares	60	1	1	1	11
Total		2431	79	93	49	327
Your RDA		—	46	—	—	—
% of Your RDA		—	172	—	—	—

[a]The RDA for vitamin A is now expressed in Retinol Equivalents (REs), but the values in food composition tables are still mostly in International Units (IUs). To make the values comparable here, use these estimates for the vitamin A RDA: 5000 IU for men and 4000 IU for women.

right). If you took in less than your RDA for a nutrient, the percentage will be less than 100; if you took in more, the percentage will be over 100.

What do the percentages mean? You have to think back to how the RDAs are derived to appreciate their significance. Since most healthy people's nutrient needs are actually below the levels recommended by the RDAs, you might very well be able to meet your need for a particular nutrient with an intake of less than 100% of the RDA. Some experts in nutrition assessment judge a diet to be probably acceptable if it contains at least 70% of the RDA values for all nutrients, although many experts do not agree on this point. (Remember, we're talking only about healthy people here; people who are ill may have higher nutritional needs.)

What is the guideline for an *upper* limit? There is no standard percentage of the RDA at which an excess amount of a nutrient can cause problems. For one nutrient, an intake of 500% (five times the RDA) could lead to difficulties if continued for months at a time. For another, there may be no negative effect from **megadoses** (often defined as ten times the RDA or more).

This disparity makes it difficult to set a limit that can be generally applied. It is important to remember that *more is not better; there is no known advantage for a healthy person to consume more than 100% of the RDA.*

megadoses—doses of a nutrient ten times the RDA or more

Sample Assessment 2.1 Analyzing a day's intake using food composition data. This food was eaten in one day by a 20-year-old woman.

Calcium	Phosphorus	Iron	Zinc	Vitamin A	Thiamin	Riboflavin	Niacin	Vitamin B-6	Vitamin B-12	Folic Acid	Vitamin C
mg	mg	mg	mg	IU	mg	mg	mg	mg	μg	μg	mg
20	61	2.1	.6	0	.26	.20	2.4	.03	0	16	0
2	1	.1	0	2	tr	tr	tr	tr	0	2	1
15	2	.3	.3	0	0	0	tr	0	0	0	0
338	410	5.6	5.2	706	.60	.48	8.6	.24	1.82	42	4
9	101	.6	.3	17	.12	.02	2.3	.22	.03	19	13
12	74	1.5	.3	27	.23	.23	2.9	.03	.03	6	1
9	46	.1	.1	0	0	0	0	0	0	0	0
3	177	.7	1.6	5	.83	.22	2.5	.34	.52	4	tr
8	78	.6	.5	0	.16	.03	2.2	.47	0	14	20
19	72	1.3	.8	766	.23	.14	1.2	.09	0	47	8
2	2	tr	tr	300	0	0	0	0	tr	tr	0
22	22	.6	.2	370	.06	.04	.2	.04	0	62	4
4	2	.1	tr	30	tr	tr	tr	tr	tr	tr	tr
149	116	.1	.5	250	.05	.20	.1	.06	.45	6	1
6	20	.4	.1	0	.02	.03	.6	.01	0	2	0
618	1184	14.1	10.5	2443[a]	2.56	1.59	23.0	1.53	2.85	220	52
1200	1200	15	12	4000[a]	1.1	1.3	15	1.6	2.0	200	60
52	99	94	88	61	233	122	153	96	143	110	87

Table 2.2 Four Basic Food Groups and Some of Their Major Nutrients

Group	Example Foods	Major Nutrients Supplied in Significant Amounts	
		By All in Group	By Only Some Foods

Fruits and vegetables	Apples, bananas, dates, oranges, tomatoes
	Broccoli, cabbage, green beans, lettuce, potatoes
		Carbohydrate
		Water
			Vitamins
			  A
			  C
			  folic acid
			Minerals
			  iron
			  calcium
			Fiber

Grain products
  (preferably whole grain; otherwise, enriched or fortified)
	Breads, rolls, bagels
	Cereals, dry and cooked
	Pasta
	Rice, other grains
	Tortillas, pancakes, waffles
	Crackers
	Popcorn
		Carbohydrate
		Protein
		Vitamins
		  thiamin
		  niacin
			Water
			Fiber
			Minerals
			  iron
			  magnesium
			  selenium

Milk and milk products	Milk, yogurt
	Cheese
	Ice cream, ice milk, frozen yogurt
		Protein
		
		Vitamins
		  riboflavin
		  B-12
		Minerals
		  calcium
		  phosphorus
		Water
			Carbohydrate
			Fat
			Vitamins
			  A
			  D

Meats and meat alternates	Meat, fish, poultry
	Eggs
	Seeds
	Nuts, nut butters
	Soybeans, tofu
	Other legumes
	  (peas and beans)
		Protein
		Vitamins
		  niacin
		  B-6
		Minerals
		  iron
		  zinc
			Carbohydrate
			Fat
			Vitamins
			  B-12
			  thiamin
			Water
			Fiber

help people evaluate and plan their diets. These plans have used as many as ten to as few as four groups. Each plan has had its enthusiasts and detractors: not one plan has satisfied everybody. Here we will briefly describe the food group plans that have been in use recently.

The *Basic Four Food Guide* is easy to remember and use because of its small number of groups. Introduced by the USDA in 1956, the plan recommends that people eat at least the stated minimum numbers of servings of fruits and vegetables, milk and milk products, meats and meat substitutes, and grain products every day to provide the foundation for an adequate diet.

The Basic Four plan was devised before scientists had studied many nutrients extensively and does not guarantee that you will get RDA levels of all nutrients. However, you are likely to come fairly close much of the time for many nutrients, especially if you eat more than the minimum recommendations. This plan emphasizes the importance of eating a variety of foods within each group, rather than repeatedly eating the same items. This is to make it more likely that you will get not only those nutrients found in all members of the group, but also those available from just some foods in each category.

The foods in each group vary in their **nutrient density;** that is, they contain variable levels of nutrients for the number of kcalories they provide. If a food has a low or moderate kcalorie value and is loaded with nutrients (broccoli is such a food), it is said to have a very *high nutrient density.* Lettuce, which is low in kcalories but relatively low in nutrients as well, has a *lower nutrient density* than broccoli. A food such as sugar-sweetened gelatin dessert, which has many kcalories and low levels of nutrients, is of the *lowest nutrient density* and is popularly referred to as "junk food."

nutrient density—a term used to describe whether a food is a good source of nutrient(s) relative to the kcalories it contains

People who are critical of the Basic Four plan point out that it does not give any guidance about consumption of many low-nutrient-density foods and beverages that people commonly eat and that are not included in the food groups—such as fats, sugary foods, and alcoholic beverages. Furthermore, there is a related issue: how do you categorize foods that are made from Basic Four items but have had so much fat and/or sugar added during processing that their nutrient density has dropped dramatically?

For example, 100-kcalories-worth of potato chips contains only one-seventh as much vitamin C as 100-kcalories-worth of baked potato, and only half the amount of many other nutrients (except fat, which is higher). Potato chips have a much lower nutrient density overall than baked potatoes. Should potato chips still be considered a serving of a vegetable?

Vegetarians may also take issue with the Basic Four food plan. For those who choose to avoid meat and milk and its products, a food plan that recommends those foods is not relevant. They object to a plan that assumes that everybody eats all kinds of foods.

Despite such criticisms, the *Basic Four Food Guide* has been widely used for decades and has taught many people how to evaluate and improve their diets. Its simplicity and adaptability continue to make it highly useful today (Derelian, 1988).

The Canadian Ministry of Health and Welfare makes very similar recommendations in *Canada's Food Guide.* These guidelines are found in Appendix B.

In 1979, USDA introduced the *Hassle-Free Guide to a Better Diet,* which reiterated many recommendations of the *Basic Four* but emphasized moderation in the consumption of foods high in fats, sugar, and alcohol. In 1986, the *Pattern for Daily Food Choices* was introduced, which suggested ranges of intake for the total diet (rather than just minimums for a foundation diet) and encouraged higher intakes of grain products, fruits, and vegetables than had been recommended previously. As before, excesses of fat, sugar, and alcohol were discouraged.

Still another food group plan is the exchange system. Described in *Exchange Lists for Meal Planning* (American Diabetes Association and American Dietetic Association, 1986), this plan consists of six lists (starch/bread, meat, vegetable, fruit, milk, and fat). Within a given list, each specified serving of food usually provides an amount of carbohydrate, protein, and fat that is comparable to that provided by every other food on the same list—therefore, each serving contains a similar number of kcalories. For example, $\frac{1}{2}$ cup of cooked broccoli or mushrooms each offers approximately 2 grams of protein, 5 grams of carbohydrate, and 25 kcalories. There is not necessarily as much uniformity within each list for other nutrients, though; vitamin and mineral contents may vary substantially from item to item. Consider, for example, that broccoli is a good source of vitamins A and C, but mushrooms are not.

People familiar with these lists find them to be a very useful tool for quickly estimating carbohydrate, protein, fat, and energy values of a food or even a whole day's intake. People with diabetes, for whom the system was originally designed, use it to help regulate their energy intake from day to day, but the system can be useful to anybody who learns it well.

The exchange lists are found in Table 2.3.

Other Dietary Recommendations In the late 1970s and throughout the 1980s, a barrage of reports containing dietary recommendations was issued by various government bodies. They reflected the growing popular commitment to self-responsibility for health and reinforced the importance of getting enough of the needed nutrients. These recommendations also addressed concerns regarding consumption of fat, sugar, sodium (a mineral found in salt and other compounds), and alcohol. They pointed out that high intakes of these substances increase some people's risk of heart and blood vessel diseases, cancer, stroke, diabetes, cirrhosis, and dental decay. (There will be more about the potential relationship between these dietary factors and diseases in later chapters.) These reports had important political ramifications, since any significant changes in eating patterns have repercussions on agricultural systems and the food processing industry as well.

The first of these recommendations was *Dietary Goals for the United States*, a report of the Senate Select Committee on Nutrition and Human Needs. Published and revised in 1977, it asserted that American eating patterns are a critical public health concern. It recommended specific reductions in fats, refined and processed sugars, cholesterol, and salt and suggested adjusting kcalorie intake to achieve desirable body weight.

Heated debate followed the release of the report, with some experts questioning whether there were adequate scientific data to substantiate that the specific levels of nutrients recommended could actually prevent or delay the stated diseases. Antagonists maintained that diets with such restrictions were unnecessary for the population as a whole. They contended that such diets should be prescribed only on a case-by-case basis, if an individual's family medical history put the person at risk for those health problems. Others said that the recommendations were difficult to translate into diets that people would eat.

Other reports making dietary recommendations at about the same time were *Healthy People: The Surgeon General's Report on Health Promotion and Disease Prevention*, which was issued in 1979, and *Toward Healthful Diets*, a 1980 paper from the Food and Nutrition Board of the National Academy of Sciences. In general, these reports agreed on the importance of variety in the

Table 2.3 Exchange Lists for Meal Planning

The six exchange lists below can be used for meal planning and evaluating food intake. Foods are grouped together on a list because they are similar in composition of energy-containing nutrients. Every food on a list has about the same amount of carbohydrate (CHO), protein (Pro), fat, and kcalories (kcal), except as noted. Any serving of food on a list can be exchanged or traded for any other serving of food on the same list.

STARCH/BREAD
Each of these equals one starch/bread serving.
(15 g CHO, 3 g Pro, trace fat, 80 kcal)

½ cup pasta or barley

⅓ cup rice or cooked dried beans and peas

1 small potato (or ½ cup mashed)

½ cup starchy vegetables (corn, peas, or winter squash)

1 slice bread or 1 roll

½ English muffin, bagel, or hamburger/hot dog bun

½ cup cooked cereal

¾ cup dry cereal, unsweetened

4–6 crackers

3 cups popcorn, unbuttered, not cooked in oil

MILK
Each of these equals one milk serving.
The calories vary for each choice.
(12 g CHO, 8 g Pro, variable fat and kcal)

1 cup skim milk (90 calories)

1 cup low-fat milk (120 calories)

8-oz carton plain low fat yogurt (120 calories)

FRUIT
Each of these equals one fruit serving.
(15 g CHO, 60 kcal)

1 fresh medium fruit

1 cup berries or melon

½ cup canned in juice or without sugar

½ cup fruit juice

¼ cup dried fruit

VEGETABLES
Each of these equals one vegetable serving.
(5 g CHO, 2 g Pro, 25 kcal)

½ cup cooked vegetables

1 cup raw vegetables

½ cup tomato/vegetable juice

MEAT AND SUBSTITUTES
Each of these equals one meat choice.
(7 g Pro, variable fat, 55–100 kcal)

1 oz cooked poultry, fish, or meat

¼ cup cottage cheese

¼ cup salmon or tuna, water packed

1 T peanut butter

1 egg (limit to 3 per week)

1 oz low-fat cheese, such as Mozzarella, ricotta

Each of these equals 2 meat choices.
1 small chicken leg or thigh

½ cup cottage cheese or tuna

Each of these equals 3 meat choices.
1 small pork chop

1 small hamburger

cooked meat, about the size of a deck of cards

½ of a whole chicken breast

1 medium fish fillet

FAT
Each of these equals one fat serving.
(5 g fat, 45 kcal)

1 t margarine, oil, mayonnaise

2 t diet margarine or diet mayonnaise

1 T salad dressing

2 T reduced-calorie salad dressing

diet, on regulation of kcalorie intake to achieve best weight, and on moderation in salt consumption. The reports reflected some differences of opinion
as to who would benefit from the restriction of sugar and fats.

Also in 1980, the USDA and the Department of Health and Human Services (formerly Health, Education, and Welfare) jointly produced *Nutrition
and Your Health: Dietary Guidelines for Americans*. These recommendations
took into account the earlier Dietary Goals and other reports and the volumi-
nous comments that had been sparked by them. They promoted a holistic
approach to nutrition rather than a disease-by-disease approach. Although
both publications reflected concern about many of the same substances, the
Guidelines were less specific in their recommendations than the Goals had
been. In 1985 and again in 1990, the Guidelines were revised. As we went to
press with this textbook, some points of the 1990 Guidelines were still under
debate, but the main points are anticipated to resemble the following:

1. Eat a variety of foods.
2. Maintain healthy weight.
3. Choose a diet low in fat, saturated fat, and cholesterol.
4. Choose a diet with plenty of vegetables, fruits, and grain products.
5. Use sugar in moderation.
6. Use salt and sodium in moderation.
7. If you drink alcoholic beverages, do so in moderation.

In 1988, *The Surgeon General's Report on Nutrition and Health* was released.
It encouraged all Americans to maintain a desirable body weight; reduce
consumption of fats, cholesterol, sodium, and alcohol; and increase consumption of complex carbohydrates and fiber. It gave additional advice for
certain groups: those without adequate fluoride in their water supply should
get fluoride elsewhere; children should limit sugars to reduce risk of tooth
decay; adolescent girls and women should increase intake of foods high in
calcium; and children, adolescents, and women of childbearing age should
consume good sources of iron.

In 1989, a committee of the National Research Council issued *Diet and
Health: Implications for Reducing Chronic Disease Risk*. This report recommended limiting intakes of fat, alcohol, and salt; maintaining moderate intake of protein; eating more sources of complex carbohydrate; maintaining
adequate intakes of calcium and fluoride; maintaining appropriate body
weight; and avoiding intakes of dietary supplements in excess of the RDA in
any one day. These practices are designed to meet overall nutritional needs
and to use what we know about the relationship between nutrition and
chronic disease to fight the leading causes of death and disability in the
developed countries: atherosclerosis (the major form of heart disease), high
blood pressure, obesity and eating disorders, cancer, osteoporosis, diabetes,
liver diseases, and dental decay.

Although many of the recommendations of the past decade may seem
redundant, they have served the important function of *consensus-building*.
And as people in many major health organizations, government agencies,
and research institutions continue to arrive at similar conclusions about the

Table 2.4 Basic Food Guide Standards for Specific Groups

| | Include at Least This Many Servings Daily | | | Suggested Daily Servings |
| | Athletes | Adult Vegetarians | | |
Basic Food Groups		Who Use Milk	Who Use Only Plant Foods[b]	Adults with Limited Budget[c]
Fruits and vegetables	Fruits/vegetables: 1 vitamin A 1 vitamin C Others to make group total of 5	Fruits/vegetables: 1 vitamin A 1 vitamin C Others to make group total of 5	Fruits: 1–4, including 1 raw vitamin C Vegetables: 4, including 2 or more dark leafy greens	Fruits/vegetables: 1 vitamin A 1 vitamin C Others to make group total of 4
Grain products	6–12 or more as needed for energy	6	Whole grain yeast bread: 4 slices Other grains: 3–5	9–12
Milk and milk products	2 or 3[a]	2 or 3[a]	0	1½
Meats and meat alternates	2	Legumes: 1 serving Nuts or seeds: 1 serving	Legumes: 2 servings Nuts or seeds: 1 serving	2

[a]Three servings for teens and through age 24; after that, 2 servings per day.

[b]Reference: Zeman, F.J. and D.M. Ney. 1988. *Applications of Clinical Nutrition*. Englewood Cliffs, N.J.: Prentice Hall.

[c]Adapted from Consumer Nutrition Division. 1983. *The thrifty food plan, 1983*. Hyattsville, MD: Human Nutrition Information Service, U.S. Department of Agriculture.

characteristics of a healthy diet, the weight of their concern may influence the food production, processing, and service industries to provide more foods that make it easier for individuals to achieve these guidelines as they select their food at home and away.

The Basic Food Guide To bring together the major concerns of these various recommendations, we have developed the Basic Food Guide, which is introduced on page 50.

The Basic Food Guide in this book was developed to build on the strengths and address some of the weaknesses of various dietary recommendations described elsewhere in this chapter. Essentially, it is a food group plan that is generally consistent with recent recommendations such as the *Dietary Guidelines* (Cronin et al., 1987), *The Surgeon General's Report on Nutrition and Health*, and *Diet and Health* (National Research Council, 1989). It also provides information about the fat, sugar, salt, and alcohol content of foods. The Basic Food Guide will be used throughout the book for describing and comparing diets.

Assessment 2.2 shows you how to analyze your diet using the Basic Food Guide. You can use it equally well for evaluating what you have already eaten and for planning what you intend to eat.

After you have done the assessments in this chapter, read *Critical Thinking 2.1* to get some additional perspectives on the results of your assessments.

The Basic Food Guide

Also note that for **grain products,** you are encouraged to use whole-grain items as much as possible; enriched and fortified products are only second best. Refined, unenriched, and unfortified products aren't even accepted as members of the group. (The effects of food processing on nutrients will be discussed in Chapter 14.)

The Basic Food Guide is a tool for quickly evaluating or planning your food intake. It recommends what kinds and amounts of foods to eat to get enough of the essential nutrients; it also gives the levels of fat, sugar, salt, and alcohol in representative foods.

The Basic Food Guide includes a page for each of the four major groups of foods. In the middle of each food group page, the minimum number of servings needed daily by an adult from that group is indicated.

As necessary, there are other important qualifying statements in the middle of the food group pages. For the **milk products** group, different intakes for various ages are recommended. For **fruits and vegetables,** note that within the minimum of five servings recommended for each day, one good source of vitamin A and one of vitamin C should be included.

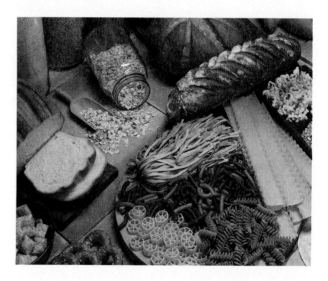

For **meats and meat alternates,** use some plant sources every week, even if you like meat well enough to eat it as your only choice from that group. The plant sources are better sources of certain substances such as magnesium (a mineral) and fiber.

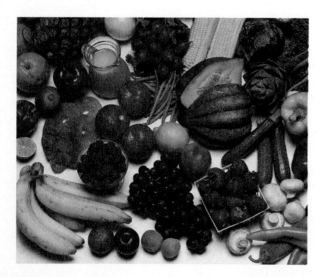

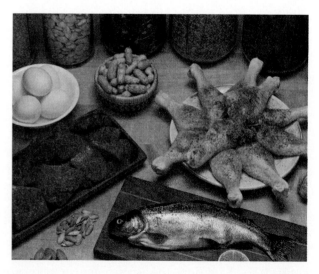

Also in the middle of each basic food group page, serving sizes for some representative foods within each group are listed. For foods that are not on the list but seem very similar to others that are found there, you can assume the same serving size.

At the bottom of each food group page are vertical columns labeled "fat," "sodium," and "added sugar." They will help you assess about how much of these substances are in some representative foods in each group. The bottom of each column represents zero, with values increasing as you ascend. Some foods from the group are placed along each column, showing the relative content of fat, sodium, or added sugar. For the sake of comparison, a specified amount of pure fat, salt, or sugar is also indicated. If you want to reduce the amounts of these substances in your diet, you can do so by eating more foods from nearer the bottom of the columns and fewer foods from higher up. In general, notice that the more processing a food has experienced, the more likely it is to have gained in fat, sodium, and/or sugar.

You can postpone forming opinions about whether you should reduce your intake of these items until after you have received more information from later chapters about what is known regarding their impact on health.

A separate page shows how to count **combination foods** such as casseroles or sandwiches. You have to mentally separate these foods into their components, identify which groups the ingredients belong to, and decide what part of a serving each represents. Some common examples are shown. Using these as guidelines, you can estimate other combination foods in your diet for yourself.

Note that the food group pages are color-coded; these colors will be used for identification purposes in tables throughout the book. For example, green denotes fruits and vegetables; whenever you see a band of green in a nutrient table anywhere in the book, the foods within the band will be fruits and vegetables.

The last page of the food group pages in the Basic Food Guide deals with **limited extras.** These are consumables that do not belong to any of the basic food groups, usually because of their very low nutrient densities. (Because of their dubious nutritional qualities, they are pictured in gray.) Nonetheless, it is reasonable to use a few servings per day if your weight allows you to eat more food than the Basic Food Guide suggests. If you need more food than that, choose more items from the basic groups.

These are the limited extras:

▶ High-fat foods: butter, cream, sour cream, cream cheese, bacon, lard and other solid shortenings, cooking oil, oil-based salad dressings, mayonnaise, margarine

▶ High sugar foods: white, brown, or raw sugar, honey, syrup, molasses, jam or jelly, soft drinks, gelatin desserts, other sweet desserts

▶ Refined, unenriched, or unfortified grain products: bread, crackers, cereals, cookies, cakes, or fried snack foods that are not made from whole, enriched, or fortified grains

▶ Alcoholic beverages (avoid during pregnancy): beer, wine, hard liquor, liqueur

▶ Foods that are low in both kcalories and essential nutrients: coffee, tea, broth, some artificially sweetened products such as soft drinks and gelatin desserts, condiments

FRUITS AND VEGETABLES

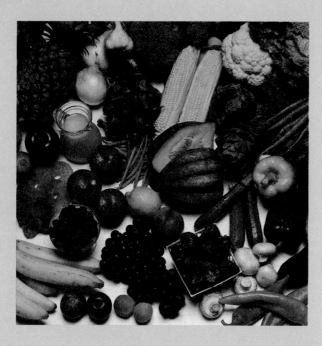

At least 5 servings daily, including

1 good source of vitamin A (apricots, broccoli, cantaloupe, carrots, pumpkin, winter squash, sweet potatoes, and spinach and other dark leafy greens)

1 good source of vitamin C (broccoli, cabbage, cantaloupe, cauliflower, citrus fruit, green pepper, kiwi fruit, strawberries)

Each of these is a serving

½ cup fresh, frozen, or canned solid product

1 medium-sized piece of fruit, e.g., apple, orange, banana

½ cup fresh, frozen, or canned juice

1 cup raw leafy vegetable

¼ cup dried fruit or vegetable

How much fat, sodium, and added sugar are likely to be found in fruit and vegetable products?
(When no serving size is specified, assume that the serving size stated above applies.)

Grams of Fat

35

30

25

20
— ⅙ of 9-inch apple pie

15

10 – 1 oz. potato chips

5 – Compare with 1 teaspoon fat
0 – { Plain, frozen fruit and vegetables
Fresh, canned fruit and vegetables

Milligrams of Sodium

1400

1200

1000
— 1 c. canned vegetable soup
800 – ½ c. sauerkraut
— 1 3¾ inch dill pickle
600 – Compare with ¼ teaspoon salt

400

200 – Many canned vegetables

0 – { Most plain frozen fruits and vegetables, canned fruit, fresh fruits and vegetables

Grams of Added Sugar

35

30 – ⅙ of 9-inch apple pie

25

20

15

10 – Fruits canned or frozen with sugar

5 – Compare with 1 teaspoon sugar

0 – { Vegetables/fruits canned without sugar
Fresh fruits and vegetables
Plain frozen vegetables

GRAIN PRODUCTS

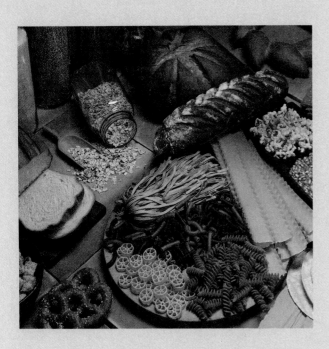

At least 6 servings daily, including at least 2 whole-grain products; otherwise enriched or fortified

Each of these is a serving

1 slice of bread or medium dinner roll

½ hamburger bun, hot dog bun, bagel, or English muffin

2½ tablespoons flour

1 ounce dry cereal

½ cup cooked cereal

3 cups popped popcorn

1 tortilla, pancake, or waffle square

½ cup cooked pasta, rice, or other grains

6 saltines, snack crackers, or 3-ring pretzels

3 graham cracker squares or small unfrosted cookies

How much fat, sodium, and added sugar are likely to be found in grain products?
(When no serving size is specified, assume that the serving size stated above applies.)

Grams of Fat
35 ———————
30 ———————
25 ———————
20 ———————
15 ———————
10 – 1 oz. fried snack foods ———
4 small oatmeal raisin cookies
5 – { Compare with 1 teaspoon fat —
Quick breads, baking powder
biscuit
0 – { Plain bread, saltines
Rice, pasta, most cereals —

Milligrams of Sodium
1400 ———————
1200 ———————
1000 ———————
800 ———————
600 – Compare with ¼ teaspoon salt —
400 – Cornflakes ———————
200 – Saltines, 1 oz. corn chips —
– Plain bread
0 – Corn tortilla ———————

Grams of Added Sugar
35 ———————
30 ———————
25 ———————
4 small oatmeal raisin cookies
20 ———————
15 – Sugar Smacks ———
10 – Frosted Mini-Wheats ———
5 – Compare with 1 teaspoon sugar —
0 – { Plain bread, tortilla,
saltines, pasta, Cheerios —

MILK AND MILK PRODUCTS

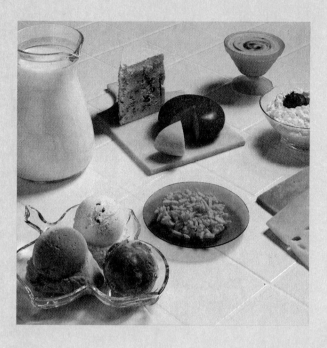

At least 2 servings (adults)

2–3 servings (children under
9 years)
3 servings (ages 9–24)

Each of these is a serving

1 cup milk or yogurt
1⅓ ounces hard cheese
2 ounces processed cheese
food
2 cups cottage cheese
1 cup sauces or puddings
made with milk
1½ cups ice cream or ice milk

How much fat, sodium, and added sugar are likely to be found in milk and milk products?
(When no serving size is specified, assume that the serving size stated above applies.)

Grams of Fat

35 ——————

30 ——————

25 ——————

20 – Ice cream ——————
    Processed cheese
15 ——————
    Cheddar cheese
10 – Ice milk ——————
    Whole milk
5 – Compare with 1 teaspoon fat ——
    2% milk
    1 cup low-fat yogurt
    low-fat cottage cheese
0 – Skim milk ——————

Milligrams of Sodium

1400 ——————

1200 ——————

1000 – 1 cup low-fat cottage cheese ——
    – Instant pudding ——————
800 – Processed cheese ——————

600 – Compare with ¼ teaspoon salt —

400 ——————
    Regular pudding from mix
200 – Cheddar cheese ——————
    – Milk ——————
0 ——————

Grams of Added Sugar

35 ——————
    Pudding
    Ice cream
30 ——————
    Fruited yogurt
25 ——————

20 ——————

15 ——————

10 ——————

5 – Compare with 1 teaspoon sugar —

0 – Milk, cheese, plain yogurt ——

MEATS AND MEAT ALTERNATES

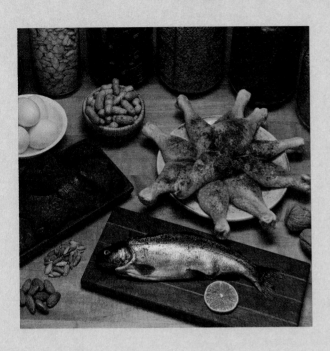

At least 2 servings daily, including plant sources several times per week

Each of these is a serving

2–3 ounces lean, cooked meat, fish, or poultry (no bone)

(a piece about the size of a deck of cards)

The following can substitute for 2 ounces of meat:

2 eggs

1 cup cooked legumes (e.g., black, garbanzo, kidney, lima, navy, pinto, soy beans; lentils; split peas)

6 ounces tofu

2 ounces (approximately $\frac{1}{2}$ cup) nuts or seeds

2 ounces (approximately $\frac{1}{4}$ cup) nut or seed butters

How much fat, sodium, and added sugar are likely to be found in meat and meat alternates?
(When no serving size is specified, assume that the serving size stated above applies.)

Grams of Fat	Milligrams of Sodium	Grams of Added Sugar
35 – 2 oz. walnuts	1400	35
30	1200	30
2 oz. roasted peanuts		25
25	1000 — 1 c. canned baked beans	
		20
20	800 – 2 oz. ham	
2 oz. bologna		15
15 – 2 oz. ham, 2 eggs	600 – Compare with $\frac{1}{4}$ teaspoon salt	
2 oz. ground beef		10 – 1 c. canned baked beans
2 oz. fried chicken	400	
10 – 2 oz. fried perch	– 2 oz. bologna	5 – Compare with 1 teaspoon sugar
6 oz. tofu	200 – 2 oz. salted peanuts	Some processed lunch meats
5 – Compare with 1 teaspoon fat	– 2 eggs	0 – { Plain cooked legumes, meat, fish, poultry, nuts
2 oz. broiled chicken (no skin)	2 oz. fried perch	
0 – Cooked legumes	0 – { 2 oz. meats, poultry, cooked legumes, tofu, nuts (all unsalted)	

COMBINATION FOODS

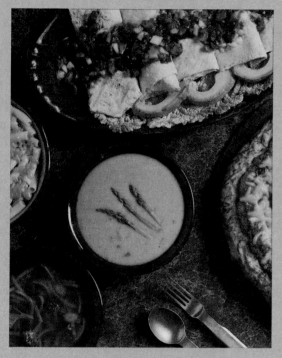

The Basic Food Guide can be used to evaluate a combination food by mentally separating it into its ingredients and estimating the amounts of basic foods present. The following examples of different types of combination dishes can be used as guidelines when you estimate similar dishes.

1 cup canned beef noodle soup

$\frac{1}{2}$ oz. meat = $\frac{1}{4}$ serving meat

$\frac{1}{4}$ c. noodles = $\frac{1}{2}$ serving grain

$\frac{1}{8}$ of 15-inch cheese pizza

$1\frac{1}{3}$ oz. cheese = 1 serving milk

pizza dough = 2 servings grain

$\frac{1}{4}$ c. vegetables = $\frac{1}{2}$ serving vegetables

1 cup canned macaroni and cheese

1 oz. processed cheese = $\frac{1}{2}$ serving milk

1 c. macaroni = 2 servings grain

2 oz. milk = $\frac{1}{4}$ serving milk

1 cup cream of asparagus or mushroom soup, made with milk

$\frac{1}{2}$ c. milk = $\frac{1}{2}$ serving milk

$1\frac{1}{4}$ T. flour = $\frac{1}{2}$ serving grain

2 T. vegetable = $\frac{1}{4}$ serving vegetable

1 cup chicken chow mein

3 oz. meat = 1 serving meat

$\frac{1}{2}$ c. vegetables = 1 serving vegetables

1 6-oz. bean burrito

$\frac{1}{2}$ c. beans = $\frac{1}{2}$ serving meat alternate

1 tortilla = 1 serving grain

How much fat, sodium, and added sugar are likely to be found in combination foods?
(When no serving size is specified, assume that the serving size stated above applies.)

Grams of Fat

35 ——————

30 ——————

25 ——————

20 ——————

    Canned cream of mushroom
15 – soup
    Bean burrito
    Canned spaghetti with meatballs
10 – Canned macaroni and cheese
    $\frac{1}{8}$ of 15" cheese pizza

5 – Compare with 1 teaspoon fat
    Canned beef noodle soup

0 – Canned beef noodle soup

Milligrams of Sodium

1400 ——————

1200 ——————

– ⎧ Canned cream of mushroom
     ⎪ soup
1000 – ⎨ Bean burrito
     ⎪ Canned spaghetti with
     ⎪ meatballs
     ⎩ Canned beef noodle soup

800 ——————

– Chicken chow mein
600 – Compare with $\frac{1}{4}$ teaspoon salt
  – $\frac{1}{8}$ of 15" cheese pizza

400 ——————

200 ——————

0 ——————

Grams of Added Sugar

35 ——————

30 ——————

25 ——————

20 ——————

15 ——————

10 ——————

5 – Compare with 1 teaspoon sugar
    Many items with tomato sauce
    Many canned soups
0 –

LIMITED EXTRAS

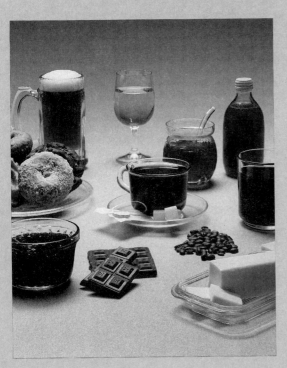

These foods are not needed for good nutrition. These foods don't contain significant amounts of nutrients. They should be used only as limited supplements rather than as mainstays of the diet.

Many of these foods have kcalories that add up quickly. If you are overweight, you can cut kcalories by eating fewer of these foods. If you are at your best weight, it is reasonable to use some of these foods daily, provided that you have included all the recommended foods as the basis of your diet.

Some items on this list have both low kcalories and low nutrient levels, such as tea, coffee, broth, low-kcalorie soft drinks, and diet gelatin desserts. Although low in most essential nutrients, they do contribute water. You can decide how much seems reasonable to consume after you have read the material on caffeine (Chapter 15), sodium (Chapter 13), and additives (Chapter 15).

Grams of sugar in sugary foods

```
40 – 12 oz. cola beverage
35
30 – ½ c. sherbet
25
20 – ½ c. gelatin dessert, 1 T. honey
15 – 1 T. syrup, ½ oz. hard candy
      1 oz. chocolate candy
10
      1 t. jam, jelly
5 – Compare with 1 teaspoon sugar
0
```

Grams of fat in fatty foods

```
20 – 1 oz. Italian salad dressing
     1 oz. French salad dressing
15 – 1⅓ oz. cream cheese
10 – 3 slices bacon, 1 oz. chocolate

5 – Compare with 1 teaspoon fat
        ⎧ 1 t. oil, 2 T. sour cream
0 –     ⎨ 1 t. butter, margarine, lard,
        ⎩   shortening, mayonnaise
```

Milligrams of sodium in salty foods

```
1400

1200

1000 – 1 T. soy sauce

 800 – 1 c. canned broth
       1 T. teriyaki sauce
       1 oz. low-kcal French dressing

 600 – Compare with ¼ teaspoon salt
 400 – 1 oz. regular French dressing
       4 green olives
 200 – 3 slices bacon
       1 T. catsup
     – 1 oz. Italian dressing
   0
```

Kcalories in refined, unenriched baked goods

```
300 – 3 oz. cheesecake
      1/16 chocolate cake with icing
250
      1 glazed donut
200 – 2 oz. brownie with icing
      1 Danish pastry
150

100 – 100 kcalories
      1 slice unenriched white bread
  0
```

Grams of alcohol in alcoholic beverages

```
35
30  Compare with 1 ounce pure alcohol
25
20 – 6 oz. wine
15 – 1½ oz. liquor
10 – 12 oz. beer
 5
 0
```

Evaluating Your Diet Using the Basic Food Guide

Assessment 2.2

If you have not already done so, familiarize yourself with the Basic Food Guide. Then, to calculate your diet with this guide, use a form such as the one shown in Sample Assessment 2.2.

Follow these steps to analyze your intake:

1. For an entire day, record all the foods and beverages you consume, along with the amounts of each. For items that are combinations, list the components separately.

2. Using the information in the Basic Food Guide, decide which groups each food belongs to (if any), and how much of a serving your intake represents. Record it in the appropriate columns. For food items that do not fit into any of the four groups, put an "x" in the column for limited extras.

3. Add the figures in each column to get subtotals for fruits and vegetables and group totals for all groups.

4. Fill in the standards for the four food groups that are appropriate for you as shown in the Basic Food Guide. Standards for athletes, some vegetarians, and people who want to eat as inexpensively as possible are shown in Table 2.4 on page 49.

5. Compare your intake to the standards. **Look only for shortages in your diet;** record them on the bottom line. If you are consistently low in your intake of foods from certain groups, you are probably getting less than you need of that group's major nutrients.

If you find that you have consumed more than the standard number of servings, do not assume that you have eaten too much. Remember, the standards are minimums, not maximums. Most people need to eat more than the standards recommend. It is smart to eat additional foods from the basic groups, rather than consuming large amounts of the limited extras.

On the other hand, if you are overly fat, you would be wise to see which columns register high. First look at how many fatty and sugary limited extras you consumed; cutting down on your intake of these foods is the best way of cutting kcalories without sacrificing important nutrients. Then check the basic foods columns. If your intake is much above the standards, you could further reduce kcalories by gradually bringing your intake down closer to the standards; don't drop below them, though, or you will shortchange yourself on essential nutrients. You can also replace some of the foods in each group that are higher in fat and sugar with other group members that have lower levels.

| Food or Beverage | Amount Eaten | Fruits and Vegetables | | | | Grain Products | Milk and Milk Products | Meat and Alternatives | Limited Extras |
		A	C	Other	Total				
	Indicate Number of Servings That Each Food Represents								
Dry cereal (enriched)	1½ oz.					1½			
Whole milk	½ c.						½		
Strawberry Pop Tart (enriched)	1					1			X
Hot dog:	1			(See following entries for bun, frankfurter & catsup)					
Bun (enriched)	1					2			
Frankfurter	1							½	
Catsup	1 T.								X
French fries	20 pcs.			2					
Orange	1 med.		1						
7-Up	12 oz.								X
Cube steak	6 oz.							2	
Mushrooms	¼			½					
Dinner roll (unenriched)	1								X
Baked potato	1 med.			1					
Butter	1 T.								X
Whole milk	1 c.						1		
Beer	12 oz.								X
Coke	24 oz.								X
Subtotals		0	1	3½	4½				
Group Totals					4½	4½	1½	2½	6
Standards		1	1		5	6	3	2	
Shortages		1	0		½	1½	1½	0	

Sample Assessment 2.2 Evaluating your diet using the **Basic Food Guide.** This illustration is based on a one-day food record of a 21-year-old man.

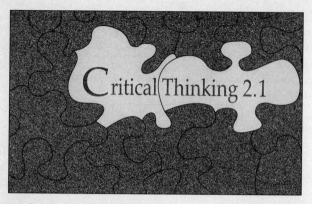

Putting Your First Assessments to Use

The situation

In this chapter, for the first of many times, you have been encouraged to evaluate your diet. How did your assessments come out? Did the results tell you that your diet is nutritious, or do you think there is need for improvement? Should you start today to make it better?

Before making a hasty decision, wait a minute. Think through your situation.

Is the information accurate and relevant?

■ The accuracy of your assessment cannot be any better than the accuracy of your record. Are you sure you recorded everything you consumed?

■ It is also important that the weights and volumes of what you consumed be correctly recorded. If you actually measured your food or had some training in estimating serving sizes, your chances of an accurate record are higher. Without practice, it can be difficult to correctly estimate portions—especially of items that vary in size and shape, such as meats; liquids and other amorphous items are also difficult to estimate.

■ If your intake on the day you recorded your diet was typical for you, your results are more likely to be relevant. If you ate less because you were not feeling well, or if you ran out of the carbonated beverage that is one of your dietary staples, your assessment will not tell you much about your usual intake.

■ If you recorded *several* typical days, including weekdays and a weekend day, your results are more likely to be relevant.

What else needs to be considered?

Let's say you have satisfied yourself that your food records are accurate and relevant; you have done the assessments correctly, and they have pointed out a few problems with your diet. Even after all that, there are more factors to take into account before making changes.

One consideration is the nature of the apparent dietary problem. If you find that your intake of a

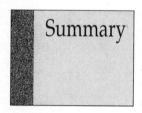

Summary

▶ Most of us alternate between overconsuming and underconsuming moderate amounts of the nutrients we need. This is normal and does not damage health. Long-term over- or under-consumption, however, can have many negative effects.

▶ There are several body-based means of measuring nutrition status. **Biochemical tests** involving the chemical analysis of blood or urine require special equipment to perform but yield relatively specific information. **Anthropometric tests** of height, weight, or skinfold thickness are easier to do but provide less specific information about nutritional status. Changes in appearance or sense of well-being may be related to nutritional status, or they may be related to another cause entirely.

▶ For most healthy people, diet analysis is more

particular nutrient is consistently very low (let's say 50% or less of your RDA), then it is a good idea to increase your intake. On the other hand, if your concern is that something in your diet is excessive, deciding what you should do will be difficult: the question is, *how much is too much?* The answer depends on the substance in question and may even depend in part on your health or family medical history; upcoming chapters will have a great deal more to say about this, nutrient by nutrient. One point that should be made immediately, however, is that people who use dietary supplements (such as vitamins and minerals) should avoid taking daily doses that exceed the RDA (National Research Council, 1989).

Another factor to consider before making dietary changes has to do with learning how to be successful at making changes: it is important to realize that because people form dietary habits over a long period of time, and because our eating habits are an important part of our identity, it is not easy to change them. Psychologists tell us that *the most successful way to make lasting changes in habits is to make small changes gradually.* This process is called behavior modification. In Chapter 9, this process and how it can be applied to diet is discussed. Assessment 9.1 gives an example of how to modify dietary behavior and increase the chances of long-term success.

What do you think?

Assuming that your assessments are accurate and valid, what should you do with the results at this point? Some options are:

- Option 1 Save them, but don't make any dietary changes until you have learned more from upcoming chapters.
- Option 2 Check Assessment 2.1 for all nutrients that frequently fall short of 70% of your RDA. Using the food composition tables in Appendices E and F, identify foods that are good sources of these nutrients and add them to your diet.
- Option 3 Put Assessment 2.1 on hold for the moment, but if Assessment 2.2 (using food groups) reveals shortfalls in your intake of some types of foods, gradually increase your consumption of foods from those groups.
- Option 4 If you are planning to make some changes now, skip ahead and read the discussion of behavior modification in Chapter 9 and Assessment 9.1 to improve your chances of success.
- Option 5 If you take nutritional supplements, check the label for what levels of nutrients they contain. Continue taking those supplements only if they do not exceed 100% of your RDA, unless you have been advised otherwise by a health care professional.

What other options do you see? Which option or combination of options makes most sense to you?

useful and practical than body-based measurements for estimating nutritional status. Diet analysis involves describing your intake of food and then analyzing it by using food composition data or a food group plan.

▶ Food group plans focus less on what specific foods were eaten and more on the general types of products consumed. Many of these plans, such as the *Basic Four Food Guide* and *Canada's Food Guide*, have been developed over the last four decades.

Such plans primarily urge people to eat enough foods of high **nutrient density** and variety to achieve recommended intakes of nutrients.

▶ More recent guidelines, such as *Dietary Guidelines for Americans, The Surgeon General's Report on Nutrition and Health,* and *Diet and Health,* have an added focus. These recommendations encourage people to modify their intake of dietary substances that are thought to be related to chronic diseases.

▶ The *Basic Food Guide,* developed for this textbook, uses the food group approach and incorporates information about the fat, sodium, and added sugar in representative foods. It includes a separate list for combination foods. The final list consists of *limited extras,* generally foods of low nutrient density that should not be consumed in excessive amounts although they can be eaten in moderation by well-nourished people who are not overweight.

References

American Diabetes Association, Inc. and the American Dietetic Association. 1986. *Exchange lists for meal planning.* Alexandria, VA: The American Diabetes Association. Chicago, IL: The American Dietetic Association.

Barrett, S. 1985. Commercial hair analysis: Science or scam? *Journal of the American Medical Association* 254:1041–1045.

Cronin, F.J., A.M. Shaw, S.M. Krebs-Smith, P.M. Marsland, and L. Light. 1987. Developing a food guidance system to implement the Dietary Guidelines. *Journal of Nutrition Education* 19:281–302.

Derelian, D. 1988. The four food groups: An instructional tool for adults. *Nutrition News* 51(no.1):1–3.

Dwyer, J.T. 1988. Assessment of dietary intake. In *Modern Nutrition in Health and Disease,* eds. M.E. Shils and V.R. Young. Philadelphia: Lea & Febiger.

Food and Nutrition Board. 1986. *What is America eating?* Washington, DC: National Academy Press.

Frisancho, A.R. 1988. Nutritional anthropometry. *Journal of the American Dietetic Association* 88:553–555.

Guthrie, H.A. 1985. Selection and quantification of typical food portions by young adults. *Journal of the American Dietetic Association* 84:1440–1444.

Hollman, P.C. and M.B. Katan. 1988. Bias and error in the determination of common macronutrients in foods: Interlaboratory trial. *Journal of the American Dietetic Association* 88:556–563.

Jarvis, W. 1989. Dubious health assessments. *Nutrition & the M.D.* 15(no.2):1–3.

Klevay, L.M., B.R. Bistrian, C.R. Fleming, and C.G. Neumann. 1987. Hair analysis in clinical and experimental medicine. *American Journal of Clinical Nutrition* 46:233–236.

Krall, E.A. and J.T. Dwyer. 1987. Validity of a food frequency questionnaire and a food diary in a short-term recall situation. *Journal of the American Dietetic Association* 87:1374–1377.

Medlin, C. and J.D. Skinner. 1988. Individual dietary intake methodology: A 50-year review of progress. *Journal of the American Dietetic Association* 88:1250–1257.

National Research Council. 1989. *Diet and health.* Washington, DC: National Academy Press.

Stark, C. 1990. A look at meat labeling: Issues and insights. *Food & Nutrition News* 62(no.1):5–6.

Surgeon General. 1979. *Healthy people: The Surgeon General's report on health promotion and disease prevention.* Washington, DC: U.S. Department of Health, Education, and Welfare (now Department of Health and Human Services).

Surgeon General. 1988. *The Surgeon General's report on nutrition and health.* Washington, DC: U.S. Department of Health and Human Services.

U.S. Congress. Senate Select Committee on Nutrition and Human Needs. *Dietary goals for the United States,* 95th Congress, 1st session, February and December 1977. Committee Print.

U.S. Department of Agriculture and U.S. Department of Health and Human Services. 1980, 1985. *Nutrition and your health: Dietary guidelines for Americans.* Home and Garden Bulletin No. 232: U.S. Government Printing Office.

Yuhas, J.A., J.E. Bolland, and T.W. Bolland. 1989. The impact of training, food type, gender, and container size on the estimation of food portion sizes. *Journal of the American Dietetic Association* 89:1473–1477.

3

Physiology for Nutrition

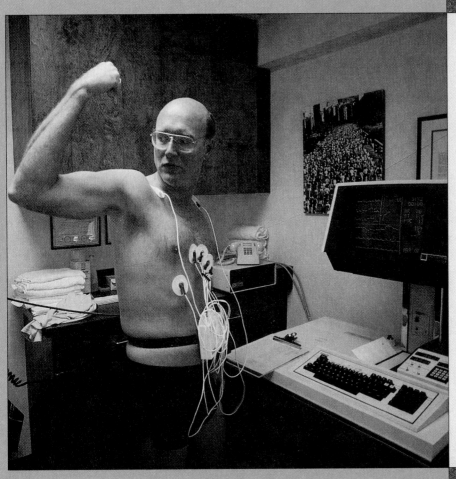

ou might think that just *eating* food should guarantee that its nutrients will become an integral part of the body. Actually, though, the body must first break food apart and then get the nutrients through several screening devices before the nutrients are usable.

Because the healthy body is so efficient at doing this, we tend to take these functions for granted. It is well worth taking an appreciative look at the carefully regulated processes and structures involved in incorporating food into the body. This information can help you understand material in upcoming chapters about what particular nutrients can do for you, and about certain abnormalities that can occur in the way the body handles nutrients.

We will discuss several processes involved in the food-using activity: digestion, which prepares food to move through the screening devices; absorption, which moves nutrients into the body's interior; circulation, which carries nutrients and oxygen to the cells and waste products from them; metabolism, during which nutrients are used; and excretion, which transports the waste products out of the body. We will also look at the cell, the entity that ultimately uses the nutrients.

In this chapter, you will become acquainted with the basic anatomy (structure) and physiology (function) of several body systems: the digestive, circulatory, and excretory systems. We will take a more detailed look at how the body handles each of the six classes of nutrients in later chapters.

Digestion Prepares Nutrients for Absorption

digestion—the process of breaking food down into substances small enough to be absorbed

absorption—the process of taking digested substances into the body's interior

alimentary canal, gastrointestinal (GI) tract—the main part of the digestive system: a hollow tube beginning at the mouth and ending at the anus

Digestion is the process of breaking food down into substances that can be absorbed. **Absorption** is the uptake of these substances into the body's interior. Both occur in the **alimentary canal** or **gastrointestinal (GI) tract.** The GI tract absorbs the digested fragments through its lining into the blood as it breaks food down into the nutrients that will eventually be used at the cellular level.

General Characteristics of the Digestive System

Many digestive organs—the mouth, salivary glands, stomach, intestines and liver, to name a few—contribute to the work of disassembling food into its various subunits. But there are special features of the system itself that enable it to carry out its unique tasks.

Shape   The main part of the digestive system consists of a hollow tube called the GI tract. The tube begins at the mouth and takes a turning and twisting route before it ends at the anus. Its entire length, if straightened

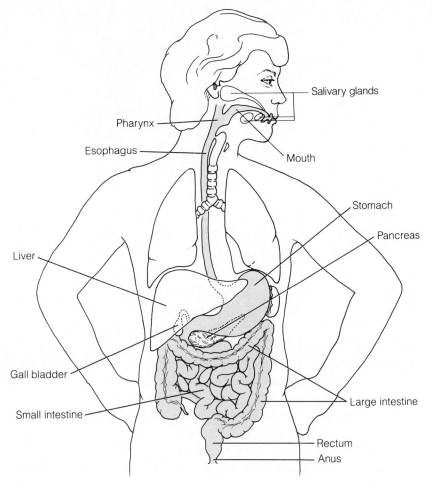

Figure 3.1 The anatomy of the digestive system.

Salivary glands

Pharynx

Esophagus

Mouth

Stomach

Pancreas

Liver

Gall bladder

Small intestine

Large intestine

Rectum

Anus

out, would be several times your height. As you look at its structure (Figure 3.1), you can see that its various specialized sections have different diameters, from the considerable width of the stomach to the rather narrow tube of the small intestine.

Lining The entire tract has a lining that can be thought of as an internal skin separating the contents of the tract from the body's actual interior (Figure 3.2). Food that is moving through the central space within the tract, called the **lumen,** is still technically "outside" your body. The lining of the tract is called the **mucosa;** it selectively allows certain types of substances to be absorbed. An important criterion in this screening process is that the materials be particles small enough to pass through the lining.

Substances that are too large to be absorbed will simply pass through the entire length of the GI tract and exit the system. For example, if a toddler swallows a small plastic button, the button will be prevented from entering his body and will simply pass through and exit the system within a few days. Similarly food fiber, the plant constituents that the human body is

lumen—the central space within which food passes through the GI tract

mucosa—the internal lining of the GI tract

Figure 3.2 The layers in the GI tract. (a) Different regions of the GI tract have many similarities in structure, even though they vary considerably in the size of the lumen (central space through which food passes) and in some other characteristics. This cross-sectional drawing shows the features the regions have in common. (b) This micrograph shows a cross section of the small intestine.

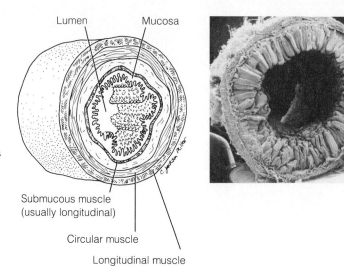

Lumen   Mucosa

Submucous muscle (usually longitudinal)

Circular muscle

Longitudinal muscle

unable to digest, will not pass through the mucosa but will travel through the tract and leave the body as solid waste.

Muscles The GI tract has many layers besides the mucosa; several of these are composed of muscles that control the progress of the contents through the tract. Longitudinal muscles run the length of the system, and others encircle it (see Figure 3.2a).

The circular muscles that occur between different areas of the tract and at the end of it are called **sphincters.** When a sphincter is relaxed, that part of the tube is open, and the contents can pass through. When a sphincter is contracted (constricted), the muscular ring is tightly closed, and forward movement through the tract is prevented. A contracted sphincter also prevents any GI contents from moving backward (up) in the tract.

Sphincter muscles are normally controlled automatically through stimulation by the nervous system. However, the last sphincter in the tract, the **anus** or **anal sphincter,** can be voluntarily controlled.

Secretions Various parts of the digestive system secrete large amounts of fluids—approximately 2 gallons per day in most people—that contain the following types of substances that assist in digestion:

1. **Mucus** is a slimy material produced by certain cells in the mucosa; it lubricates the tract, keeping the lining moist and allowing food to move more readily through the system, as well as coating the lining to protect it from some of the tract's harsher secretions.
2. Chemical compounds are produced that have a particular acidity or alkalinity needed for digestion.
3. **Enzymes,** which are proteins that speed up the rate of biochemical reactions in the body, are produced in various parts of the digestive system to help in the breakdown of food. Names of enzymes can often be recognized by their "-ase" endings—for example, prote*ase*, an enzyme

sphincters—circular muscles between different sections of the GI tract that help to regulate the passage of materials

anus (anal sphincter)—the last sphincter in the GI tract; can be voluntarily controlled

mucus—slimy material produced by the mucosa

enzymes—proteins that speed up biochemical reactions

that acts on protein; lip*ase,* an enzyme that acts on lipid (fat); and amy*lase,* an enzyme that acts on starch.

4. **Hormones,** which are chemical messengers produced in one region of the body and targeted to affect a process at some other body site, influence many aspects of digestion. Names of hormones often end in "-in" or "-ine"—for example, epinephr*ine,* gastr*in,* secret*in.*

hormones—chemical messengers produced in one region of the body that affect a process in another region

Transit Time The amount of time it takes from ingestion of a food until its solid waste leaves the system is called the **transit time.** Normally, transit time is from 24 to 72 hours in a healthy individual, although remnants of the residue of a given meal may remain in the system for a week or more. Factors that can influence the rate of transit, either speeding it up or slowing it down, include the content of the diet, medications, emotions, physical activity, and various illnesses. If transit time is much faster than normal, diarrhea results; if it is much slower, constipation occurs.

transit time—the time that elapses between ingestion of food and elimination from the body of the solid waste that results from food

Maintenance The innermost lining of the GI tract, which directly contacts food, is renewed every two to three days. This replacement is necessary because even though there are mechanisms to protect the mucosa from damage, the digestive secretions and the movement of food through the tract cause wear and tear.

Phases of Digestion and Absorption

Just as the different sections of the GI tract vary in structure, they also vary in function. Thus it's logical that digestion and absorption represent a series of coordinated phases and responses that together accomplish the task. Let's look at these steps.

Cephalic Phase: Sometimes the First Step in the Process *Cephalic* means "pertaining to the head"; just thinking about food can initiate digestive processes. If you see food, smell it, or even hear sounds associated with it, you may sense your digestive processes beginning, even though you have not eaten anything. Your stomach may growl, and your saliva and other digestive juices may flow more copiously in anticipation. In some instances, the responses of the GI tract can be as active as if the food had actually been eaten (Mattes and Mela, 1988).

These sensations may make you *want* to eat, but your body does not necessarily *need* food when you experience them.

The Mouth: Point of Entry When food enters the mouth, the digestive system becomes undeniably active. With your teeth, you cut, grind, and mash food, making it easier to swallow and more accessible to the various digestive substances it will encounter along the way.

In addition, the presence of food stimulates the flow of saliva, the watery mucus produced in the mouth. Saliva not only lubricates the upper part of the GI tract, but also moistens dry foods and turns them into a cohesive wad. In addition, saliva contains the first of many enzymes involved in digestion: amylase. Amylase begins the breakdown of starch, a form of carbohydrate. Saliva functions even after food has been swallowed by rinsing the surface of the teeth, which helps prevent their decay. The amount of saliva that is produced and swallowed throughout the day probably totals 1 to $1\frac{1}{2}$ quarts (Marieb, 1989).

pharynx—section of the GI tract just beyond the mouth

The Pharynx: Origin of the Swallow   The **pharynx,** located just beyond the mouth, is a common pathway for both the digestive and respiratory systems. It is part of the GI tract for food and part of the airway for breathing. When it is being used for food, openings to the other portions of the airway are normally closed by muscles controlled automatically by the nervous system.

Because it contains the muscles for swallowing, the pharynx's special function in digestion is to move food along to the next region of the tract, the esophagus.

esophagus—passageway that conducts food from the pharynx to the stomach

peristalsis—rhythmic waves of involuntary muscular contraction that move food in the proper direction through the GI tract

The Esophagus: The Stomach Connection   The **esophagus** is a conduit between the pharynx and the stomach. Once food is in this structure, it is moved along by rhythmic waves of muscular contraction that are automatically controlled by the nervous system. This involuntary digestive muscular activity is called **peristalsis;** it occurs in every region of the GI tract from the pharynx to the rectum. Usually gravity, too, plays a role in helping move foods down the esophagus, but peristalsis can accomplish the task by itself if you are not in an upright position.

At the bottom of the esophagus is a sphincter that relaxes to allow food to pass into the stomach but then closes to prevent digestive juices and food from moving back into the esophagus. Sometimes this sphincter does not stay tightly closed while food is being mixed with digestive juices in the stomach, and part of the stomach contents wash back up into the lower part of the esophagus. Since the stomach juices contain chemicals that are irritating to the lining of the esophagus, repeated contact causes pain that is referred to as "heartburn," although it has nothing to do with the heart. This sphincter is also open during vomiting.

The Stomach: Mixer and Reservoir   The stomach is the pouchlike enlargement in the GI tract that has the elasticity to accommodate from 1 to 2 quarts of food and fluid. Although one of its important functions is simply to hold what has been eaten until the lower portions of the tract are ready to receive and process its contents, it also has several unique roles.

chyme—slushy mixture of food and digestive juices produced in the stomach

• **Mixing Activity**   Peristaltic contractions in the stomach are very strong. The muscles squeeze and churn the contents, mixing digestive juices with the food particles. The slushy blend that results is called **chyme.**

• **Secretions**   The stomach produces digestive juices that contain strong hydrochloric acid and enzymes that act on protein to begin its digestion. The production of these juices is stimulated by the presence of food in the stomach. Emotions can either increase or decrease these secretions: when people feel aggressive, resentful, angry, hostile, sad, afraid, or depressed, the rate at which these substances are produced may either speed up or slow down.

Since the tissues of the stomach are composed of protein, it would seem as though they should be vulnerable to digestion by their own gastric (stomach) juices. However, under normal circumstances the tough material and tight construction of the stomach lining prevent self-digestion. Furthermore, the mucus produced there sets up a protective barrier. In most cases, these features of the stomach also protect it against damage from acids in food (which are generally weaker than stomach acid anyway) and from spices in foods. A study done in Texas showed that two spicy Mexican-style meals consumed one day by 11 out of 12 normally healthy people produced no significant stomach damage observable the next day (Graham et al., 1988). However, these fail-safe mechanisms can break down if the stomach frequently produces excessive amounts of acid, and/or the stomach is unusually vulnerable to its acid. Known irritants such as alcohol, caffeine, and tobacco can provoke or worsen the situation (Harvard Medical School, 1986). Drugs can also be powerful irritants: in the Texas study cited above, 11 of 12 people showed significant damage the next day from having taken a total of six aspirin tablets with bland (non-irritating) meals the previous day. If irritation eventually wears deep into the lining, a **peptic ulcer** results. (This term is also often used for ulcerations that occur in the esophagus or in the small intestine as well as in the stomach; more on this shortly.)

• **Absorption**   Little absorption takes place through the stomach. Two common substances can be absorbed without being digested first—water and alcohol—and they are absorbed from this site in only small amounts. (Some drugs can also be absorbed through the stomach.)

• **Emptying**   Chyme is emptied from the stomach over a period of several hours; it is released from the stomach into the small intestine at intervals when the sphincter between them is relaxed. The rate at which the stomach empties depends on a number of factors. Consistency of the material influences emptying: liquids leave the stomach more rapidly than solids do. The macronutrient composition also makes a difference: in pure form, carbohydrates leave the fastest, proteins leave next, and fats the most slowly. Since most consumables are mixtures of macronutrients, their emptying time depends on the relative nutrient content of each. Not surprisingly, the volume of what has been eaten is also a factor: a huge meal takes longer to empty than a smaller one.

Stomach (or gastric) emptying is regulated more by the small intestine than by the stomach itself, although both are involved. When chyme contacts the intestinal mucosa, hormonal messages based on the compo-

peptic ulcer—open sore in the lining of the esophagus, stomach, or small intestine, produced in susceptible individuals by acidic digestive juices and/or other irritants

sition of the chyme are sent back to the sphincter at the lower end of the stomach; this controls when and how much chyme will be released. The nervous system can also prompt the opening or closing of the sphincter, depending on how distended the small intestine is, and on various chemical factors.

Emotions may affect emptying as well, either slowing or hastening it. A physician who x-rayed the stomachs of college football players found that on game days, the players' stomachs took two to four hours longer to empty, presumably because of stress (Mirkin and Hoffman, 1978).

The Small Intestine: Scene of the Major Action In a length of approximately 10 feet, your **small intestine** accomplishes the major work of digestion. It divides most of the carbohydrates, proteins, and fats into small units, and then absorbs them. It also absorbs the substances that are small enough to pass through the lining without digestion: water, vitamins, minerals, and alcohol.

small intestine—longest section of the GI tract, performing the major work of digestion and absorption

• **Secretions** In addition to the enzyme-containing digestive juices produced by the intestinal mucosa, secretions from two organs connected to the tract also enter the intestinal lumen. The **liver** is a large multifunction organ that filters blood and processes and stores various body substances. It produces **bile,** a solution that is stored in the **gall bladder** until it is needed. Bile is necessary for the digestion of fat. Because fat is not soluble in water, it would be likely to form a glob in the midst of the watery material; but bile acts to keep fat **emulsified** (divided into small droplets) after intestinal muscular activity mechanically breaks it apart. This makes the fat more accessible to enzymes for digestion and absorption.

liver—organ that produces bile; performs many metabolic functions

bile—liquid produced in the liver and stored in the **gall bladder** until needed for fat digestion in the small intestine

emulsified—dispersed in small droplets through another substance with which the dispersed material ordinarily does not mix

The **pancreas** also has several functions, one of which is to produce secretions that contain alkali, which neutralizes the hydrochloric acid in the chyme. (If this process fails, or if the amount of stomach acid is excessive, a peptic ulcer can develop here. The section of the small intestine in which ulceration is most often seen is the part immediately below the stomach called the *duodenum;* therefore an ulcer here is more specifically called a *duodenal ulcer.*) In addition, the pancreas produces various amylases, proteases, and lipases.

pancreas—organ producing secretions that neutralize the acidity of the chyme and enzymes that help to digest macronutrients

• **Mechanical Activity** Two kinds of muscular activity take place in the small intestine to mix and move the contents. Peristalsis, as in other areas, is evident here. In addition, circular muscles constrict at intervals to produce a "sausage-link" effect. After the contents between the contracted muscles have been mixed for a time, the muscles relax, and then other muscles constrict to form a new series of "links"; these are called **segmentation contractions.**

segmentation contractions—intermittent constrictions of circular muscles that produce "segments" of intestine whose contents are mixed for a time before new segments are formed

• **Absorption** The structure of the lining of the small intestine equips it perfectly for its additional critical role of absorbing the end-products of digestion. Millions of thin, flexible fingerlike projections extend from the lining, giving the effect of a terrycloth-lined tube. Called **villi** (singular:

villi—thin, fingerlike projections of the intestinal mucosa that extend into the lumen, greatly increasing the surface area for absorbing nutrients

villus), these projections waft about in the intestine, ready to absorb digested macronutrient particles, water, vitamins, and minerals.

Projecting from the villi are even smaller strands called **microvilli,** which enlarge surface area further (Figure 3.3.). It is estimated that this convoluted construction multiplies the intestinal surface area by 600 times what it would have been if the intestine were smooth. If the absorptive surface could be flattened out, it would measure approximately 200 square meters (Ganong, 1989), an area equivalent to the size of a tennis court. (The estimates of other physiologists vary.) After the nutrients have been absorbed, they are distributed to the body's cells via circulation, which will be described later in this chapter.

microvilli—microscopic projections from the villi that increase the intestine's absorptive surface area even further

The small intestine of a healthy person does a thorough job; it is here that 90% or more of the carbohydrate, fat, and protein that were consumed are digested and absorbed. The absorption of vitamins and minerals from the small intestine is less predictable, since absorption of these nutrients is influenced by the presence of other food constituents. Water is also absorbed here, a function that is shared with the large intestine.

large intestine (colon, bowel)—last major section of the GI tract, serving as a collecting chamber for solid waste, a home for bacteria, and an absorption site for water and certain minerals

The Large Intestine: Absorber and Reservoir It may seem there is nothing left for the **large intestine (colon** or **bowel)** to do after the small intestine has played its major role. However, several important functions are performed by this section of the digestive tract.

- **Collection** The large intestine serves as a collecting chamber for solid waste, which it holds until the feces are excreted. Of all the regions of the digestive system, food spends the longest time here, often 24 hours or more.
- **Holding and Harboring of Bacteria** Because peristalsis and segmentation contractions move contents more slowly through the colon, bacteria

Figure 3.3 The villi of the small intestine. (a) The left side of this illustration represents a cross section of the small intestine, showing how the villi project into the lumen. The right side is a magnification of two villi, showing their microvilli. These projections greatly enlarge the absorptive surface beyond what it would be if the lining were smooth. (b) The micrograph shows the microvilli on a single villus.

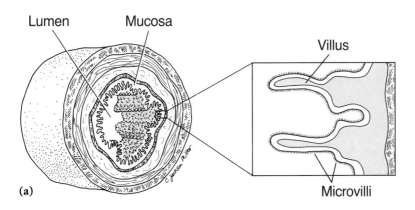

(a)

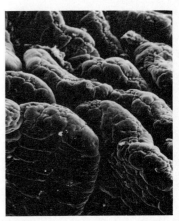

(b)

have an opportunity to become established and to flourish. Their population is impressive: the number of bacteria in the GI tract is estimated to be more than ten times the number of cells in the human body (Savage, 1987).

Bacteria act on the portions of food that have not yet been digested and absorbed by the human system. Some of the products of the breakdown are used by the bacteria for their own sustenance. Others are available to the person after absorption from the colon: recent research suggests that up to 10% of the kcalories a person absorbs may come via this route (McNeil, 1984).

Another benefit of these bacteria is that they produce some vitamins during the course of their own metabolism that seem to be partially absorbed by the body. Small amounts of the B vitamins and vitamin K are thought to be obtained in this way.

As bacteria metabolize food, they produce gas as one of their waste products. If the amount is small, it causes no symptoms; however, if a great deal of gas accumulates, it is emitted through the anus.

• **Absorption**   The colon offers the body its last chance to absorb much of the remaining water and the elements sodium and chloride. If the colon fails to do this, diarrhea results. Normally, however, there is substantial reclamation of these materials before the solid waste is excreted.

• **Defecation**   The solid waste, called **feces** or **fecal material,** is excreted when the anal (rectal) sphincter at the end of the colon is relaxed; this process is called **defecation** or **laxation.** In babies, it is automatic and

feces, fecal material—solid waste excreted from GI tract; consists of bacteria, food residue, water, digestive secretions

defecation, laxation—evacuation of feces from the colon

Table 3.1 Summary of Processes That Mix or Move the GI Contents

Location	Process
Mouth	Chewing
Pharynx	Swallowing
	Peristalsis
Esophagus	Peristalsis
Stomach	Peristalsis
	Absorption of small amounts of water and alcohol
Small intestine	Peristalsis
	Segmentation contractions
	Absorption of water, vitamins, minerals, alcohol, and digestion products from carbohydrates, lipids, and proteins
Large intestine	Peristalsis
	Segmentation contractions
	Absorption of water, sodium, chloride, some B vitamins, and products of bacterial metabolism
Rectum	Peristalsis
	Defecation

Table 3.2 Summary of Secreted Agents That Help Break the Macronutrients Apart in the GI Tract

Location	Agents Acting on Carbohydrate	Agents Acting on Fat	Agents Acting on Protein
Mouth	Amylase in saliva		
Stomach			Hydrochloric acid Protease
Small intestine	Amylase from pancreas	Bile produced by liver	Protease from pancreas
	Enzymes from mucosa that complete carbohydrate digestion	Lipase from pancreas Enzymes from mucosa that complete fat digestion	Enzymes from mucosa that complete protein digestion
Large intestine	(Here bacteria carry out their own chemical processes on remaining nutrients.)		

uncontrolled; as children mature, they learn to recognize the sense of fullness in their rectum and to temporarily delay defecation. In adults, any frequency of laxation from three times per day to three times per week is considered normal.

What is considered a comfortable and convenient frequency of laxation varies with each individual. Even cultural patterns influence expectations to a certain extent; the "once a day" standard that many Americans think is best is not the only healthy pattern. When an unusually long time passes between one defecation and the next, people sometimes use a **laxative** to expedite the process.

laxative—a medication that promotes defecation

You have now taken a tour through the GI tract. Table 3.1 summarizes these processes by reviewing the regions of the canal in which the mixing, moving, and absorbing activities occur. Table 3.2 summarizes the body's digestive secretions that act on carbohydrate, fat, and protein and tells where they have their effects on the macronutrients. We will next focus on the microscopic unit that *needs* the nutrients—the cell.

The Cell Is Where Nutrients Are Used

The **cell** is the smallest, simplest unit of living matter. It is within the cell that the most basic life processes take place, including the release of energy from nutrients. All living animal cells have certain structural and functional similarities. Figure 3.4 illustrates these:

cell—the smallest, simplest unit of living matter

• A thin, *selectively permeable cell membrane,* which encloses and protects the contents by controlling what substances come into and go out of the cell.

Figure 3.4 The cell. Animal cells have certain structural similarities, which are pictured.

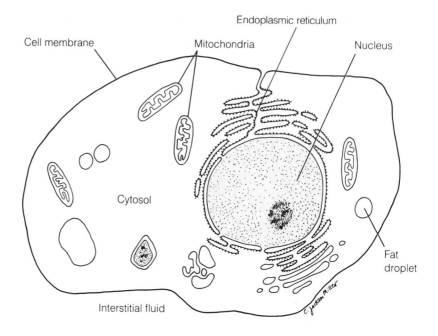

• *Cytosol,* the fluid that fills the cell and in which all the cell bodies are suspended.
• A *nucleus,* which contains genetic information that enables new cells of the same type to form by division from the original.
• *Mitochondria,* small bodies within the cell in which energy production takes place.
• An *endoplasmic reticulum,* a network of channels involved in synthesis of protein and fatty materials.
• Various other types of small bodies that make or store protein or fat, and still others that destroy materials for which there is no further need.

Although a cell is microscopic, its importance cannot be overestimated. Some organisms are single cells that are able to function independently; bacteria and yeasts are examples. More complex organisms—like you—consist of millions of interrelated specialized cells that function together.

When cells are grouped together in a more complex life form, they are seldom so tightly packed that their membranes touch each other. Rather, there are spaces between the cells called interstitial spaces, which are filled with **interstitial fluid.** You have seen interstitial fluid when it has oozed from a minor abrasion or a scrape in your skin that was not deep enough to cause bleeding. This same fluid has a role to play in nutrition that will be described soon.

interstitial fluid—fluid that fills the spaces between cells

Building a Body from Cells

tissue—similar cells united to perform a particular function

When many cells of the same type are grouped together to perform a similar function, they are collectively referred to as a **tissue.** The body's tissue types are muscular, nervous, connective (for binding together and supporting body structures), and epithelial (for coverings and linings, such as the skin or the lining of the GI tract).

Several tissues combine to form **organs,** which are capable of more complex physiological processes; the stomach, for example, is an organ made up of epithelial, muscular, and nervous tissues. Several organs combine into **systems,** such as the digestive system, and function cooperatively to accomplish a major physiological purpose. Systems, then, unite into a total **organism.**

This variety and interdependence among the functions of cells make the body not only extremely complex, but also very versatile and able to adapt to different conditions.

Sustaining Cells Through Metabolism

As mentioned early in this book, the chemical processes that take place in the living cell are referred to by the umbrella term *metabolism*. A regular supply of nutrients is essential for metabolism to take place.

Metabolic reactions occur all the time in every living cell. Synthesis reactions build up new substances that will become part of the body's structure or will be used to help it function; these metabolic processes are collectively referred to as **anabolism.** Simultaneously, breakdown reactions dismantle other materials into smaller units; this is referred to as **catabolism.**

Although both are occurring in all cells at the same time, anabolism and catabolism may take place at different rates at different times or in different cells. During periods of growth—such as childhood, pregnancy, muscle building, and healing—synthesis outstrips breakdown. At other times, such as during illness or injury, breakdown predominates.

Circulation Delivers Nutrients Where They Are Needed

The primary function of the circulatory system is to deliver to all of the body's individual cells the nutrients and oxygen they need to derive energy for living. Equally important and simultaneous roles of the circulatory system are to carry various cellular products to other sites in the body and to carry the waste products of metabolism away from the cells for disposal. The lymphatic system also plays a role in channeling nutrients to the body's cells.

General Characteristics of the Circulatory System

The **circulatory system** is a closed, continuous network of elastic blood vessels in which the body's 4- to 6-quart blood supply cycles repeatedly. The

organ—a specialized body part composed of various types of tissues that work together to perform a particular function or functions

system—a set of interdependent organs that together perform a function that none could do alone

organism—any individual living thing, whether plant, microorganism, or animal; the most complex forms consist of a set of interdependent systems that together sustain life

anabolism—the combining of simpler substances into more complex substances by a living system

catabolism—the breakdown of complex substances into simpler substances by a living system

circulatory system—closed, continuous network of blood vessels in which blood cycles repeatedly throughout the body

heart provides the power that keeps this vital fluid pulsing throughout the body nonstop from before birth until death.

The Heart The heart is the pump that keeps blood moving through the circulatory system. It is composed of strong muscles that normally contract and relax 50 to 90 times per minute when the body is at rest.

The vessels that enter and leave the heart are few in number but large in size, since the body's entire blood supply is channeled through them.

Two Loops There are two loops through which the body's blood is routed: one that circles between the heart and the lungs (the pulmonary circuit), and one that connects the heart to all the other parts of the body (the systemic circuit). Each circuit is powered by a different side of the heart, as shown in Figure 3.5.

Here's what happens in the pulmonary circuit:

1. Blood is pumped from the right side of the heart to the lungs through a network of branching blood vessels.
2. In the lungs, where the vessels are especially small and permeable, the blood releases carbon dioxide (a waste product of cellular activity) to be exhaled and takes in oxygen from the newly inhaled air.
3. The blood returns to the left side of the heart.

The following takes place in the systemic circuit:

1. Blood is pumped from the left side of the heart to all areas of the body through a network of branching blood vessels.
2. Where the vessels are very small and permeable, oxygen and nutrients move out through the vessel walls, and carbon dioxide and other cellular metabolic products pass into the blood.
3. The blood returns to the right side of the heart.

This sequence is repeated with every heartbeat from before birth until death.

Names of Vessels Although the blood vessels form a continuous system, they are called by different names depending on where they are in the circuit. The large vessels that carry blood away from the heart are called **arteries.** They divide into many branches in order to distribute blood to different areas of the body.

After each branching, they are more numerous and smaller in diameter. Small arteries are called *arterioles*, and the very smallest versions, through which the exchange of nutrients from the blood supply and wastes from body cells finally occurs, are called **capillaries.** The network of tiny blood vessels that serves a given region of the body is its capillary bed.

(You can imagine how numerous the blood vessels need to be to have a capillary close to every body cell—every cell of skin, bone, nerve, muscle,

arteries—vessels that carry blood away from the heart

capillaries—smallest blood vessels, through which exchange of nutrients from the blood supply and wastes from body cells occurs

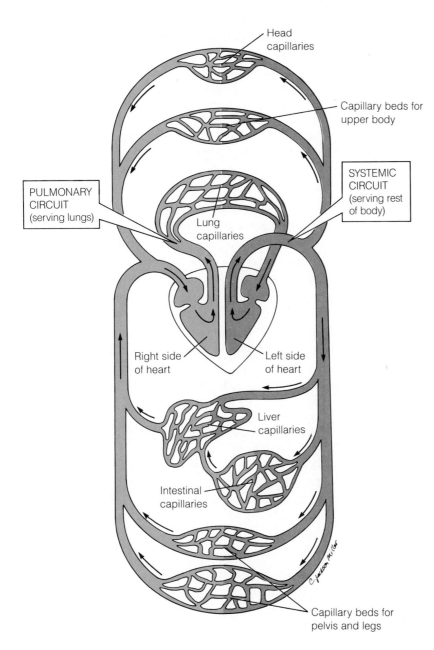

Head
capillaries

Capillary beds for
upper body

SYSTEMIC
CIRCUIT
(serving rest
of body)

PULMONARY
CIRCUIT
(serving lungs)

Lung
capillaries

Right side
of heart

Left side
of heart

Liver
capillaries

Intestinal
capillaries

Capillary beds for
pelvis and legs

Figure 3.5 Schematic diagram of circulation. This drawing represents the route blood takes through the two circuits that begin and end at the heart. (Note that in anatomical drawings, the right and left sides are pictured as though you were looking at the body from the front.) Red indicates blood that is richer in oxygen; blue is for blood carrying more carbon dioxide.

and so on. You have approximately 60,000 miles of blood vessels within you to accomplish this!)

Now to complete the circuit: blood returns toward the heart through *venules*. These merge to form **veins,** large venules that funnel blood back into the heart.

How do nutrients make their entry into this system? Answering that question requires looking at the capillary bed in the part of the circuit that serves the small intestine.

veins—vessels that carry blood to the heart

The Route Taken by Nutrients Entering the Bloodstream

Recall that nutrients are absorbed into the villi in the small intestine. There are capillaries in each villus, as shown in Figure 3.6, which are ready to take up nutrients that are absorbed.

Capillaries take in mostly water-soluble nutrients. Many of the digested nutrients that are absorbed into the circulatory system need more modification before they can be used by the body's cells. For this reason, the venous blood leaving the small intestine goes to the liver, where such changes can be made.

The liver is the body's major metabolic clearinghouse. In the liver, many nutrients are made more suitable for circulation, energy production, or storage. Some nutrients remain in the liver; others resume their journey via the veins back to the heart.

As these veins merge with those returning from other body areas, the blood they are carrying mixes, and the nutrients are distributed through it. The dissolved nutrients keep recycling in the blood as described here and as shown in Figure 3.5: from the heart to the lungs, then back to the left side of the heart, which pumps them to all regions of the body.

Getting the Nutrients into Cells

When nutrients are distributed via the circulation to all of your capillary beds, they are able to move through the thin selectively permeable capillary membranes into the interstitial fluid (Figure 3.7). From the interstitial fluid, the nutrients are absorbed through the individual selectively permeable cell membranes into the interior of the cells.

Figure 3.6 The villi and their blood vessels. Each villus is laced with a network of capillaries that take in nutrients absorbed during digestion.

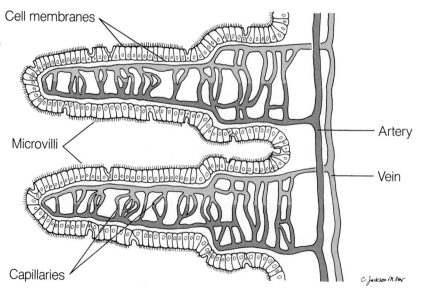

While they are taking in nutrients, the cells are simultaneously releasing wastes and other products of their metabolism into the interstitial fluid. Many of these products are then absorbed back into the capillaries and thereby into the general circulation. In a later section, we will describe how the body gets rid of wastes.

Distributing Blood to Various Body Regions

The volume of blood that is channeled to each of the body's various regions is determined largely by the amount of blood that is *needed* there at any given time. When the body is at rest, the heart typically directs to the abdomen about half of the total amount of blood it pumps; approximately one-sixth goes to skeletal muscle (muscle that is attached to bone); and the rest is shared by the heart, brain, skin, and other organs (Ganong, 1989). This distribution is adequate to meet resting needs. However, if a person is engaged in strenuous physical activity, as much as seven-eighths of the blood supply may be directed to the active skeletal muscles, which are in immediate need of oxygen and nutrients for energy production.

If a person has recently eaten a large meal, a greater-than-normal portion of the blood supply will be committed to the intestines in order to pick up the nutrients that are absorbed. If you eat a large meal shortly before strenuous exercise, your skeletal muscles and GI tract will both need a greater blood supply at the same time. These increased demands cannot both be met fully and simultaneously. It is possible, therefore, that physical performance and digestion may be temporarily impaired. (Eating just a *small* amount is not likely to interfere with physical performance, though.) For this reason it is not a good idea to eat a large meal within three hours of intense physical activity.

A Sidekick for the Circulatory System: The Lymphatic System

The **lymphatic system** is a second system of vessels that serves the body; it carries lymph, the clear fluid formed from interstitial fluid, which filters into tiny lymphatic vessels. These vessels constitute a one-way network that eventually funnels lymph from all over the body into two large lymphatic vessels that empty into major veins returning to the heart (Figure 3.8). This system drains surplus fluid away from the tissues, which would otherwise become swollen.

It is the lymphatic vessels that serve the small intestine that have an important role in nutrition. Besides collecting lymph, they also absorb and transport some of the nutrients that the blood capillaries in the villi do not carry. Figure 3.9 shows how these small lymphatic vessels, called **lacteals,** fit into the total absorption scheme. The lacteals take in mainly fatty products of digestion and carry them through this network, merging with larger and larger lymphatics until they join major veins.

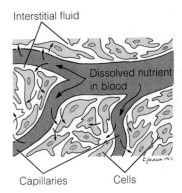

Figure 3.7 The route taken by nutrients from the capillaries to the cells. Nutrients are carried by the circulation to all regions of the body. They pass through the selectively permeable capillary walls into the interstitial fluid, and from there into the cells.

lymphatic system—one-way system of vessels; one function is to absorb and transport certain nutrients; eventually empties into the circulatory system

lacteals—small lymphatic vessels in the villi

Figure 3.8 Schematic drawing of the lymphatic system. This system carries lymph (which has been filtered from interstitial fluid) and nutrients (which have been picked up in the small intestine). Both enter the bloodstream where the lymphatic system connects with major veins near the heart.

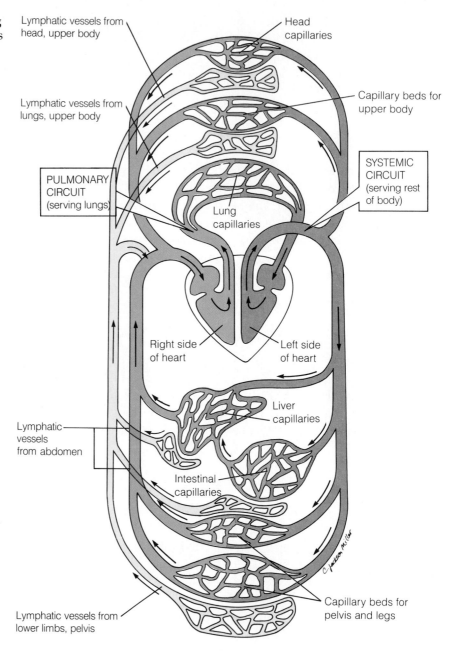

Lymphatic vessels from head, upper body

Head capillaries

Lymphatic vessels from lungs, upper body

Capillary beds for upper body

PULMONARY CIRCUIT (serving lungs)

SYSTEMIC CIRCUIT (serving rest of body)

Lung capillaries

Right side of heart

Left side of heart

Liver capillaries

Lymphatic vessels from abdomen

Intestinal capillaries

Lymphatic vessels from lower limbs, pelvis

Capillary beds for pelvis and legs

Excretion of Waste Products Occurs via Several Routes

To round out the picture of how the body uses nutrients, it is appropriate to mention the means by which the body disposes of substances for which it has no further use. As discussed in the section on the digestive system, solid waste is excreted from the body as feces. When it leaves the body, some

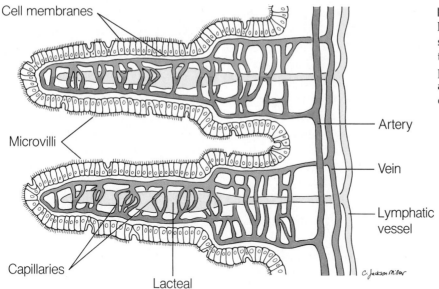

Cell membranes

Microvilli

Capillaries

Lacteal

Artery

Vein

Lymphatic vessel

C. Jackson Miller

Figure 3.9 Lacteals. Each villus in the small intestine, besides housing capillaries, contains a lacteal. For the most part, the lymphatic system absorbs the fatty products of digestion.

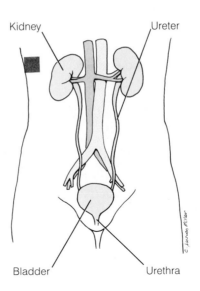

Kidney

Ureter

Bladder

Urethra

C. Jackson Miller

Figure 3.10 The urinary system and some neighboring structures. The two kidneys are the body's chief organs for cleansing its internal fluids of soluble waste and excreting surplus water and nutrients. Ureters carry the urine to the bladder for storage until it is excreted through the urethra.

water is also lost, since plant fiber and bacteria in the feces hold a certain amount of water and take it out with them.

Several other routes exist by which water and soluble substances leave the body. The greatest amount of water exits the body via the **urinary system.** As the body's blood supply continuously flows through the capillaries of the kidneys, much of the water and many of the dissolved substances (solutes) in the blood pass from the capillaries into the functional units of the kidneys, which are called *nephrons.* The role of the nephrons is to filter waste products out of the blood. Most of the water and solutes are reabsorbed back

urinary system—system that filters wastes out of the blood and excretes them in the urine

into the bloodstream from the nephron; those that are not reabsorbed become urine. This process is under strict hormonal control to ensure that the body keeps adequate water and other substances to support its life processes. The urine is collected and held in the urinary bladder until it is excreted (Figure 3.10).

perspiration—loss of water due to sweating or evaporation from body surfaces

Perspiration, body water loss due to sweating or surface evaporation, is another route by which water and some minerals leave the body. Although everybody loses some moisture through the skin every day, the amounts lost in this way by different people and on different days are extremely variable. (More on this in Chapter 4 [on water].)

Along with the carbon dioxide they exhale, people also lose some water vapor through the capillaries of the lungs. The amounts lost in this way are proportional to the rate at which a person breathes. For example, when you are exercising hard, you lose much more carbon dioxide and water by this route than you would if you were at rest. You will also lose more via the lungs when you first arrive at a high altitude, because you need to breathe more often to get enough oxygen into your body.

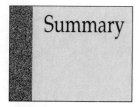

Summary

▶ **Digestion** is the process of breaking food down into substances small enough to be taken into the body's interior. This intake process is called **absorption.**

▶ The main part of the digestive system consists of a hollow tube called the **alimentary canal** or **gastrointestinal (GI) tract.** Its many specialized sections vary in diameter, but all sections have a **lumen** (space through which food passes) and a **mucosa** (inner lining). Longitudinal and circular muscles—some of the latter called **sphincters**—control the passage of material from one section of the tract to the next. **Mucus, enzymes,** and **hormones** are secreted at various points along the way to assist in digestion.

▶ The amount of time food spends in the tract **(transit time)** is affected by diet, drugs, emotions, physical activity, and state of health.

▶ Digestion and absorption have several phases, and each section of the tract has its own functions to perform. (1) Food is ground in the mouth. (2) The **pharynx** moves food into the **esophagus,** where involuntary muscular contractions called **peristalsis** transport the food to the stomach. (3) The stomach is very active in digestion, attacking food both mechanically and chemically to produce a slushy blend called **chyme.** (4) Digestion continues in the **small intestine** with the aid of secretions from other organs. The **liver** produces **bile,** which **emulsifies** fats (divides them into small droplets), and the **pancreas** produces digestive enzymes and substances that help to neutralize the acid in the chyme. Most of the absorption process also occurs in the small intestine, whose **villi** and **microvilli** project into and expose an enormous surface area to the chyme. (5) The **large intestine** collects solid waste, provides a home for bacteria, and absorbs water and some minerals.

▶ The **cell** is the smallest, simplest unit of living matter and is the site at which the absorbed nutrients are used. In addition to their nucleus, cytoplasm, mitochondria, and endoplasmic reticulum, all cells are surrounded by a selectively permeable membrane that controls what substances can enter or leave it. Cells in the body are often separated by small spaces filled with **interstitial fluid.** Cells grouped together to perform a similar function are referred to as a **tissue;** tissues combine to form **organs;** organs that cooperate to perform a major physiological task compose a **system;** and several interrelated systems make up an **organism.**

▶ The chemical processes collectively referred to as metabolism take place at all times in every living cell. Synthesis and breakdown reactions may take place at different rates at different times or in different cells.

▶ The **circulatory system** delivers nutrients and oxygen to all the body's cells. It is powered by the heart, which moves blood through a closed system of blood vessels. One section of the system loops between the heart and the lungs, and the other section circles between the heart and all other parts of the body. **Arteries** carry blood away from the heart; **veins** carry blood back to it; and the exchange of nutrients and wastes takes place across the walls of the smallest vessels, called **capillaries.** Nutrients enter the bloodstream through the capillaries of the small intestine.

▶ The **lymphatic system** is a one-way network of vessels that carry lymph as well as some nutrients. The nutrients are picked up at the villi by small vessels called **lacteals.**

▶ Excretion of waste products occurs via several routes. Solid waste is excreted from the body as feces. Most water leaves the body by way of the **urinary system,** which also has the job of filtering waste products out of the blood. Additional water is lost by **perspiration,** and by exhalation of water vapor from the lungs.

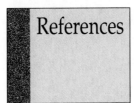

References

Ganong, W.F. 1989. *Review of medical physiology.* Norwalk, CT: Appleton & Lange.

Graham, D.Y., J.L. Smith, and A.R. Opekun. 1988. Spicy food and the stomach. *Journal of the American Medical Association* 260:3473–3475.

Harvard Medical School Department of Continuing Education. 1986. Ulcer drugs—old and new. *Harvard Medical School Health Letter* 11(March):1–4.

McNeil, N.I. 1984. The contribution of the large intestine to energy supplies in man. *American Journal of Clinical Nutrition* 39:338–342.

Marieb, E.N. 1989. *Human anatomy and physiology.* Redwood City, CA: The Benjamin/Cummings Publishing Company.

Mattes, R.D. and D.J. Mela. 1988. The chemical senses and nutrition: Part II. *Nutrition Today* 23:19–25.

Mirkin, G. and M. Hoffman. 1978. *The sportsmedicine book.* Boston: Little, Brown and Company.

Savage, D.C. 1987. Factors influencing biocontrol of bacterial pathogens in the intestine. *Food Technology* 41:82–86.

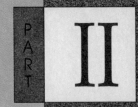

P A R T

II

MACRONUTRIENTS: BUILDING BLOCKS AND ENERGY SOURCES

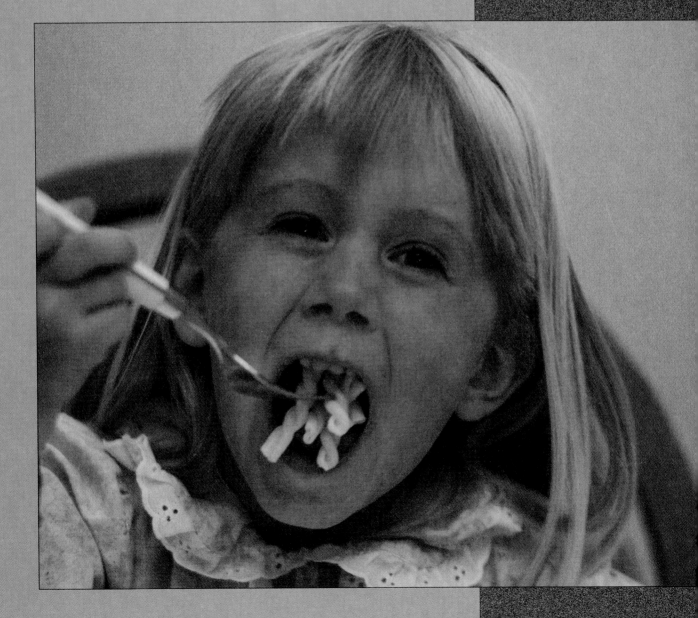

Water: Not to Be Taken for Granted

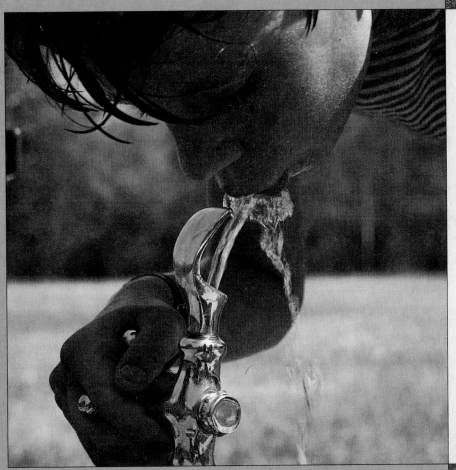

In This Chapter

- Water Is the Largest Body Constituent and Has Many Functions
- Many Systems Help Maintain Hydration and Regulate Distribution
- Dehydration Has Serious Consequences
- Water Is Available From Three Sources
- Recommendations Suggest Healthy Levels of Fluid Intake

W ater. There's no doubt that we take it for granted. Maybe that's because we have such easy, inexpensive access to it almost all of the time; we seldom feel deprived of it.

But you can probably remember some occasions when you were short of water. You became thirsty and, if you didn't have any fluids handy, you probably felt quite uncomfortable—or even desperate—until you found a way to quench your thirst.

We have such a drive to replace lost water because it is crucial to our survival: we would die if we had to go without it for more than a few days, whereas we can last for weeks without other essential nutrients. If a person gets lost in a desolate area, there's much more reason to be concerned about finding a source of water than about finding food. What is it that makes our **hydration** (water status) so crucial to our well-being?

hydration—referring to the presence of water

Water Is the Largest Body Constituent and Has Many Functions

You get a sense of why this substance is so important when you know how much of the body is water: water accounts for 60% of the body weight for the typical young adult male and 50% for the young adult female (Randall, 1988).

Water is found throughout the body. Fluids such as blood plasma (the watery portion without blood cells) and interstitial fluid are over 90% water, and the cytosol within cells also contains a considerable amount of water.

Figure 4.1 Percentage of water in various body tissues. The percentage of water in most body tissues is fairly predictable, although the proportion of water in fat tissue varies within a range, as shown.

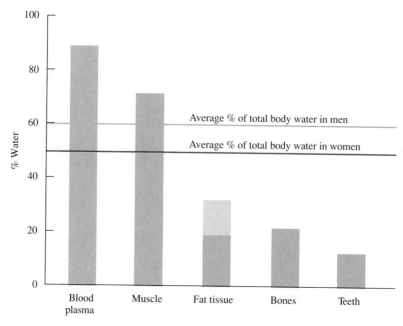

This means that every kind of tissue contains water, although not in the same proportions: muscle tissue is almost 72% water by weight, bones are about 25% water, teeth about 10% water, and fat tissue varies from 20–35% water (Figure 4.1). From the information depicted on the graph, you can see that individuals can differ from one another in the exact percentage of body water they have, depending on the relative amounts of the different types of tissues they contain. A person who has a higher-than-average proportion of body fat, which contains relatively little water, is likely to have a lower percentage of body water than thinner people of the same age. Body composition also explains why the average woman, who has a higher proportion of body fat than the average man, has a lower percentage of body water.

Age makes a difference too: a newborn infant may consist of as much as 75% water. By the time a child is a year old, water content is close to 60%. But what does water actually *do* in the body?

Medium in Which Reactions Happen

Many biochemical reactions can take place only if the reacting compounds are dissolved in water: water is the critical biochemical **solvent** (liquid that can hold dissolved substances). Because this is true, almost all body water contains **solutes** (dissolved substances); no body fluid is 100% water.

Many chemicals, when they are dissolved in water, dissociate (break apart) into electrically charged particles called **ions** or **electrolytes.** Certain electrolytes such as sodium and potassium have a great deal of influence on body water balance—that is, how water is distributed in the body. This will be discussed more thoroughly shortly.

When a solution has an excess of positively charged hydrogen ions (H^+), the solution is **acidic.** When a solution is capable of binding hydrogen ions, it is **basic** or **alkaline.** For example, when negatively charged hydroxyl ions (OH^-)—which are capable of binding H^+—are in excess, the solution is basic. When there are equal numbers of H^+ and negative ions that can bind with H^+, the solution is **neutral.** Water itself (H_2O or HOH) is an example of a neutral substance, since a small portion of its molecules dissociate into equal numbers of H^+ and OH^- ions.

The **pH scale** is a measure of the concentration of hydrogen ions in solution. Figure 4.2 shows a pH scale; 7 is the neutral value, with values below 7 being acidic and values above 7 being alkaline.

The body is very sensitive to changes in pH. Blood and lymph are normally maintained within a very narrow range around 7.4, just slightly basic. If the pH varies by only a few tenths of a pH unit, the normal functioning of many body systems can be interrupted. It is not surprising, then, that your body has a number of mechanisms that help to maintain a constant pH; these are called **buffers.** Several nutrients participate in buffer systems; we will discuss them in Chapter 8 (on proteins) and Chapter 13 (on minerals).

solvent—liquid in which substances can be dissolved

solutes—substances dissolved in water or another solvent

ions, electrolytes—particles that carry an electrical charge in solution

acidic solution (acid)—one containing an excess of positively charged hydrogen ions (H^+)

basic (alkaline) solution—one containing an excess of negatively charged ions that can bind H^+

neutral solution—one containing equal numbers of H^+ and negatively charged ions that can bind H^+

pH scale—a measure of the concentration of hydrogen ions (H^+) in solution

buffer—chemical substance or system that minimizes changes in pH by releasing or binding hydrogen ions

Participant in Biochemical Reactions

hydrolysis—chemical breakdown process in which water is one of the reacting substances

There are also situations in which water itself is one of the reacting compounds. For example, in the process of digestion, when carbohydrates, fats, and proteins are broken into smaller units in preparation for absorption, water participates in the splitting process, which is called **hydrolysis,** by contributing its own components to the new compounds. Figure 4.3 illustrates how this occurs.

Medium of Transport

Some body fluids outside of cells have as their major function the task of carrying substances around in the body. Blood is the prime example of a nutrient- and/or waste-transporting body fluid (as was discussed in Chapter 3 and shown in Figure 3.5); interstitial fluid and lymph (Figure 3.8) are other examples. In addition, water-based secretions of the GI tract carry digestive enzymes to where they are needed.

Lubricant and Cushion

Some body fluids serve as lubricants that enable solid materials to slide against each other. Examples are saliva, which promotes easier movement of food through the upper part of the digestive tract, and tears, which allow the eyeballs to rotate smoothly in their sockets. Synovial fluid is a thick liquid encapsulated within many joints; it provides a protective cushion for the tissues of the joint.

Temperature Regulator

Another key function of water is to help control body temperature. This is important because there is a rather narrow range of internal temperatures in which human life processes can continue. If a person's temperature, which is normally around 98.6°F (37°C), falls below about 80°F (27°C) or rises above 108°F (42°C), death is likely to result. These values are for oral temperatures; the actual internal (or core) temperatures are approximately 1°F (0.6°C) higher.

Water is involved in temperature control in several ways. One property of water is that it does not change temperature as readily as some other substances do in response to environmental temperature changes. Therefore, the body maintains its normal temperature more easily with water than it would if it were filled with other fluids. Blood and interstitial fluid, because of their high water content and wide distribution throughout the body, are very important in keeping its core temperature stable.

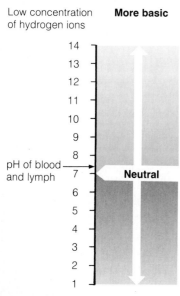

Figure 4.2 The pH scale. The measure of strength of acids and bases.

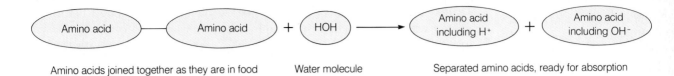

Amino acid — Amino acid + HOH → Amino acid including H⁺ + Amino acid including OH⁻

Amino acids joined together as they are in food   Water molecule   Separated amino acids, ready for absorption

Sometimes, though, either internal factors (such as an increasing body temperature resulting from vigorous physical activity) or external factors (such as very hot or very cold environmental temperatures) may threaten the consistent internal temperature of the body. In these cases, various mechanisms help body fluids moderate the changes in body temperature or even bring it back toward normal.

For example, if you are in a very cold environment without adequate clothing and your body temperature is beginning to fall, your body conserves heat by constricting (narrowing) the blood vessels near the skin surface. This causes less blood to be circulated near the surface, thereby slowing the loss of heat from the blood. Conversely, if you are overheated, blood vessels of the skin dilate, bringing a larger volume of blood near the surface where it loses some heat to the environment. At the same time, you may exude fluid from the skin—*perspiration*—the evaporation of which results in further loss of heat.

Figure 4.3 Hydrolysis: an important biological function of water. In this example, two amino acids (the units that compose proteins) are split and the water itself is divided between the two new units. This type of reaction is involved in the digestion of carbohydrates, fats, and proteins.

Many Systems Help Maintain Hydration and Regulate Distribution

In order for water to carry out the functions described above, there needs to be enough water in the body, and it needs to be distributed properly. A number of mechanisms help maintain hydration and regulate the distribution of water in the body.

Thirst

Your sense of thirst plays an important role because it prompts you to take in water when it is needed—in fact, before you have lost 1% of your body weight as water. Thirst occurs when receptors in the brain (in the region called the *hypothalamus,* which controls many basic body functions) are stimulated in response to certain physiological changes. If there is a reduction in the volume of your body fluids, or if there is an increase in the concentration of substances dissolved in the blood, or if the mucosa of your mouth and pharynx become dry, then these receptors are stimulated and you become thirsty (Ganong, 1989; Marieb, 1989).

There is also a mechanism that signals when you have had enough water and should stop drinking, but it is not very well understood. It appears to be located in the GI tract, because our sense of thirst is inhibited before ingested water has reached the blood stream (Marieb, 1989).

Although these mechanisms ordinarily work quite well to help healthy people maintain body water balance, they can be inadequate in certain circumstances. During illness, for example, people may not drink enough to meet their needs for water; it may be that the discomforts associated with their condition override their perception of thirst or lead to a premature sense of satiety (satisfaction). Similarly, when people have been exercising hard and sweating heavily for a long period of time, they are unlikely to drink enough to restore their losses. Also, elderly people may have a blunted sense of thirst (RDA Subcommittee, 1989).

We will consider these situations again later in the chapter when we discuss what deliberate steps people can take to assure themselves of meeting their fluid needs.

Absorption of Water from the Gastrointestinal Tract

Once water has been consumed, it needs to be absorbed before it can do its work in the body.

Water does not need to be broken down into smaller units prior to absorption. The first site in the GI tract at which it can be absorbed is the stomach. Actually, only a minute amount is absorbed here, but this is notable nonetheless because so few substances can be absorbed at all from this organ.

Over 80% of water is absorbed by the villi of the small intestine (Ganong, 1989). The remainder goes through to the large intestine, where much of what remains is reclaimed. Ninety-eight percent of the water contained in all of the fluids that enter the GI tract, including both dietary sources and fluids secreted into the tract from the body, is eventually absorbed (Ganong, 1989).

Distribution into Intracellular and Extracellular Volumes

Once absorbed, water is distributed between two general locations: inside and outside body cells. The water inside all body cells is collectively referred to as the **intracellular volume** or compartment; the water outside cells is called **extracellular.**

Extracellular water, the smaller volume, includes the watery portion of blood (plasma), interstitial fluid and lymph, gastrointestinal fluids, fluids contained within the spinal column and eyes, tears, and the synovial fluid that cushions the joints.

Figure 4.4 shows the normal apportionment of the approximately 42 liters of total body water into these two compartments in a typical 70-kg male.

Implications of Changing Volumes   It is important that adequate water volume be maintained in both of the two compartments: there are negative consequences if either one gets depleted.

intracellular volume—refers to body water contained within cells

extracellular volume—refers to body water outside cells

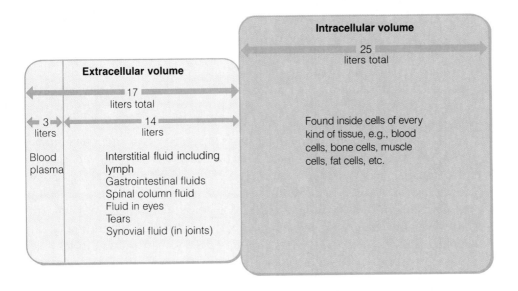

Figure 4.4 Body fluids. Intracellular and extracellular volumes in an average 154-pound male. (Note: total body fluid varies with body size and composition.)

If intracellular fluid is decreased, cellular metabolism, including energy production, may not take place efficiently. If extracellular fluid is decreased, blood volume drops; this means that less oxygen can be delivered to body cells. In addition, body temperature rises because the heat produced by metabolic processes is being absorbed by a smaller volume of fluid, which is less able to get rid of the surplus heat. This jeopardizes the functioning of the brain, the circulatory system, skeletal muscles, and every other body system.

Factors Involved in Internal Fluid Movement To understand what can cause changes in compartment volumes, it is necessary to focus on cell membranes, which divide the intracellular and extracellular compartments.

In Chapter 3, it was mentioned that water can pass easily through the selectively permeable membranes that enclose body cells. When equal volumes of water move through these membranes in both directions, there is no change in compartment volumes.

Sometimes, however, more water passes through in one direction than the other, resulting in changes in the volumes. To understand why this can occur, remember that there are various substances dissolved in body fluids that the selectively permeable cell membranes will not allow to pass through them. This means that some solute particles accumulate on one side of the cell membrane, resulting in a higher concentration of particles per volume of solution on that side.

Such an imbalance in compartment volumes is temporary. A basic principle of physiology is that a solvent (usually water) moves through membranes to equalize the concentration of particles in solution on the two sides. Therefore, when there is a greater concentration of solute on one side of a membrane than on the other, more water will move across the membrane

osmosis—movement of solvent across a selectively permeable membrane to equalize the concentration of the solute on the two sides

to the side with the greater concentration of solute. This process is called **osmosis.** Osmosis results in an increase in the volume of water on one side of the membrane and a decrease in the volume of water on the other side (Figure 4.5).

Several kinds of particles in the body cannot readily pass through selectively permeable membranes. Dissolved protein is one. In a healthy, well-nourished individual, protein concentrations usually remain stable on both sides of the cell membrane. As a result, protein normally does more to *maintain* than to *change* intracellular volumes.

Substances other than protein are more likely to pass through membranes and therefore to produce fluid shifts. Two of these are the positively charged electrolytes potassium and sodium. The great majority of the body's potassium ions are located inside body cells, whereas the sodium ions are found mostly outside cells. The ions are held in these respective compartments because a mechanism in the cell membrane, called the sodium–potassium pump, actively transports potassium through the cell membrane into the cell but ejects sodium, segregating it in the extracellular fluid. If the concentration of positive ions like potassium inside the cell differs from the concentration of positive ions like sodium outside the cell, there will be a water shift in the direction of the greater concentration of ions.

Many other dissolved materials besides sodium and potassium are segregated largely to one side of the cellular membrane or the other. For example, negatively charged chloride and bicarbonate ions are mainly outside the cell and, along with sodium, influence extracellular volume. On the other hand, positively charged magnesium and negatively charged sulfur- and phosphorus-containing complexes help maintain the intracellular volume.

Figure 4.5 How osmosis affects fluid volumes in a simple model.

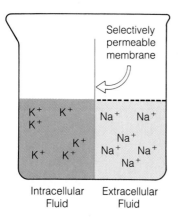

Intracellular Fluid   Extracellular Fluid

When ions (represented here by potassium [K$^+$] and sodium [Na$^+$]) are equally concentrated in the intracellular and extracellular fluid, the volumes of water are equal on both sides of the selectively permeable membrane.

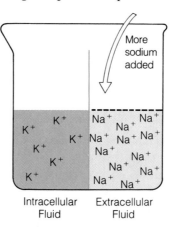

Intracellular Fluid   Extracellular Fluid

When more sodium is added to the extracellular fluid, the concentration of ions becomes higher in that compartment.

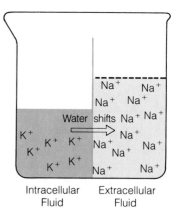

Intracellular Fluid   Extracellular Fluid

To equalize the concentrations, water moves through the selectively permeable membrane by osmosis from the compartment where ions are less concentrated to the compartment where they are more concentrated. The volumes of both compartments change in the process.

Excretion of Water

Water leaves the body by four routes: via the kidneys as urine; via the GI tract in the feces; via the skin as perspiration; and via the skin and lungs as **insensible losses,** which occur as water evaporates from body cells that are in contact with dryer surrounding air. As water losses occur by the latter three routes, and as fluid intake fluctuates, the kidneys adjust the amount of urine produced to maintain a healthy hydration status.

insensible loss—a loss that occurs without it being perceived

Typically, the healthy body loses 2 to 3 liters of fluid per day by all routes combined. Figure 4.6 indicates what proportions are lost by each of the four routes, but there is tremendous variability in these values from person to person, and from day to day. Even environmental factors can have a big impact on water losses. In the mountains, for example, insensible losses are much higher than at sea level. This is due to the low humidity of the atmosphere at altitude and a person's increased rate of respiration (Askew, 1989).

In addition to their role in water excretion, the kidneys also regulate the body's electrolyte status to maintain **homeostasis** in regard to body fluids. The kidneys can produce urine ranging from dilute (with only low levels of electrolytes present) to quite concentrated (with much higher levels of one or more electrolytes). A number of hormones are involved in regulating these processes.

homeostasis—maintenance of the body's normal internal environment, accomplished by biochemical control mechanisms

For example, when electrolytes are becoming too concentrated in the blood, the hormone *antidiuretic hormone (ADH)* causes the kidneys to excrete proportionately less water and more electrolytes. When sodium ions in body fluids are beginning to fall (or potassium is relatively in excess), a complex set of hormonal mechanisms involving the hormone *aldosterone* causes the kidneys to hold back sodium that would ordinarily have been excreted in the urine; and since water follows sodium, when sodium is resorbed, water is also retained (Marieb, 1989).

Let's take a look at some examples of these mechanisms at work.

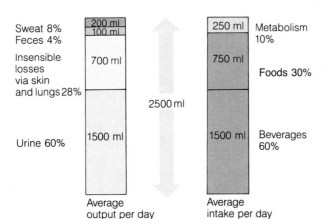

Figure 4.6 Major routes of water output and intake. When total output and intake are in balance, the body is adequately hydrated. The volumes shown are typical for the moderately (not extremely) active adult.

Sweat 8%
Feces 4%

Insensible losses via skin and lungs 28%

Urine 60%

200 ml
100 ml
700 ml
1500 ml

2500 ml

250 ml Metabolism 10%
750 ml   Foods 30%
1500 ml Beverages 60%

Average output per day

Average intake per day

Examples of Fluid Regulation

If you eat some unusually salty food, the salt (which is a compound made of sodium and chloride) will be absorbed and will appear in your blood and interstitial fluid as sodium and chloride ions. Since the concentration of the sodium ions in the interstitial fluid and blood is likely to be higher than that of the positive ions like potassium inside the cell, water will move by osmosis from inside the cells to the interstitial fluid until the concentrations of the ions in the water on both sides of the membrane are equalized. You will become thirsty, and your body will produce ADH. Soon after this, as sodium and chloride ions circulate through the kidneys, the kidneys will gradually discard the surplus ions and water via the urine. Working together, these mechanisms help restore homeostasis.

The physiological changes that occur as you perspire during heavy exercise also demonstrate fluid shifts. When you sweat, you lose water from your interstitial fluid. You also lose a small amount of sodium and chloride, but this amount is much less than the proportion of water you lose. Your remaining interstitial fluid contains a higher concentration of ions than your intracellular fluid does; this causes water to move mainly from your body cells into the interstitial spaces to equalize the concentration. At the same time, the loss of fluid volume causes you to become thirsty and simultaneously sets in motion complex hormonal mechanisms that cause the kidneys to withhold electrolytes and water from the urine.

Diarrhea is another condition that puts hormonal mechanisms to work. When fecal material moves through the colon too quickly for the usual amount of electrolytes (and water) to be absorbed, body sodium levels decrease, and aldosterone prompts the kidneys to reclaim sodium and, consequently, water that would otherwise have been released in the urine. This mechanism is usually sufficient to correct for fluid and electrolyte losses if the diarrhea is not severe or prolonged and if the person is able to drink and eat. However, as the next section points out, this is not always the case.

Dehydration Has Serious Consequences

Sometimes the conditions affecting water intake and/or output are so severe that mechanisms designed to maintain hydration are not equal to the task. In such cases, the body becomes dehydrated, and body functions are impaired. At worst, death occurs.

For example, many infants and young children in the developing countries get diseases that cause diarrhea. (Many of these diseases are caused by drinking water that came from supplies contaminated with disease-causing microorganisms.) As fluid and electrolyte losses continue, the child is often unwilling or unable to consume sufficient fluids or food, and dehydration proceeds rapidly. At losses of 10–20% of body water, death results; millions

CHAPTER FOUR
Water: Not to Be Taken for Granted 97

of infants and young children die annually from such diseases. Simple solutions that replace water, electrolytes, and other substances can change the outcome: in 1987, it was estimated that at least half a million children were saved by such *oral rehydration therapy* (UNICEF, 1988).

Even in healthy people, various degrees of dehydration can occur; this is a common problem for the endurance athlete. With moderate sweating, individuals generally produce 1 to 2 liters of sweat per hour (Pivarnik, 1989), but in warm weather some athletes have been found to produce more than 2 liters (4 pounds) of sweat per hour (Costill, 1986). When you consider that the stomach can only accommodate about 1 liter per hour, you can see that even when a person drinks as much fluid as possible along the way, a fluid deficit is likely to occur. The Slice of Life gives examples of net losses of weight that people have experienced owing to losses of water during extended physical activity.

Slice of Life

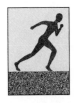

Fluid Losses During Physical Activity

People who exercise for extended periods can experience substantial fluid losses. Here are some examples of amounts of body water lost by people in particular situations:

■ Juan, who uses his bicycle regularly for transportation in town during the week, likes to head out of the city on pleasant weekend afternoons to "open up" on the rolling country roads. In a ride of several hours, it is not uncommon for him to lose 3–5 pounds, even though he drinks the contents of his water bottle (and sometimes several refills) along the way.

■ Cindy, an enthusiastic volleyball player, easily loses 2 pounds of body fluids during a couple of hours of vigorous play with friends. She usually wears a medium-weight sweat suit when playing outside in spring and fall when temperatures are in the 50s and 60s.

■ Craig, a 235-pound university football linebacker, lost 9 pounds playing in the spring game. The temperature rose into the 80s that afternoon; other factors promoting fluid loss were the heavy pads and clothing that he wore. Joel, a 290-pound defensive tackle, lost 15 pounds in the same game.

■ Bill, a lean and fit man in his thirties, lost 3 pounds while playing 1½ hours of nonstop recreational basketball on an indoor court where the temperature was maintained at approximately 65°F. He was dressed in shorts and a lightweight T-shirt.

■ Karen, a women in her forties, ran a 20-mile race one morning when the temperature was over 70°F. Although she drank fluids at every water stop along the course, downed a couple of cups of juice at the finish, and sipped on a huge root beer during the ride home, she weighed 6 pounds less when she got home than she had weighed before the race.

If you were to engage in these activities under similar circumstances, your fluid losses would not necessarily match those in the examples above; individual variability plays a big role in fluid loss.

Remember: such body water losses will—and *should*—be regained quickly by drinking generous amounts of fluids. Do not confuse water loss with fat loss. ▼

Loss of water weight is a problem to the person who is competing, because when you lose as little as 2% of your normally hydrated body weight because of water loss, your physical performance will be impaired (Saltin and Costill, 1988). For example, when a 150-pound person loses about 3 pounds of body water, performance is likely to start deteriorating.

One study quantified the effects of a 4% loss of water-weight in young men who had sweated in a sauna: their muscular endurance decreased by about 30% (Torranin et al., 1979). Even four hours after they had drunk enough water to restore their body weight, their muscular endurance was not back to normal; it takes time for ingested water to make its way to all the body cells that need it. This fact has particular implications for wrestlers, who sometimes deliberately dehydrate themselves to make their weight classes, and then expect to be at top strength within a couple of hours after drinking some water. It doesn't work.

Table 4.1 identifies consequences of various levels of fluid deficit.

Water Is Available from Three Sources

The body functions best if its fluid losses are replaced promptly. You can rightly assume that beverages are a major source of water. What may be less obvious is that almost all solid foods contribute water as well. In fact, some "solid" foods have a higher weight percentage of water than some liquids. Table 4.2 demonstrates this.

When average dietary intakes are evaluated in large dietary surveys, it is found that beverages usually account for more than half of the 2–3 liters that are taken in daily, and foods account for less than half. However, these values can vary considerably with food and beverage choices. An additional smaller amount comes from within the body itself: when carbohydrates, fats, and proteins are metabolized to produce energy, they also yield carbon dioxide and water. Figure 4.6 shows typical volumes of water supplied daily from the three sources. This chapter's Nutrition for Living points out some of the influences food and beverage intakes can have on each other.

Are some fluids better than others? Water itself is an excellent choice; but if you prefer another beverage, there are a couple of things to consider. If

Table 4.1 Adverse Effects of Dehydration

% Body Weight Loss

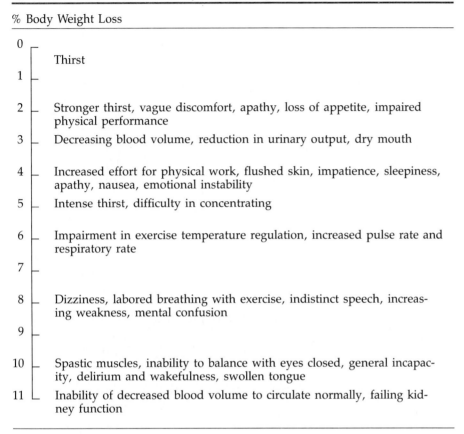

% Body Weight Loss	Effect
0–1	Thirst
2	Stronger thirst, vague discomfort, apathy, loss of appetite, impaired physical performance
3	Decreasing blood volume, reduction in urinary output, dry mouth
4	Increased effort for physical work, flushed skin, impatience, sleepiness, apathy, nausea, emotional instability
5	Intense thirst, difficulty in concentrating
6	Impairment in exercise temperature regulation, increased pulse rate and respiratory rate
8	Dizziness, labored breathing with exercise, indistinct speech, increasing weakness, mental confusion
10	Spastic muscles, inability to balance with eyes closed, general incapacity, delirium and wakefulness, swollen tongue
11	Inability of decreased blood volume to circulate normally, failing kidney function

References: 1) Askew, E.W. 1989. Nutrition and performance under adverse environmental conditions. In *Nutrition in Exercise and Sport*, eds. J.F. Hickson and I. Wolinsky. Boca Raton, FL: CRC Press, Inc. 2) Greenleaf, J.E. 1982. The body's need for fluids. In *Nutrition and athletic performance: Proceedings of the conference on nutritional determinants in athletic performance*, ed. W. Haskell, J. Scala, and J. Whittam. Palo Alto, CA: Bull Publishing Company.

you are primarily thinking about what *volume of water* you can get from various beverages, there is not much difference between them: most beverages are approximately 90% water by weight. However, some beverages contain substances that increase urine production and consequent body water loss. Caffeine (found primarily in coffee, tea, and some carbonated beverages) and alcohol (in beer, wine, whiskey, and others) have a **diuretic** effect. Consequently, beverages with high concentrations of these chemicals are less desirable water sources than beverages that don't contain such chemicals or that have low concentrations of them. Furthermore, caffeine and alcohol have other effects on the body that you may want to limit or avoid; these are discussed in Chapters 15 and 18.

diuretic—increasing the excretion of urine

Another consideration in choosing a beverage is what nutrients it contains besides water. For example, fruit juices contain carbohydrates and possibly vitamins A and/or C; milk beverages contain protein, carbohydrate, calcium, phosphorus, riboflavin, and other nutrients; and sugared carbon-

Table 4.2 Percentage of Water in Some Foods

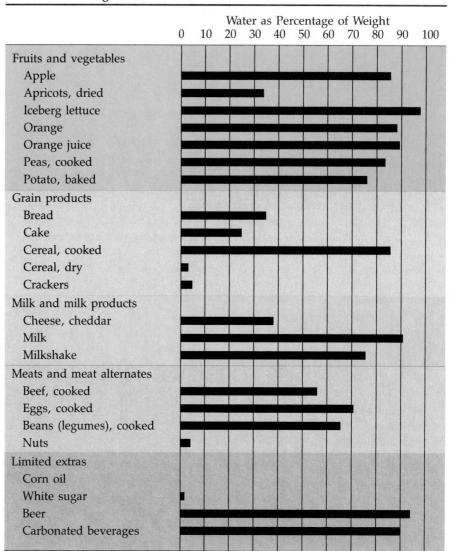

	Water as Percentage of Weight

ated beverages and fruit-flavored drinks contain considerable levels of carbohydrate. Therefore, beverages can make a substantial nutritional contribution to the day's intake; they need to be considered for their energy and nutrient values as well as their water content.

In recent years, certain trends in purchased beverage consumption have developed. Overall intake is up, with gains in soft drinks, fruit juices, and fruit drinks; declines have been seen in the consumption of coffee, tea, and milk. In the 1980s, the per capita consumption of soft drinks surpassed that of milk; in fact, it exceeded the consumption of milk and fruit juices *combined* (National Food Review, 1988). The per capita intake of milk has been declining slightly, while the intake of carbonated beverages has been rising at a faster rate.

The popularity of bottled water has increased significantly. The reason seems to have less to do with nutrition than with the general public's concerns about possible contamination of public and private water supplies. Although Chapter 15 deals extensively with toxicants in our food supply, it seems appropriate to discuss the quality of drinking water here. Critical Thinking 4.1 addresses this issue.

Recommendations Suggest Healthy Levels of Fluid Intake

There are various guidelines for getting the right amount of fluid. Sometimes thirst alone is not enough to keep us aware of our body's need for water. To achieve healthy levels of water, we need to understand how our diets and activity levels play a part in either supplying water to or depleting it from our systems. In this section we will discuss various guidelines for maintaining the right amount of fluid in our bodies.

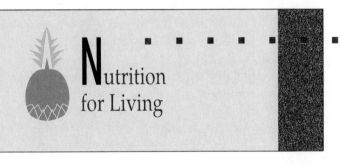

Nutrition for Living

Evaluating Your Water Needs

How can the food and drink you consume make a difference to the amount of water you need? Here are some points to take into account:

■ Whole-grain products and food with added fiber call for extra fluid intake because cereal fiber—which is excreted in the feces—absorbs many times its weight in water, and that water leaves the body with the solid waste. In light of these facts, it is advisable to consume extra fluids with dry high-fiber foods and supplements such as bran.

■ If you eat a lot of fruits and vegetables, you get a substantial amount of fluid from them. Even though some water is retained by the fiber of the produce, most of the generous amount of water in fruits and vegetables is absorbed into the body. From five servings of fresh, canned, or frozen fruits and vegetables, you get approximately $\frac{1}{2}$ liter of water.

■ Eating especially salty foods calls for drinking extra fluid along with them since you need water to excrete excesses of salt from the body. That's hardly a secret—your sense of thirst tells you to have something to drink with cheese and crackers or a fast-food entrée.

■ Alcoholic beverages—especially those with a relatively high alcohol concentration such as whiskey or brandy—can lead to dehydration. This helps explain why many people have a dry mouth the morning after a party. Less alcohol and more mixer can lessen the likelihood of dry mouth . . . and will lessen the dehydration of all other body tissues at the same time.

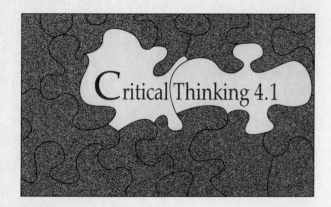

Is Bottled Water Better?

The situation

The radio is playing as you are getting ready for work. "Is your drinking water pure?" the advertisement asks. "Join the thousands who are now using Brady's Bottled Water. . . ." Although you have heard the ad many times before, this time it gives you a moment's pause. You have a flashback to a news item you saw on TV a few nights ago, in which residents of a local community raised questions about the quality of their water supply. When you went grocery shopping the next day, you noticed that a considerable amount of shelf space was devoted to bottled water. You had regarded the increasing interest in bottled water as largely a fad, but now you are beginning to wonder.

Is the information accurate and relevant?

- The ad insinuates that water, to be drinkable, should be *pure*. Absolutely pure water is almost nonexistent, although if water is distilled and deionized, it comes close; furthermore, many of the dissolved and suspended substances in natural water do not affect its safety, and some even give it sought-after flavors. It is important, however, for water to be *safe;* that is, the levels of potentially harmful dissolved and suspended substances it contains need to be lower than levels that are known to cause harm.
- Although the vast majority of public water supplies meet the standards established by the Safe Drinking Water Act of 1974 (amended in 1986), there *is* increasing concern about water quality. The U.S. Geological Survey and the Environmental Protection Agency (EPA) have been doing extensive testing of water supplies, and Congress has given the EPA a timetable for setting limits on additional chemicals not dealt with in the earlier legislation (Tufts Diet and Nutrition Letter, 1989).
- It is true that the use of bottled water has grown considerably in recent years. Between 1976 and 1987, the purchase of bottled water increased almost four-fold (Environmental Nutrition, 1988; Putnam, 1989). Currently, the industry grosses over $100 million per year in the United States.

What else needs to be considered?

In order to think through this issue, it is important to have some information both about typical drinking water supplies and about bottled water.

In the United States, approximately half the population uses public water supplies that come from surface water—that is, from rivers, streams, reservoirs, and lakes (American Council on Science and Health, 1989). The other half uses water that comes from underground sources, called groundwater, which is from either a public water supply or a private well.

It is possible for either surface water or groundwater to become contaminated. In the developing countries, where many citizens do not have access to clean public water and adequate sewerage systems, *pathogenic (disease-carrying) organisms* from contaminated water cause millions of deaths per year. The World Health Organization has stated, "The number of water taps per 1000 persons is a better indication of health than the number of hospital beds" (Myers, 1984).

In developed countries, 98% of citizens have

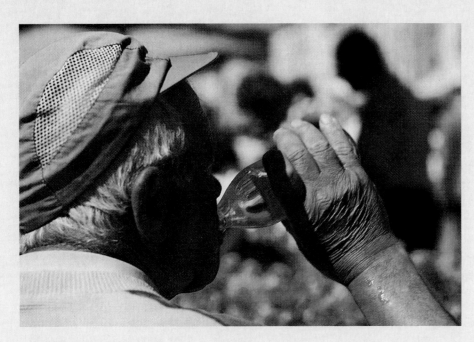

Increasing popularity of bottled water. Bottled water is not necessarily purer or safer than tap water, but it may offer advantages to some.

access to clean water (Myers, 1984). In the United States, the Environmental Protection Agency (EPA) sets standards for public water supplies, with accompanying regulations and defined treatment techniques. These standards encompass both microbial contaminants and other pollutants. Standards for substances believed to be carcinogenic are generally placed at a level that would cause a one-in-a-million cancer risk over a 70-year life span (American Council on Science and Health). For people who have their own wells, public health officials recommend testing at least yearly for microbial safety and for any other contaminants that seem likely, based on the source of supply. Some local and state public health departments will do such tests (usually for a fee); if not, they can recommend reputable laboratories (Baumeister, 1990).

Based on EPA standards, public water supplies are regularly monitored for safety; those that require treatment generally are subjected to coagulation or filtration and then the water is chlorinated. If tests reveal problems, the water utility is required to give public notice both via the public media and by direct mail to all users. New private wells need to be tested to be sure the water is free from pathogens, and subsequent annual testing is recommended.

Contamination can occur from various sources. Substances used in *agriculture* can run off into surface water or seep into groundwater, potentially reaching levels that are unacceptable. The substances of major concern are nitrates (nitrogen-containing compounds from both natural and chemical fertilizers), herbicides, and insecticides (National Research Council, 1989). Pollutants from *petrochemical industries, mining,* and *manufacturing* can also be a problem: these include such substances as hydrocarbons (e.g., crude oil, gasoline, and creosote) and heavy metals. Creative cleanup approaches, such as enhancing conditions that encourage naturally occurring microbes to break down hydrocarbon pollutants (Knox, 1988), are being researched.

Another substance of concern is lead. Although it is possible for lead to be present in surface or groundwater supplies, the cause of excessive lead in water is likely to be closer to home. If lead is present in household water pipes or solder or in the service lines from public water mains, small amounts can dissolve into water moving through those pipes. It is more likely that lead will leach into water if the water is hot, if it is acidic, and if it stands in the pipes for several hours (e.g., overnight or all day). Various means of protecting

Continues

against this problem have been enacted or proposed. Some states now require that the plumbing and solder in new construction be lead-free and that public water supplies have their pH adjusted to at least 8 (mildly alkaline) (Raloff, 1989). Although plumbing in older homes would seem to provide the greatest risk, mineral compounds can form on the inside of the pipes over time, actually setting up a physical barrier between the potential source of lead and the water; therefore, older plumbing is not necessarily more risky. The only way to determine if there is a problem is to have the water tested. When you draw a water sample for a test, follow the instructions carefully; the lead content of water that has been standing in pipes for several hours can be substantially different from the amount present after the water has been running for 2–3 minutes (Wisconsin Department of Natural Resources, 1988).

Now for a few facts about bottled water. The U.S. Food and Drug Administration is responsible for setting the standards for bottled water, and they have adopted identical standards to those the EPA has set for public water supplies; the only additional proviso is that the bottling conditions must be sanitary. Therefore, water can be bottled from ordinary public supplies; sometimes it is filtered, flavored, deionized, or carbonated to change the taste. Tests have shown that bottled waters are not always in compliance with standards; in a test of 37 brands of domestic and imported mineral waters bought off the shelves in Chicago and Pittsburgh, 24 had one or more substances that were not in compliance with the drinking water standards in the United States (Allen et al., 1989).

What do you think?

Should you use bottled water instead of the water you consume now? As you think through these options, consider whether your choice would be different if you currently use water from a public supply or from a private well.

■ Option 1   Without having your tapwater tested, you use bottled water as a precaution for all drinking and cooking purposes.

■ Option 2   You have your tapwater tested. If it meets water safety standards, you decide to use it and to enjoy a variety of bottled waters (e.g., flavored, carbonated) on occasion.

■ Option 3   You have your water tested for substances for which you think there may be some risk; if the water exceeds standards for safety, you use bottled water or use one of the following options.

■ Option 4   If tests indicate that lead is a problem after water has been standing in pipes but not after several minutes of running the water, you "flush" the pipes by leaving the tap open for 2–3 minutes after water has been standing for several hours; you use bottled water after long periods of disuse but not at other times; you install an approved treatment device or have your plumbing replaced.

■ Option 5   If tests indicate that other chemicals are a problem, you ask the testing agency whether there are filtering systems that will reduce the levels to within acceptable limits and you install such recommended systems.

■ Option 6   You forget the issue if there are no reports of problems regarding water quality in your area.

Do you see other options, or reasonable combinations of options, that are acceptable to you?

Consume Water in Proportion to Kcaloric Expenditure

The 1989 RDA recommends that moderately active, healthy people (including the elderly) should consume from 1 milliliter (ml) to 1.5 ml of water per kcalorie expended (RDA Subcommittee, 1989). This amounts to at least 1 liter (approximately 1 quart) of fluid from all sources per 1000 kcalories used. People on low-kcalorie diets should note that this standard applies to kcalories *expended*, not to kcalories taken in; therefore, *you should drink at least as much fluid while on a weight reduction diet as you did before.*

Infants routinely need 1.5 ml of water per kcalorie. Not only do their cells have a higher water content, but their immature kidneys also require more fluid in order to remove metabolic wastes.

These standards based on energy usage are not likely to meet the needs of a person who has been extremely physically active; for these individuals, the following two guidelines are more appropriate.

Replace Weight of Water Lost

This guideline is useful for people who are very physically active. An afternoon of tennis, a day of vigorous outdoor work, a long hike or run, or a sports team practice session are all activities for which this recommendation is appropriate. It simply involves weighing yourself (without clothing) in advance of the period of activity and again afterwards. For every pound lost, you should drink 2 cups of fluid. Pace the drinking at whatever rate is comfortable for you, such as 1 cup every 15 minutes or so, until you have restored the entire amount.

This deliberate approach is warranted because, as mentioned earlier, your sense of thirst alone is not likely to prompt you to rehydrate completely after a period of heavy sweating. In fact, if you rely in such cases only on thirst to tell you how much fluid is needed for rehydration, you will probably take in only about half the needed amount in the first 24 hours (Saltin, 1978). It may take as long as three days to replace the fluid lost in one day of heavy sweating unless you drink more than thirst prompts you to consume.

Successive days of such activity without deliberate replacement of water lead to progressive dehydration, which has resulted in the tragic, easily preventable deaths of some athletes. Because players often do not pay attention to their own needs in this regard, coaches should weigh their players daily. If a player has not replaced most of the fluid losses from the previous practice day, that player should be prohibited from participating again until he or she has done so.

You may have been mentally protesting during this discussion that body weight losses also reflect fat that was lost owing to such strenuous activities, and therefore it should not be necessary to drink so much that the person's original weight is restored. Although it is true that fat is lost, the weight of the fat lost during any vigorous activity of a few hours' duration is very

Figure 4.7 Replacing lost body fluids. This skier is attempting to restore water she has lost through perspiration and respiration.

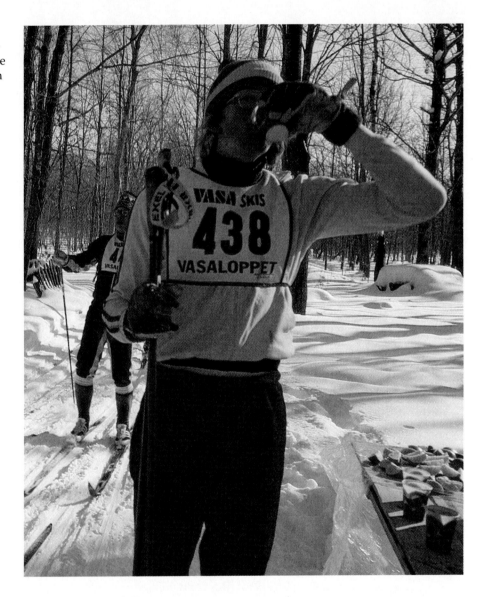

small compared to the weight of the water lost. As an extreme example, most runners of average size lose *less than a pound of body fat during a marathon* (26 miles, or several hours of running) but can easily perspire between 10 and 20 pounds of fluid during that experience. Therefore, weight loss is indeed a suitable approximate measure of water loss.

"Replace Ahead," During, and After Heavy Sweating

Although it is impossible to "replace" water before you lose it, in a practical sense it seems to help. People who *pre*hydrate and/or consume water *during* exercise can delay the physiological problems associated with dehydration (Figure 4.7).

If exercise goes on for a long time, though, often people cannot keep up with their losses. Recommendations about hydration for physical endurance activities, then, are compromise measures that will achieve only partial rehydration; the rest must be completed after the activity. Table 4.3 outlines a typical suggested program for the athlete. The military services have a rule of thumb for fluid intake while working in hot environments: an average-sized man should drink 1 liter of water in the morning, 1 liter at each of 3 meals, and 1 liter before any period of sustained activity (Askew, 1989).

Table 4.3 Amounts of Water Needed for Extended Physical Activity

When to Drink	How Much to Drink
Before activity	
2 hours before	2–3 cups of water
10–15 minutes before	2 cups of cold (40–50°F) water
During activity	
Every 10–15 minutes	$\frac{1}{2}$–1 cup of cold water
After activity	
Every 15 minutes, or at comfortable intervals	1 cup of fluid (continue until 2 cups have been consumed for every pound lost)

Drinking *cold* water (40–50°F) shortly before and during activity is suggested because cold water increases the motility of the stomach and it leaves the stomach faster than warmer water. This hastens its absorption and its beneficial effects (Fink, 1982). Water at the temperatures and volumes suggested in Table 4.3 does not appear to cause stomach cramps. Such distress is more likely when larger volumes are consumed (Costill, 1986).

Notice that *water* is recommended in preference to other fluids. That is because it is the most critical substance needed in extra amounts during exercise, and it may be better absorbed without the addition of other materials. Beverages with very high sugar contents are known to be retained longer in the stomach than plain water would be, thereby delaying the absorption of the water (American Dietetic Association, 1987). For events that exceed $1\frac{1}{2}$ hours of continuous, vigorous activity, however, some intake of carbohydrate can be useful; Chapter 6 will discuss this more fully.

Some endurance athletes wonder about the need for drinks that contain the electrolytes sodium, chloride, and potassium. Actually, your body does not lose much potassium during exercise. Sodium and chloride are present in sweat but in lesser concentrations than are present in body fluids; because their relative concentration in body fluids actually *increases* while you are perspiring, there is ordinarily no need for athletes to be concerned about them while they are exercising. This will be discussed more fully in Chapter 13 (on minerals).

A very few athletes may experience problems because of a combination of decreased levels of body electrolytes and high intakes of water (Coleman,

1988): these are *superendurance* athletes who compete continuously for 6 hours or more. An ultramarathon runner, for example, consumed 20 liters of fluid during 8½ hours (62 miles) of running; another took in 24 liters in 10½ hours. After hours of heavy perspiration and copious water intake, their body fluids were unusually dilute in sodium, and they experienced apparent "water intoxication" requiring hospital treatment (Frizzell et al., 1986; Saltin and Costill, 1988).

Experts estimate that the healthy human body can cope with intake of approximately 20 liters of water per day (Barr and Costill, 1989), but beyond that level, the kidney's ability to produce urine is likely to be exceeded. It is very rare for anyone—even the most conscientious superendurance athlete— to consume this much fluid, but the above examples demonstrate the axiom in nutrition that even substances as critical to our well-being as water will produce toxicity if consumed in excessive quantities.

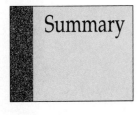

Summary

▶ Though the average person devotes little thought to his or her **hydration,** water is crucial to survival. It is the largest body constituent, normally accounting for half or more of body weight and comprising some proportion of every tissue.

▶ Aside from its structural functions, one of water's most important roles is as a biochemical **solvent.** Many types of **solutes,** including charged particles called **electrolytes,** are dissolved in body water. An **acidic solution** contains an excess of positively charged hydrogen ions (H^+), and a **basic solution** contains an excess of negatively charged ions that can bind H^+. A solution containing equal numbers of H^+ and negative ions is **neutral.** The **pH** of a solution is a measure of its H^+ ion concentration, which is given on a scale from 1 (very acidic) to 14 (very basic). The body is extremely sensitive to changes in pH, and several nutrients participate in **buffer** systems that help maintain it at the proper level.

▶ Water also participates in certain metabolic reactions such as **hydrolysis** (a type of breakdown reaction), acts as a transport medium and lubricant, and helps to regulate body temperature.

▶ Water must be present in the right places as well as in the right amounts. It enters the body through the digestive system (mainly via the small intestine), and once absorbed becomes part of either the **intracellular** or **extracellular compartment.** Water moves between the two compartments across cell membranes. The process of movement, which results in an equal concentration of water on both sides of the membrane, is called **osmosis.** Given sufficient time, a healthy individual can compensate for the effects on water balance of eating an unusually salty food or losing a great deal of water in perspiration, provided that enough water is consumed to make up for the losses.

▶ As essential as water is, like all other nutrients it has a beneficial range of intake. Although it would be difficult to consume too much unintentionally, deliberate extreme overconsumption is both possible and harmful.

▶ Water is lost by four routes: (1) urine excretion, (2) **insensible loss** and perspiration (both involving evaporation of water from the skin), (3) exhalation of water vapor, and (4) excretion in the feces. The amounts of water lost by these routes can vary considerably; for example, prolonged strenuous exercise increases water loss through perspiration as well as respiration.

▶ If body water losses exceed intake, progressive dehydration occurs with accompanying penalties. If your normal body weight decreases by as little as 2% because of water loss, your physical performance will be impaired. Greater losses have even more serious consequences, and at 10–12% of body weight lost as water, death will result.

▶ Water is available from three sources: (1) beverages, (2) foods, and (in much smaller amounts) (3) the body's own metabolic processes.

▶ Usually, you can meet your needs for water by drinking to satisfy thirst. However, in situations of unusual loss, deliberate replacement is advised.

References

Allen, H.E., M.A. Halley-Henderson, and C.N. Hass. 1989. Chemical composition of bottled mineral water. *Archives of Environmental Health* 44(no.2):102–116.

American Dietetic Association. 1987. Position of the American Dietetic Association: Nutrition for physical fitness and athletic performance for adults. *Journal of the American Dietetic Association* 87:933–939.

Askew, E.W. 1989. Nutrition and performance under adverse environmental conditions. In *Nutrition in exercise and sport*, eds. J.F. Hickson and I. Wolinsky. Boca Raton, FL: CRC Press, Inc.

Barr, S.I. and D.L. Costill. 1989. Water: Can the endurance athlete get too much of a good thing? *Journal of the American Dietetic Association* 89:1629–1635.

Baumeister, R. 1990. Personal communication. Madison, WI: Chief, Public Water Supply Section, Wisconsin Department of Natural Resources.

Coleman, E. 1988. *Eating for endurance.* Palo Alto, CA: Bull Publishing.

Costill, D.L. 1986. *Inside running.* Indianapolis, IN: Benchmark Press, Inc.

Environmental Nutrition. 1988. Bottled waters making big splash with more than 700 varieties on market. *Environmental Nutrition* 11(no.5):4–5.

Fink, W.J. 1982. Fluid intake for maximizing athletic performance. In *Nutrition and athletic performance: Proceedings of the conference on nutritional determinants in athletic performance*, ed. W. Haskell, J. Scala, and J. Whittam. Palo Alto, CA: The Bull Publishing Company.

Frizzell, R.T., G.H. Lang, D.C. Lowance, and S.R. Lathan. 1986. Hyponatremia and ultra-marathon running. *Journal of the American Medical Association* 255:772–774.

Ganong, W.F. 1989. *Review of medical physiology.* Norwalk, CT: Lange.

Knox, C.E. 1988. What's going on down there? *Science News* 134:362.

Marieb, E.N. 1989. *Human anatomy and physiology.* Redwood City, CA: The Benjamin/Cummings Publishing Company.

Myers, N. 1984. *GAIA: An atlas of planet management.* New York: Doubleday.

National Food Review. 1988. Food consumption. *National Food Review* 11(no.2):2–8.

National Research Council. 1989. *Alternative agriculture.* Washington, DC: National Academy Press.

Pivarnik, J.M. 1989. Water and electrolytes during exercise. In *Nutrition in exercise and sport*, eds. J.F. Hickson and I. Wolinsky. Boca Raton, FL: CRC Press, Inc.

Putnam, J. 1989. Food consumption. *National Food Review* 12:1–9.

Raloff, J. 1989. EPA proposes new rules to get the lead out. *Science News* 134:118.

Randall, H.T. 1988. Water, electrolytes, and acid-base balance. In *Modern nutrition in health and disease*, eds. M.E. Shils and V.R. Young. Philadelphia: Lea & Febiger.

RDA Subcommittee. 1989. *Recommended dietary allowances.* Washington, DC: National Academy Press.

Saltin, B. 1978. Fluid, electrolyte, and energy losses and their replenishment in prolonged exercise. In *Nutrition, physical fitness, and health.* International series on sports sciences, volume 7, eds. J. Parizkova and V.A. Rogozkin. Baltimore: University Park Press.

Saltin, B. and D. Costill. 1988. Fluid and electrolyte balance during prolonged exercise. In *Exercise, nutrition, and energy metabolism*, eds. E.S. Horton and R.L. Terjung. New York: Macmillan Publishing Company.

Torranin, C., D.P. Smith, and R.J. Byrd. 1979. The effect of acute thermal dehydration and rapid rehydration on isometric and isotonic endurance. *The Journal of Sports Medicine and Physical Fitness* 19:1–9.

Tuft's Diet and Nutrition Letter. 1988. Is there anything that is still safe to eat? *Tuft's Diet and Nutrition Letter* 6(no.6)3–6.

UNICEF. 1988. Oral rehydration therapy. *UNICEF annual report 1988*. NY: UNICEF Headquarters.

Wisconsin Department of Natural Resources (DNR). 1988. Lead in drinking water. Madison, WI: Wisconsin DNR.

5

Energy Sources and Uses

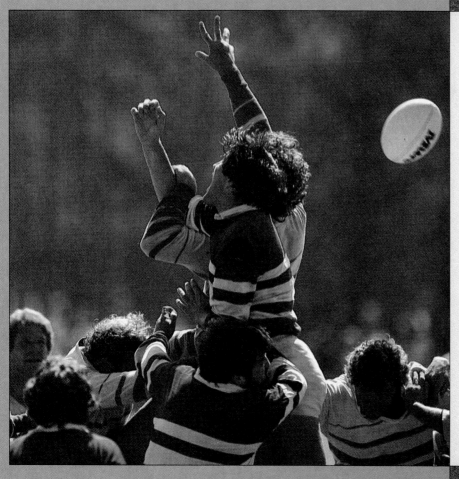

M ost people think of energy as the commodity they need to be vigorously active—to run with the family dog, dunk a basket-ball, race a bicycle, swim, bounce on a trampoline. There is no question that such activities use energy—and lots of it. However, energy is also needed by a person sitting quietly in a rowboat waiting for the fish to bite or by someone sleeping in front of the TV. That is because energy is used continuously to carry out the basic processes that keep people alive. The amount of energy needed for such maintenance processes in a day is approximately the same amount of energy needed to walk 20–25 miles (Astrand, 1988). From this, you can see that most people use more energy for the life-sustaining functions than for physical activity.

energy—the capacity to do work, measured in kcalories; the power to affect physical changes

Energy is expressed in several forms in the body. Movement exemplifies mechanical energy. Energy that powers metabolic reactions is chemical energy. The tiny electrical impulses generated by nerve cells represent electrical energy. Heat produced by the body is thermal energy; most body energy ultimately takes this form.

As you know, people get their energy from food. Most people have at least a general idea of how much energy (how many kcalories) various foods provide, but what they may not know is that the amount of energy available from foods depends directly on how much of the macronutrients protein, fat, and carbohydrate is in them. Alcohol also furnishes energy. Foods differ markedly in their energy values because they have different levels of these substances.

This chapter provides an overview of getting and spending energy. It is a useful introduction to Chapters 6–8, which deal separately and in greater detail with carbohydrate, fat, and protein.

Human Energy Is Described in Kilocalories

kilocalories (kcalories, kcal)— units in which energy is measured

Energy is commonly measured in units called **kilocalories,** which are abbreviated **kcalories** or **kcal** in this book. A kcalorie is the amount of heat required to raise the temperature of 1 kilogram of water one degree Celsius (1°C).

Even energy that does not immediately take the form of heat is described in kcalories. Energy intake and energy output are both expressed in kcalories: we talk about food providing a certain number of kcalories, and about various activities using a particular number of kcalories. (The *calorie* used in the study of physics is only $\frac{1}{1000}$ as large as the *kcalorie* used here.)

The metric system also quantifies energy in kilojoules. There are 4.18 kilojoules in 1 kilocalorie. However, since the kcalorie is the more familiar descriptor, we have used that term throughout this book.

There Are at Least Three Ways the Body Expends Energy

Scientists know about three general purposes for which the body uses energy: to support life-sustaining functions, for physical activity, and for internally processing food that has been consumed. There may be an additional way in which energy is expended—in response to extreme environmental factors. Let's discuss each of these expenditures individually.

Life-Sustaining Functions

Continuously throughout life, every body expends energy for the activities that keep it alive. These activities include breathing; producing heartbeats; maintaining body temperature and muscle tone; and the functioning of the glands, cells, and nervous system. Collectively, these life-sustaining processes are referred to as **basal metabolism,** and the amount of energy required to maintain them for a specified unit of time is called the **basal metabolic rate (BMR).** To actually measure a person's BMR, it takes very specialized equipment and precise conditions. Because the protocol for determining BMR is difficult and inconvenient, it is seldom done except in very specialized research. Basal metabolism usually accounts for 60 to 70% of the typical North American's daily energy expenditure.

Data collection for research on energy use is now likely to be done under somewhat less stringent conditions, producing a value called the **resting metabolic rate (RMR)** or resting energy expenditure (REE). If you had your RMR measured, you would need to rest quietly in a comfortable environment for several hours following a meal and physical activity; under such circumstances, your energy use might be slightly higher because it could include a small amount of energy used for purposes other than basal activities. RMR usually accounts for 65 to 75% of total daily energy expenditure.

Most people will never have a BMR or RMR test done on themselves, but research on others has provided data from which formulas for *estimating* RMR have been derived; one of the simpler methods of calculating RMR will be shown in Assessment 5.1.

A number of individual factors affect a person's basal energy needs; they are discussed in the paragraphs that follow. As you read, note that several of these factors involve two general variables: how much lean body mass a person has (including muscle, which typically represents 35–40% of body weight) and whether the amount of that tissue is changing. Additionally, you should note that certain internal organs are responsible for a disproportionate amount of basal energy usage: the liver and brain, which account for only 4% of a person's body weight, are responsible for 40% of the RMR

basal metabolism—all the metabolic processes that must take place continuously to sustain the life of an animal

basal metabolic rate (BMR)—the number of kcalories required to maintain life-sustaining activities for a specified amount of time; requires very specific conditions for exact measurement

resting metabolic rate (RMR)—the number of kcalories used during a specified amount of time at rest; usually a slightly higher value than BMR due to measurement under less stringent conditions

(Owen, 1988). Therefore, especially once a person has reached adulthood, the fairly consistent energy usage of these organs exerts a certain stabilizing effect on the RMR.

Body Size A tall, large person usually has a higher BMR than a short, small person. The different BMRs reflect the different total amounts of lean tissue each body contains. There may not be much difference in BMR between a fat person and a thin person of the same height, though, because fat tissue is not very active metabolically and does not use much energy.

Age Since people increase their mass of lean tissue as they progress from infancy through adolescence, the number of kcalories used for basal processes increases during the growth years. The growth process itself increases the BMR further: BMR is high during the growth spurts of the toddler period and adolescence.

Once a person has achieved full size, lean body mass and BMR decrease gradually by anywhere from 2% to 3% per decade (RDA Subcommittee, 1989).

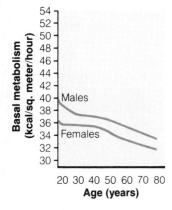

Sex Males generally have higher BMRs than females of the same age and size. This is mainly because males usually have proportionately more lean tissue than females have. There may be hormonal influences as well. Some recent research suggests that women's basal needs may be lower than previously thought (Owen, 1988).

Figure 5.1 illustrates the effects of both sex and age after physical maturity.

Figure 5.1 The effect of sex and age after maturity on BMR. This graph shows that males usually have a higher BMR than females. Growth during the early years of life raises BMR; aging beyond maturity results in a gradual decline in the energy used for internal processes. (Adapted from Guyton, A.C. 1981. *Textbook of medical physiology.* Philadelphia: W. B. Saunders Company.)

Growth When body tissue is added, whether it is protein or fat, energy is required to synthesize the tissue—energy that is over and above the energy value of the material itself. The average energy cost is about 5 kcalories per gram of growth tissue gained (RDA Subcommittee, 1989).

Health Status A person who is physically fit generally has a higher BMR than one who is not. This reflects the larger muscle mass in the person who exercises.

The BMR of a person who is losing weight (very quickly) often decreases; this is one reason why people who are on severe kcalorie-restricted diets lose weight more slowly after they have been dieting for a while. The decreased BMR may persist even after the person has finished dieting and is simply maintaining weight (Elliott et al., 1989). The BMR of a starving person may be as much as 30% lower than that of the same person before deprivation. Chapter 10 points out that this is a serious criticism of "crash" dieting: it can result in a situation that leads to weight regain.

Fever raises the BMR. For every Fahrenheit degree above normal temperature, BMR is about 7% higher; for every Celsius degree of fever, there is almost a 13% increase in BMR (Heymsfield and Williams, 1988). Injuries and surgery also increase basal needs; extensive burns can double a person's energy requirement.

Thyroid Hormone Level The thyroid hormone *thyroxin* is a metabolic accelerator. If your body produces less thyroxin than most people's, your metabolic processes are slower, a fact that is reflected in a lower BMR. On the other hand, people who produce an overabundance of thyroxin have higher basal metabolic rates as a result.

If low or high thyroxin production interferes with a person's health, either situation can usually be corrected by medical intervention. Fortunately, both conditions are unusual.

Pregnancy During pregnancy, maternal and fetal growth raises the woman's BMR above its prepregnant level. This will be considered in more detail in Chapter 16.

Individual Variation Some people use more (or less) energy for basal metabolic activities than would be expected, taking into consideration the factors just listed. It is not uncommon to find variation of as much as 20% in either direction; even greater differences have been observed. These variations seem to have a strong genetic component (Poehlman and Horton, 1989).

Physical Activity

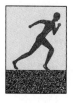

The second largest use of energy, typically, is for physical activity. This is the only aspect of energy expenditure over which you have very much control. Because most energy used for physical activity is converted to heat, this component of energy use is referred to as the **thermic effect of exercise.**

The amount of energy a person uses for physical activity can vary markedly from one day to the next. This contrasts with BMR, which isn't likely to be much different from day to day. The proportion of energy most people use for physical activity is 20–30% of total kcalories, although the manual laborer or serious athlete would use a higher proportion.

Three factors influence the amount of energy you use for physical activity: the type of activity you engage in, the length of time you do it, and your body weight.

Type of Activity Activities that use a larger amount of muscle mass use more energy. For example, walking requires more energy than sitting and typing because more large muscles are involved in walking. The intensity of an activity also has a direct influence on energy usage: running, even though it involves many of the same muscle groups as walking, uses more energy per unit of time because the stride is longer and more frequent. Table 5.1 and Figure 5.2 give examples of how much energy is expended during various activities. Note that these values are for activity alone and do not include energy that is simultaneously being expended for basal needs.

thermic effect of exercise (TEE)— the number of kcalories expended above RMR as a result of physical activity

Table 5.1 Energy Cost of Some Activities

Activity	kcal/kg/minute	Activity	kcal/kg/minute
Bicycling (racing)	0.127	Painting outside	0.057
Bicycling (leisurely)	0.042	Playing ping-pong	0.073
Canoeing (leisurely)	0.024	Piano playing	0.018
Carpentry	0.045	Rowing in a race	0.267
Cleaning (light)	0.030	Running (5½ min/mile)	0.269
Cooking	0.015	Running (7 min/mile)	0.208
Dancing (fast)	0.148	Running (9 min/mile)	0.173
Dancing (slowly)	0.050	Sewing (hand or machine)	0.007
Dishwashing	0.017	Singing (loud)	0.013
Dressing, personal care	0.025	Sitting (writing)	0.007
Driving a car	0.015	Skating	0.058
Eating	0.007	Skiing (cross-country, level)	0.099
Field hockey	0.114	Skiing (cross-country, uphill)	0.254
Grocery shopping	0.040	Sleeping	0
Football	0.112	Squash	0.192
Garage work (repairs)	0.046	Standing (relaxed)	0.008
Golf	0.065	Stock clerking	0.034
Gymnastics	0.046	Swimming (2 mph)	0.132
Horseback riding (walk)	0.023	Tennis	0.089
Horseback riding (gallop)	0.112	Violin playing	0.010
Judo	0.175	Volleyball	0.030
Knitting	0.012	Walking (3 mph)	0.039
Laboratory work	0.018	Walking (3 mph, carrying 22 lb)	0.046
Laundry (light)	0.022	Walking (4 mph)	0.057
Lying still, awake	0	Walking downstairs	0.012 kcal/flight
Painting inside	0.014	Walking upstairs	0.036 kcal/flight

Compiled from data published by Taylor and McLeod, 1949; Durnin and Passmore, 1967; McArdle et al., 1981; and Passmore and Durnin, 1955. Values have been modified to eliminate energy expended for BMR and the thermic effect of food (discussed later in the chapter). Since values for the same activity vary from one source to another, these values are unavoidably less precise than they appear.

Do not discount the effect that even small movements can have on overall energy usage; one researcher has estimated that *fidgeting* can cost 100–800 kcalories per day (Ravussin, 1986).

Duration of Activity Time is the second factor to be considered in calculating energy expenditure. Obviously, the longer an activity is continued, the more energy will be used.

It is sometimes difficult to estimate how much time is actually involved in an activity if it is performed only intermittently. For example, people who spend eight hours during the day at a downhill ski area may spend only a couple of hours skiing, considering time spent in lift lines, on lifts, and in the chalet.

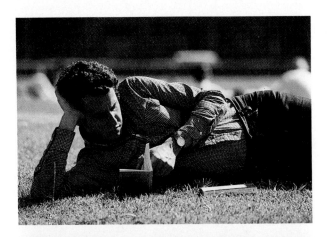

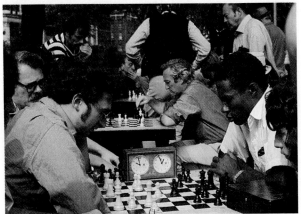

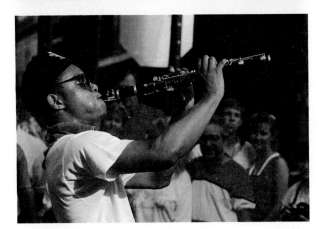

Figure 5.2 Energy cost of various activities. These activities use different amounts of energy. (a) The person lying still uses no energy for activity. (b) The chess players use about 30 kcalories per hour for their slight activity. (c) The musician probably uses double that amount, depending on how much he moves as he plays. (d) Folk dancers may use 500 kcalories per hour. (e) The runners use the highest amount of energy: a 154-pound person running 7-minute miles uses almost 900 kcalories per hour for the activity alone.

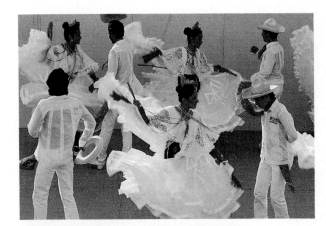

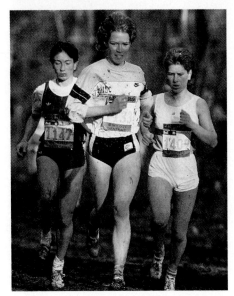

Body Weight   Body weight also influences energy expenditure. The heavier a person is, the more energy he or she expends in moving that mass. This means that if you and a friend who is larger exercise together, your friend uses more energy than you while performing the same exercise at the same intensity for the same length of time.

In theory, you could calculate your total day's energy expenditure from physical activity by keeping a careful diary of your activities in 5-minute intervals, multiplying those times by the appropriate figures from Table 5.1, and summing them; but such records are very difficult to keep accurately.

Biological Processing of Food

For decades, researchers have known that a certain expenditure of energy is required for the physiological processes of digestion, absorption, transport, and for the storage of food and its nutrients. That is, your body uses a small amount of energy for processing food internally before you have access to the larger amount of energy the food contains . . . just as it takes a small investment of money to make big money.

thermic effect of food (TEF)—the number of kcalories expended (at rest) above RMR during the several hours following a meal; caused by the energy demands of digestion, absorption, transport, and storage

These processes usually occur within six hours following a meal, and the production of heat as a by-product is called the **thermic effect of food** (an outdated term for the concept is *specific dynamic effect*). Approximately 6–10% of the energy in the food a person consumes is used for internal processing of food.

Extreme Dietary and Environmental Factors

In recent years, scientists have taken interest in the fact that under certain circumstances, there is greater energy expenditure than the three factors discussed so far would lead you to expect.

Some people, when they take in much more energy than they expend for basal functions, physical activity, and the body's biological processing of food, seem to have a mechanism for dissipating a portion of the surplus kcalories. Instead of gaining the amount of body fat that would be predicted from the extra kcalories consumed, their bodies expend some of the extra kcalories as additional heat. One researcher suggests that this occurs particularly when the surplus kcalories come from carbohydrate; surplus kcalories are less likely to be dissipated as body heat when they are consumed as fat. In addition, surplus kcalories from fat are more likely to result in extra fat on the body (Poehlman and Horton, 1989). (Other people apparently do not have this mechanism; they convert most of their surplus energy—whatever the source—into body fat. Theoretically, this conversion could explain some cases of obesity.)

Scientists regard the dissipation of extra kcalories as heat as an instance of **adaptive thermogenesis.** The term suggests that the body adapts energy expenditure to changing conditions (in this case, to the excessive energy intake and composition of the food eaten) by producing heat but no real "work."

Another instance in which adaptive thermogenesis may occur is in response to environmental cold. It is well known that hibernating animals maintain a steady body temperature in spite of the fact that environmental temperature may vary considerably. Such heat production is called *nonshivering thermogenesis.* It is not known whether this phenomenon also occurs in humans.

Some scientists theorize that adaptive thermogenesis may occur in animals whose bodies contain, in addition to the usual white fat tissue, a second type of fat called *brown fat* (Kinney, 1988). It is brown because it contains a much larger number of mitochondria, the cellular structures in which much of the body's energy is produced. Although brown fat is known to exist in animals that hibernate and in newborn human infants, it is not yet known whether human adults retain this tissue or how much they might have.

Figure 5.3 summarizes the relative amounts of energy used in a 24-hour period for the functions of basal metabolism, the thermic effect of exercise, the thermic effect of food, and for adaptive thermogenesis.

The next section suggests ways of estimating how much energy you use.

There Are Several Ways to Estimate Your Daily Energy Needs

A number of methods have been suggested for estimating how many kcalories a person is likely to use all together for basal metabolic activity, physical activity, and the body's processing of food. The three methods we show here vary in their ease of use and in their accuracy.

RDA Estimate

The RDA committee has collected data on typical daily kcaloric usage by people of different ages and sex; they appear in Table 5.2. The committee departed in this instance from its usual method of establishing an RDA, that is, in establishing recommendations to meet the needs of most of the population. Rather, it cited *median* values for energy intake recommendations, noting that values for adults are based on light-to-moderate activity levels as

adaptive thermogenesis—energy expended by an animal in response to extreme environmental conditions; produces heat but no "work"

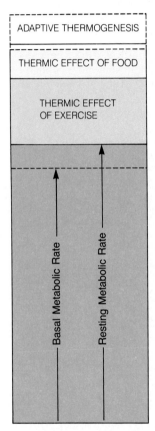

Figure 5.3 Total energy expended in 24 hours. This is a representation of 24-hour energy expenditure in a relatively inactive person. The amount of energy attributed to adaptive thermogenesis is tentative; an exact measure must wait until we know more about this means of energy expenditure. (Adapted from Danforth, E. 1985. Diet and obesity. *The American Journal of Clinical Nutrition* 41:1132–1145.)

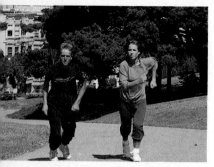

Variation in daily energy expenditure. These people, although they may be involved in the same activities throughout a day, expend different amounts of energy.

performed by people of the body weights referenced in the table. If your body size is substantially different from that stated in the table for your category or if you are much more or less physically active, your energy usage may differ from that suggested. Even if you appear to be similar to the reference person, your energy expenditure might vary by 20% in either direction.

Table 5.2 Median Heights and Weights and Recommended Energy Intake[a]

Category	Age (years) or Condition	Weight (kg)	Weight (lb)	Height (in)	Average Energy Allowance (kcal)[b] Per kg	Average Energy Allowance (kcal)[b] Per day[c]
Infants	0.0–0.5	6	13	24	108	650
	0.5–1.0	9	20	28	98	850
Children	1–3	13	29	35	102	1,300
	4–6	20	44	44	90	1,800
	7–10	28	62	52	70	2,000
Males	11–14	45	99	62	55	2,500
	15–18	66	145	69	45	3,000
	19–24	72	160	70	40	2,900
	25–50	79	174	70	37	2,900
	51+	77	170	68	30	2,300
Females	11–14	46	101	62	47	2,200
	15–18	55	120	64	40	2,200
	19–24	58	128	65	38	2,200
	25–50	63	138	64	36	2,200
	51+	65	143	63	30	1,900
Pregnant	1st trimester					+0
	2nd trimester					+300
	3rd trimester					+300
Lactating	1st 6 months					+500
	2nd 6 months					+500

[a] Adapted from *Recommended Dietary Allowances,* 10th edition, 1989, with permission of the National Academy Press, Washington, DC.

[b] In the range of light to moderate activity, the coefficient of variation is ±20%.

[c] Figure is rounded.

Calculated Estimate of Energy Usage for One Day

Many formulas, some complex and others not so complex, have been developed for estimating kcalories expended in a day. Assessment 5.1 presents less intricate formulas that you can use to yield rough approximations of energy used for basal activities, physical activity, and your body's processing of food. Even though the results are just estimates, the fact that the calculations involve data specific to you is likely to improve their accuracy over the tabular estimates.

Record of Typical Energy Intake

A final means of estimating your daily energy usage is to determine what your typical daily kcaloric intake is. Energy intake and expenditure are roughly equivalent values, provided you are neither gaining nor losing weight and provided your activity level is fairly constant from day to day.

As a result, if your weight and activity level are quite stable, you can get an idea of how much energy you use daily by keeping diet records for several consecutive typical days, calculating their energy content, and then averaging them. (The next section describes how to calculate the energy content of various foods.)

Now that we have considered how a person expends energy, let's discuss the source of that energy: food.

A Food's Energy Value Depends on Its Content of Protein, Fat, and Carbohydrate

You can calculate how much energy is obtainable from a food if you know how many grams of protein, fat, carbohydrate, and/or alcohol it contains. (Water, vitamins, and minerals provide no energy, but have other valuable functions.) When you know those amounts—and we will suggest sources of that information shortly—you can calculate the energy value of each constituent by multiplying it by the following values:

- 4 kcalories per gram of protein
- 9 kcalories per gram of fat
- 4 kcalories per gram of carbohydrate
- 7 kcalories per gram of alcohol

Scientists have found that these values are reasonable averages of the actual energy yielded in the body by these substances from various food sources. The energy value of the whole food, then, is the sum of the kcaloric values of its constituents. Figure 5.4 shows these values for 1 cup of fruit-flavored yogurt.

Energy Nutrients That Occur in Foods of the Basic Groups

Table 5.3 shows the level of protein, fat, carbohydrate, and alcohol contained in some representative foods from each of the basic food groups. You can see that foods vary widely in their composition. Even within a food

Figure 5.4 Calculating the energy value of a food of known composition.

FOOD	*1 cup fruit-flavored yogurt*		
	Protein (g)	Fat (g)	Carbohydrate (g)
Enter the composition of the food	10	3	43
Multiply by kcal/g of nutrient to get kcal from each nutrient	× 4 40	× 9 27	× 4 172
Total the kcal	40 +	27 +	172 = 239

Table 5.3 Energy Sources in Some Representative Foods[a]

Foods	Serving Size	Protein (g)	Fat (g)	Carbohydrate (g)	Alcohol (g)
Fruits and vegetables					
Peach, fresh	1 medium	1	tr	**10**	0
Lettuce, romaine	1 cup	1	tr	**1**	0
Mashed potato with milk	½ cup	2	1	**19**	0
Grain products					
Bread, whole wheat	1 slice	3	1	**16**	0
Toast, whole wheat	1 slice	3	1	**15**	0
Cornflakes, plain	1¼ cups	2	tr	**24**	0
Cornflakes, sugared	1¼ cups	2	tr	**46**	0
Popcorn, air popped	3 cups	3	tr	**18**	0
Diary products					
Milk, whole, 3.3% fat	1 cup	8	8	**11**	0
Milk, 2% fat	1 cup	8	5	**12**	0
Yogurt, plain, made from low-fat milk	1 cup	12	4	**16**	0
Meats and meat alternates					
Chicken, breast, roasted, no skin	3 oz	**27**	3	0	0
Chicken, breast, batter fried	3 oz	21	**11**	8	0
Ground beef, broiled	3 oz	21	**16**	0	0
Peanuts, oil roasted	½ cup	20	**36**	14	0
Great northern beans, cooked	1 cup	14	1	**38**	0
Combination foods					
Cheese pizza	⅛ of 15"	15	9	**39**	0
Limited extras					
Brownie with icing	0.9 oz	1	5	**15**	0
Beer	12 oz	1	0	14	**13**
Carbonated fruit-flavored drink	12 oz	0	0	**42**	0

[a]The value for the constituent that provides the largest number of kcalories is in bold print.

group, there is considerable variation in the levels of energy nutrients. For example, fruits and vegetables vary widely in their carbohydrate content. Meats and meat alternates, although they all have high protein levels, have different fat and carbohydrate contents.

In Table 5.3, the energy nutrient that is responsible for the greatest number of kcalories in each food is in bold print. Because fat and alcohol furnish more kcalories per gram than carbohydrate or protein, they can be the largest contributors of energy without being the heaviest components.

Energy Nutrients Shown on Food Composition Tables

Appendices E and F list the energy, nutrient content, and kcaloric values for hundreds of foods. Sometimes the number of kcalories shown per serving of food will not exactly match the values you will get when you calculate them as described earlier. The discrepancy is due to the slight differences in conversion factors used to calculate the values in the appendices. The appendix values are more accurate, but your calculated values are close, usable estimates.

Energy Nutrients Shown on Nutrition Labels

Nutrition labels are another source of information about energy nutrients in foods. As of this writing, the only foods required to carry a nutrition label are those that make a nutrition claim (such as "low sodium") or foods to which nutrients have been added. Many other products also carry a nutrition label although it is not mandatory for them to do so; more foods will be required to carry them in the future.

The top part of a nutrition label must specify the number of grams of protein, carbohydrate, and fat contained in each serving of food and the number of milligrams of sodium per serving. This part of the label must also tell the serving size on which these values were based and how many servings of product are in the whole container. The nutrition label also states the energy value per serving, rounded to the nearest 10 kcalories. Figure 5.5 is an example of a nutrition label.

Assessing the Percentage of Kcalories Furnished by Protein, Fat, and Carbohydrate in Your Diet

When you have food composition data for the foods you have eaten, it also is possible to determine what percentage of your total kcaloric intake for a day came from each of the energy nutrients. This is of interest because a number of dietary guidelines for good health are expressed in these terms.

There seems to be a growing consensus among health agencies and pro-

Estimating Kcalories Used in 24 Hours

Use a form similar to that in Sample Assessment 5.1 to do these calculations.

1. Estimating RMR

a. Convert your body weight to kilograms by dividing your weight in pounds by 2.2 lb/kg.
b. In Table A, below, identify which sex and age range you belong to, and copy the adjacent equation for estimating your RMR into the appropriate space of your assessment form.

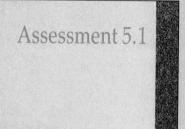

Assessment 5.1

Table A Equations for Estimating RMR from Body Weight

Sex and Age Range (years)	Equation to Derive RMR in kcal/day
Males	
0–3	$(60.9 \times wt^a) - 54$
3–10	$(22.7 \times wt^a) + 495$
10–18	$(17.5 \times wt^a) + 651$
18–30	$(15.3 \times wt^a) + 679$
30–60	$(11.6 \times wt^a) + 879$
>60	$(13.5 \times wt^a) + 487$
Females	
0–3	$(61.0 \times wt^a) - 51$
3–10	$(22.5 \times wt^a) + 499$
10–18	$(12.2 \times wt^a) + 746$
18–30	$(14.7 \times wt^a) + 496$
30–60	$(8.7 \times wt^a) + 829$
>60	$(10.5 \times wt^a) + 596$

[a]Weight in kilograms

Source: RDA Subcommittee. 1989. *Recommended dietary allowances*. Washington, DC: National Academy Press.

c. Enter your kg weight into the equation for "wt" and do the calculation; it yields an estimate of the number of kcalories you expend per day for RMR.

2. Estimating energy expenditure for RMR plus the thermic effect of exercise (TEE)

a. Estimate how many hours you spend per day at the various activity levels in Table B in Sample Assessment 5.1, and enter the number of hours for each in column 1. The sum of the values in column 1 must be 24 for the hours in a day.

b. Multiply each number in column 1 by the adjacent value in column 2; figures in column 2 represent how many multiples of a person's RMR are used per hour for *RMR plus activities in this category.* Enter these values in column 3; they are weighted factors that take into account both the nature of the activity and the amount of time you spend doing such activities.

c. Sum the values in column 3, and divide it by 24. This factor represents your average overall use of energy for RMR plus activity for the day.

d. Multiply your RMR (the value you derived in 1c) by the overall factor (from 2c above); the product is an estimate of the number of kcalories you use per day for RMR and activity combined.

3. Estimating energy expenditure for the thermic effect of food (TEF)

TEF accounts for approximately 10% of a person's total energy use. You can get a reasonable estimate by calculating 10% of your energy use for RMR plus TEE (from 2d above).

4. Estimating total energy expenditure

Total daily energy expenditure is the sum of the values for RMR, TEE, and TEF. (It is not possible to estimate energy expenditure for adaptive thermogenesis.) If you are a woman who is pregnant or lactating, you must include an additional amount to cover the energy demands of those conditions (see Sample Assessment 5.1).

Sample Assessment 5.1 Estimating kcalories used in 24 hours (The 3 examples below are color-coded to show calculations for Ann, Trent, and Sally.)

Example 1: | Ann. | Ann is a student on a large campus. On class days, she usually concentrates on her coursework; for a break, she visits with friends. As she considers her usual activities and how they would be divided into the categories in Table B, she makes this list:

sleeping = 8 hours

lying down watching TV = 1 hour

sitting in class, standing in labs, eating, talking with friends, or studying = most of the day (She figures it would be easiest to estimate other activities first, and assume that these activities take the remainder of the day.)

carrying book bag while walking = 1 hour

walking around at home, fixing meals, cleaning up = 1.5 hours

Example 2: Trent. Trent is a student and is on the basketball team. Each weekday, in addition to dealing with his coursework, he spends three hours at practice; of that time, about two hours are spent on the court doing drills and playing. His time for the whole day is usually spent as follows:

sleeping = 7 hours

sitting in class, standing in labs, eating, talking with friends, or studying = most of the day (He figures this "by difference," as Ann did.)

carrying book bag while walking = 1.5 hours

basketball = 2 hours

Example 3: Sally. Sally is a student who works a fast-food job part-time. Despite her busy schedule, she participates in an hour of aerobics several times a week because she enjoys it and it helps her maintain fitness and feel good; she averages her aerobics time as .5 hour per day. She makes this activity list:

sleeping = 7 hours

sitting in class, standing in labs, eating, talking with friends, or studying = most of the day (by difference)

carrying book bag = 1.5 hours

work = 2 hours

aerobics = .5 hour

fixing meals, cleaning up = .5 hour

1. weight (wt) in kilograms (kg) = $\dfrac{\text{wt in pounds (lb)}}{2.2 \text{ lb/kg}}$

$$\text{kg wt} = \dfrac{\text{lb}}{2.2 \text{ lb/kg}} = \underline{\quad} \text{ kg}$$

$\dfrac{134 \text{ lb}}{2.2 \text{ lb/kg}} = 61 \text{ kg}$	$\dfrac{170 \text{ lb}}{2.2 \text{ lb/kg}} = 77 \text{ kg}$	$\dfrac{120 \text{ lb}}{2.2 \text{ lb/kg}} = 55 \text{ kg}$

RMR = (____ × ____) + ____ = ____ kcal/day

Note: First multiply the numbers *within the parentheses;* then add the number outside the parentheses.

(14.7 × 61) + 496 = 1393 kcal/day	(15.3 × 77) + 679 = 1857 kcal/day	(14.7 × 55) + 496 = 1305 kcal/day

2.

Table B: Activity Levels

Activity category	Col 1: est. hrs/day	Col 2: RMR + TEE factor	Col 3: weighted factor	Col 1	Col 3	Col 1	Col 3
Resting Sleeping, reclining	9	1.0	9.0	7	7.0	7	7.0
Very light Seated and standing activities with little locomotion	12.5	1.5	18.8	13.5	20.3	13	19.5
Light Walking @ 2.5–3 mph, carpentry, housework, child care, golf, food service jobs	1.5	2.5	3.8	0	0	2	5.0
Moderate Walking @ 3.5–4 mph, carrying load, cycling, skiing, tennis, dancing	1	5.0	5.0	1.5	7.5	2	10.0
Heavy Walking uphill with load, felling trees, basketball, football, soccer	0	7.0	0	2	14.0	0	0
	24	TOTAL	36.6	24	48.8	24	41.5
		AVERAGE PER HOUR	1.5		2.0		1.7

RMR × average per hour = kcalories used for RMR + TEE/day

1393 × 1.5 = 2090 kcal/day	1857 × 2.0 = 3714 kcal/day	1305 × 1.7 = 2219 kcal/day

3. TEF = (RMR + TEE) × .1 = _____ kcal/day

2090 × .1 = 209 kcal/day	3714 × .1 = 371 kcal/day	2219 × .1 = 222 kcal/day

4. TOTAL = (RMR + TEE) + TEF + * = _____ kcal/day

*Women in the last two trimesters of pregnancy add 300 kcalories; lactating women add 500 kcalories.

2090 + 209 = 2299 kcal/day TOTAL	3714 + 371 = 4085 kcal/day TOTAL	2219 + 222 = 2441 kcal/day TOTAL

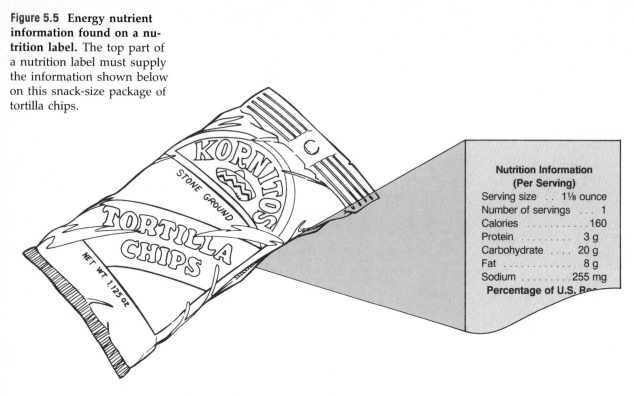

Figure 5.5 Energy nutrient information found on a nutrition label. The top part of a nutrition label must supply the information shown below on this snack-size package of tortilla chips.

Nutrition Information
(Per Serving)
Serving size . . 1⅛ ounce
Number of servings . . . 1
Calories 160
Protein . . . . 3 g
Carbohydrate . . . . 20 g
Fat . . . . 8 g
Sodium . . . . .255 mg
Percentage of U.S. R

fessional organizations that the optimal proportion of energy from each of the energy nutrients is as follows:

Nutrient	Recommended proportion of total energy intake
Fat	30% or less
Protein	10–15%
Carbohydrate	55% or more

Assessment 5.2 shows how you can calculate values for your own diet.

Food Energy Not Needed Immediately Is Stored in the Body

Even though our *use* of energy is continuous, our energy *intake* is not. It is not necessary to eat nonstop in order to have energy, because the body can store energy for later use.

Conversion and Storage of Energy Nutrients

The body does not necessarily store energy in the same form as it occurred in the food you consumed. For example, although *some* dietary carbohydrate is stored in the body as carbohydrate, even more may be converted to fat. The dispensation of incoming energy sources depends on many factors, such as current energy needs and reserves.

Fate of Dietary Carbohydrates   **Sugars** and **starches** are the major forms of dietary carbohydrates. When they are digested, absorbed, and processed by the body, their predominant product is the simple sugar **glucose.** Some of this glucose is used to maintain normal levels in the blood; blood glucose is one of the body's most readily available sources of energy.

After a meal, however, there is usually more glucose available than is needed for maintaining a normal blood glucose level. Some of the extra amount is used to produce **glycogen,** a much more complex substance composed of hundreds of glucose units linked together. Glycogen in animals is the counterpart of starch in plants. Glycogen is stored in limited amounts in the liver and skeletal muscles.

The glucose that still remains is converted into fat, a very different substance from the carbohydrate from which it originated. Once it has been converted into fat, for the most part it cannot be converted back into glucose.

Fate of Dietary Proteins   Food protein components are also quite versatile. If the body has an urgent need for energy that cannot be met in other ways, some protein components can be converted into other compounds (including glucose) and used for energy. However, protein components are best used when reassembled into body proteins, the substances that are the primary components of skeletal muscles and vital organs. There is a limit to how much body protein will be produced; body protein increases especially during growth and/or a deliberate muscle-building program. If both of these needs have been met and there are still more protein components in the body, then parts of them are converted into fat. Once these components have been converted into fat, they cannot be converted back into essential protein components.

Fate of Dietary Fats   Dietary fat is the most predictable substance of the lot. Its absorbed components can follow either of two routes. They can be hydrolyzed into intermediate components and then used for energy, or they can be reassembled in the form of body fat. The body has a greater capacity for fat storage than for storage of any other energy source.

Fate of Dietary Alcohol   If alcohol has been ingested, it is usually used quickly for energy production. Whatever is not metabolized rapidly is converted into fat.

Figure 5.6 summarizes these interconversions. You can see that your body is well designed for survival: a surplus of energy from any source can be converted into body fat as a hedge against future scarcity.

sugars—simple forms of carbohydrate

starches—complex forms of carbohydrate consisting of sugar units linked together

glucose—a simple sugar; a common product of dietary carbohydrate digestion, and a readily available energy source

glycogen—a complex carbohydrate consisting of glucose units linked together; serves as a storage form in animals

Figure 5.6 The body's options for generating and storing energy. Since energy is essential for life, our chances of survival are increased by the body's ability to obtain energy from different dietary constituents. Here, boxes represent breakdown products from the diet and intermediate compounds of metabolism; ovals represent storage forms for energy nutrients in the body.

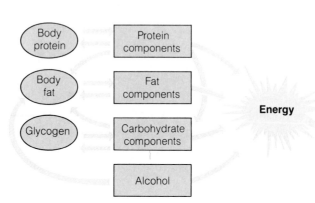

Calculating the Percentage of Kcalories from Protein, Fat, and Carbohydrate in a Day's Intake

Here's how to calculate the percentages of kcalories you derive from each energy nutrient for a day:

1. Keep a 24-hour food record on as typical a day as possible, using a form similar to that shown in the sample. List all foods and beverages consumed. (Add a column if you also consumed alcohol.)

2. Use Appendices E and/or F to find the protein, fat, and carbohydrate contents of those foods; adjust the values to correspond to the amounts of food you consumed; and enter the values in the appropriate columns. For example, if you drank 2 cups of milk, and the appendix gives values for 1 cup, you will have to double all values as you record them.

3. Figure the sum for each column.

4. Multiply the sum for each column by the energy value per gram of each nutrient.

5. Total the kcalories from all nutrients. If you consumed an alcoholic beverage, you can determine how many kcalories the alcohol provided by subtracting the kcalories provided by the beverage's protein, fat, and carbohydrate from the total kcalories in the beverage.

6. Divide the kcalories from each energy substrate by the total kcalories consumed; this yields a decimal fraction.

7. Multiply each decimal fraction by 100 to get the percentages; round each to the nearest percent.

Assessment 5.2

Food or Beverage	Amount Eaten	Protein (g)	Fat (g)	Carbo-hydrate (g)
Pork sausage, 2 small links	2 oz.	6	8	tr
Boiled egg	1	6	5	1
Buttermilk	1 cup	8	2	12
Hash browned potatoes	½ cup	3	9	22
Banana	1 med.	1	1	27
Cracked wheat bread	1 slice	2	1	13
Butter	1 T.	tr	12	tr
Honey	1 T.	tr	0	17
Swiss cheese	2 oz.	16	16	2
Whole milk	1 cup	8	8	11
Roast beef, lean only	3 oz.	23	12	0
Baked squash	1 cup	2	2	21
Butter	1 T.	tr	12	tr
Enriched noodles	1 cup	7	2	37
Cracked wheat bread	1 slice	2	1	13
Butter	1 T.	tr	12	tr
Popcorn, oil, salt	2 cups	2	6	12
Unsweetened canned grapefruit juice	1 cup	1	tr	22
Ice cream	1 cup	5	14	32
Totals **Multiply by kcal/g of nutrient** **to get kcal from each nutrient**		92 × 4 368	123 × 9 1107	242 × 4 968
Total the kcal		368 +	1107 +	968 =	2443
Divide nutrient kcal by total kcal **which yields a decimal fraction**		÷ 2443 0.15	÷ 2443 0.45	÷ 2443 0.40
Multiply by 100 to get percent		15%	45%	40%

Sample Assessment 5.2 Calculating the percentage of kcalories from protein, fat, and carbohydrate in a day's intake

Typical Energy Reserves in the Body

Carbohydrate and fat are the two primary substances that the body uses for energy; the body uses a much smaller proportion of protein for energy. While it might seem logical that the body must contain large amounts of both carbohydrate and fat and only a small amount of protein, that's not the way it is.

First consider carbohydrate stores. You usually have only about 20 grams of glucose (less than an ounce) in your entire blood supply and interstitial fluids at any given moment; but glycogen, which can be broken down into glucose very quickly when needed, is more generously available. You have approximately 100 grams of glycogen in your liver (which can be used for functions anywhere in the body) and about 400 grams in the cells of various muscles (which can be used only by the muscles in which it is located). All this carbohydrate together represents about 2000 kcalories.

Fat is much more plentiful. Although there is tremendous variation, the average young man's body ranges from 12–16% fat by weight and the average young woman's body is between 22% and 26% fat. A man who weighs 154 pounds and is 15% fat has approximately 23 pounds of body fat (almost 10,500 grams), which has an energy potential of roughly 94,500 kcalories. (Compare that to the potential kcalories available from carbohydrate.)

Typically, protein constitutes about 15% of a man's body weight and somewhat less of a woman's. However, only a portion of it is available for energy production. Because your skeletal muscles, your heart, and other vital organs are made largely of protein, you cannot survive if your body breaks down a lot of it.

Table 5.4 summarizes these energy resources in the typical adult male.

So far we've described energy balance in regard to the whole body. To understand the rest of our discussion of energy, it will be helpful for you to have a general understanding of what happens in an individual cell, the biological unit in which energy is actually generated and used.

What Happens in Body Cells During Energy Production

The processes by which energy is derived from carbohydrate, fat, and protein are regulated by enzymes. Just as enzymes are needed to digest these substances from the diet, enzymes are critical to the metabolic processes within cells that release energy from **energy substrate.**

energy substrate—any material that yields energy through enzymatic processes

For example, when carbohydrate is metabolized, it undergoes various enzyme-mediated changes that transform it into intermediate compounds. A glucose molecule, which contains six carbon atoms, is split into two 3-carbon units in a series of reactions; these are the reactions that constitute the process called **glycolysis.** Glycolysis occurs in the cytosol of the cell,

glycolysis—process in which body cells metabolize glucose without oxygen

Table 5.4 Likely Amounts of Stored Energy Sources in a Typical 70-kilogram (154-lb) Adult Male

	Approximate Grams Present	Potential Kcal Available
Carbohydrate[a]		
Glucose in blood and interstitial fluids	20	80 ⎫
Glycogen		⎬ 2080
Liver	100	400
Skeletal muscles	400	1600 ⎭
Fat (assuming 15% of body weight)	10,500	94,500
Protein (assuming 15% of body weight)	10,500	[b]
Total		~97,000

[a] From Ganong, W.F. 1989. *Review of medical physiology*, p. 244. E. Norwalk, CT: Lange Medical Publications.

[b] Although the body contains a substantial amount of protein, it is generally not much used for energy. If extreme and prolonged duress cause it to be used in significant amounts for energy, the body can withstand the loss of only about half of its protein before death will result (Hoffer, 1988).

without the use of any oxygen from the air; therefore, it is referred to as **anaerobic oxidation.** During glycolysis, **lactic acid** can be produced. The process of glycolysis is the first stage in the production of energy from glucose (Figure 5.7).

Several steps in the process of glycolysis (as well as in other energy-yielding reactions to be discussed shortly) involve a compound called **adenosine triphosphate** or **ATP;** it is the "energy currency" of the body. The bonds that hold phosphate units to the ATP molecule are high-energy bonds. When a unit of phosphate is split from ATP, this energy is released or "spent," and **adenosine diphosphate** or **ADP** results. ATP is spent, for example, during two of the reactions required for splitting glucose into 3-carbon units.

In other steps of glycolysis, ATP is *regenerated* from ADP. Some of these steps involve intermediate vitamin-containing compounds called **coenzymes,** which are critical to ATP production. The *yield* of ATP from anaerobic glycolysis is slightly more than the amount *used* during the process; it amounts to 2 molecules of ATP. In a subsequent process called *electron transport*, however, more ATP is produced for a total net gain of 8 molecules of ATP (Smith et al., 1983).

The anaerobic process of glycolysis is only the beginning of energy production from glucose. Next, the 3-carbon units produced by glycolysis move from the cytosol into the mitochondria of the cell. The energy-producing reactions that occur in the mitochondria ultimately involve oxygen and are therefore called **aerobic** oxidation.

In the mitochondria, the 3-carbon units are modified into activated 2-carbon units (the third carbon is converted to carbon dioxide and released). In the process, more vitamin-containing coenzymes are formed that ultimately lead to the production of ATP.

anaerobic—referring to the absence of oxygen

oxidation—energy-producing metabolic processes

lactic acid—metabolic product of glycolysis that can build up in muscles and be accompanied by fatigue

adenosine triphosphate (ATP)—a compound that acts as energy "currency"; energy is released when a phosphate unit is split off and **adenosine diphosphate (ADP)** is formed

coenzyme—a molecule, usually containing a vitamin, that unites with a protein to form an enzyme

aerobic—referring to the presence of oxygen

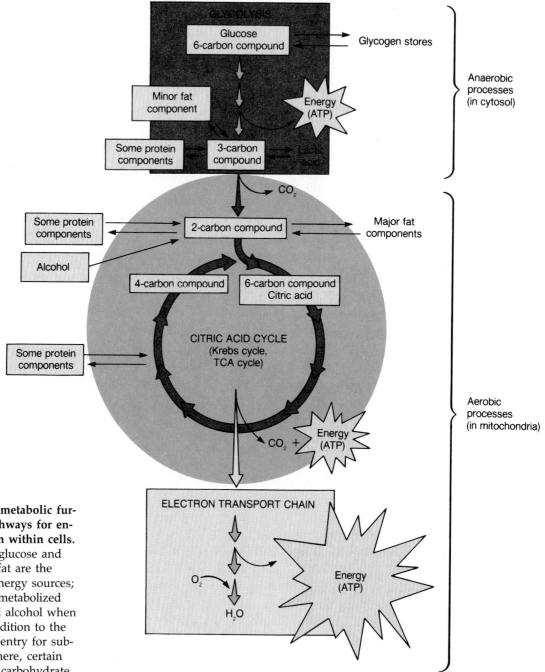

Figure 5.7 The metabolic furnace: some pathways for energy production within cells. Carbohydrate (glucose and glycogen) and fat are the body's major energy sources; protein is also metabolized for energy, and alcohol when available. In addition to the main points of entry for substrates shown here, certain components of carbohydrate, fat, and protein can enter via less-used pathways. Anaerobic and aerobic processes produce very different amounts of energy. All together, anaerobic and aerobic oxidation of one molecule of glucose usually yields 38 units of ATP.

The activated 2-carbon units then enter a series of nine enzyme-controlled reactions called the **citric acid cycle** or the **tricarboxylic acid (TCA) cycle** for chemicals created in the process. (It was originally named the **Krebs cycle** for the scientist who defined this sequence of cellular reactions; Hans Krebs won a Nobel prize in 1937 for having done so.)

To begin the cycle (Figure 5.7), an activated 2-carbon unit combines with a 4-carbon unit to form a larger compound, citric acid. In the subsequent reactions of the cycle, one-by-one the carbons and oxygen from the original glucose molecule are split off until all have been converted to carbon dioxide.

As the carbon and oxygen from the original glucose molecule are being dispensed with, hydrogen from the glucose is taken up by vitamin-containing coenzymes and shuttled into another important set of reactions, the **electron transport chain.** Here, the electrons from hydrogen are transferred from one compound to another and combined with oxygen, producing large amounts of ATP and water in the process.

All together, the reactions of glycolysis, the citric acid cycle, and the electron transport chain produce 38 units of ATP from one molecule of glucose. Of this, by far the greatest amount was produced by aerobic oxidation; only 2 of these units were produced solely by glycolysis.

What about the other energy nutrients? Are there separate pathways by which the body produces energy from them?

The answer is that components of protein and fat make use of the same pathways by which carbohydrate is metabolized. Components of protein can be metabolized via both aerobic oxidation (the citric acid cycle) and anaerobic oxidation (glycolysis), but most components of fat can be metabolized only via the citric acid cycle. The citric acid cycle is involved in the metabolism of all energy nutrients and alcohol, although their components enter the pathways at various steps in the sequence.

Why is it useful for you to know what is happening at the cellular level when your major interest is to understand the energy needs of the whole body? We have exposed you to this biochemistry because it becomes relevant as we look at the next important energy issue—how the proportion of energy produced from the different energy nutrients at any given time varies with the circumstances. If you keep in mind what you learned in this close-up of the individual cell, it will help you to understand what happens in the whole body.

citric acid cycle, tricarboxylic acid (TCA) cycle, or **Krebs cycle**—a sequence of biochemical reactions that are key to aerobic energy production

electron transport chain—a series of reactions in which the hydrogen atoms released during glycolysis and the reactions of the citric acid cycle combine with oxygen to form water, releasing energy in the process

The Proportions of Carbohydrate, Fat, and Protein Used for Energy Production Are Influenced by Various Factors

The proportion of energy furnished by carbohydrate, fat, and protein has important implications. For example, if you want to lose body fat, it helps to know what factors favor the metabolism of fat. If you want to participate in endurance athletic activities such as long-distance swimming or bicycling, you benefit from knowing how to use more fat and less carbohydrate, since the small amount of carbohydrate in the body can be the limiting factor in how long you can continue before you feel exhausted.

This is not to say that metabolism is completely driven by factors that you can manipulate or that there is no "usual" pattern of utilization of carbohydrate, fat, and protein.

When you are at physical rest, your body derives similar amounts of energy from carbohydrate and fat. The popular belief that carbohydrate is "all used up" before fat is metabolized is not the case; carbohydrate and fat are used simultaneously for energy production. When you are physically active, however, various circumstances are likely to bring about a shift in the proportion of energy derived from carbohydrate and fat—or even protein. These factors are discussed in the sections that follow.

Amount of Oxygen Available

The amount of oxygen available to body cells affects the proportions of fat and carbohydrate that will be used for energy production. Remember what you learned in the close-up of energy metabolism in the cell: *the utilization of fat always requires oxygen, but carbohydrate can be utilized with or without oxygen.*

When you exert yourself physically to the extent that you are gasping for breath after a couple of minutes, you feel as though you cannot get enough oxygen to sustain the job. That is exactly the case: you cannot sustain the activity by aerobic oxidation. Your oxygen-starved cells must produce additional energy anaerobically (by glycolysis). Power lifting and sprints of swimming or running are examples of activities in which this occurs; they are called *anaerobic activities*. When you exercise anaerobically, you depend primarily on carbohydrate.

During anaerobic activity, the chemical *lactic acid* is produced. When lactic acid builds up in muscles that are strenuously exercised—and it does so very quickly during intense activity—you feel fatigued. For this reason, you can sustain anaerobic oxidation for only a minute or two at a time. Your fatigue is not from using up your carbohydrate; you still have an ample supply. Rather, the accumulation of lactic acid lowers the pH of your muscle and reduces its ability to contract; this is likely to be the cause of muscle tiredness (Saltin and Gollnick, 1988). You recover gradually, as lactic acid is metabolized aerobically while you rest.

In contrast, if the activity is not so intense, your body depends more heavily on aerobic oxidation (the citric acid cycle). That means you can use fat as well as carbohydrate as an energy source. When you exert yourself physically for an extended period at a comfortable pace—the pace at which most people walk, jog, swim, dance, bicycle, and cross-country ski—the activity is referred to as an *aerobic activity*. Fat is the mainstay of aerobic activity, although it can never be the exclusive source of energy; a small amount of carbohydrate must always be involved in fat oxidation.

Although the terms *aerobic activity* and *anaerobic activity* imply that their energy comes exclusively from aerobic or anaerobic oxidation, *all* activities actually involve some energy input from both aerobic and anaerobic oxidation.

Many activities involve alternate periods of intense (anaerobic) and less intense (aerobic) activity. Tennis, wrestling, and basketball are examples of such activities.

Duration of Activity

You metabolize proportionately more fat and less carbohydrate as you prolong an aerobic exercise session. As you begin aerobic activity, the initial demand for more energy is met largely by the metabolism of carbohydrate. Gradually, as your body adapts to the continuing need for this higher level of energy production, the metabolism of fat furnishes a larger and larger proportion of the energy. After approximately a half-hour of continuous exercise at a moderate pace, fat becomes the predominant energy source.

State of Training

Your state of training affects the proportions of fat and carbohydrate that are used for energy production. The better your physical conditioning, the greater the proportion of fat you will use during exercise. The less-trained person uses relatively more carbohydrate (Saltin and Gollnick, 1988).

Typical Diet Composition

The composition of your diet also makes some difference in the proportions of nutrients you use for energy. The more carbohydrate you habitually consume, the larger the fraction of carbohydrate you will use while exercising. Conversely, people who routinely consume diets with lower levels of carbohydrate will metabolically adapt to using a smaller proportion of carbohydrate (Saltin and Gollnick, 1988). Such adaptation takes place over a period of several weeks.

Scarcity of Fat and/or Carbohydrate

There are some times when the body cannot produce enough energy from carbohydrate and fat to meet immediate needs. During these times, body protein is sacrificed to produce energy. Instances when this is likely to occur are during starvation (including starvation from extreme weight-reducing diets); during physical activities that are demanding, continuous, and last over an hour (for example, long-distance bicycle racing or running); and during the first couple of weeks of a rigorous athletic regimen undertaken by an untrained person (Lemon and Nagle, 1981).

Now that you have been introduced to the roles of carbohydrate, fat, and protein in energy production, the next three chapters will acquaint you with other important functions of these nutrients.

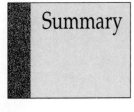

Summary

▶ **Energy** intake and output are both commonly measured in **kilocalories (kcalories, kcal);** 1 kcalorie is the amount of heat needed to raise the temperature of 1 kilogram of water 1°C.

▶ The body uses energy for at least three types of functions. (1) **Basal metabolism** refers to all the processes that must take place continuously to sustain life. The number of kcalories required to maintain these processes for a specified amount of time is called the **basal metabolic rate (BMR);** it accounts for 60–70% of a typical North American's daily energy expenditure. It is influenced by such factors as body size, age, sex, and general health. A slightly higher value, the **resting metabolic rate (RMR)** is often used as an approximate measure of BMR. (2) Physical activity is the only form of energy expenditure over which you have much control, and unlike BMR it can vary markedly from day to day. Factors influencing the **thermic effect of exercise** are the type of activity you engage in, the length of time you engage in it, and your body weight. (3) The body also uses energy to process food; since heat is given off while this occurs, this is referred to as the **thermic effect of food.** About 6–10% of the energy a person consumes is used for this purpose. (4) Extreme environmental factors may increase the body's expenditure of energy. Intake of excessive kcalories and environmental cold may cause extra energy utilization, which is referred to as **adaptive thermogenesis.**

▶ Energy usage tables, calculations of energy usage, and records of energy intake can all provide estimates of your daily energy needs.

▶ A food's energy value depends on its content of the energy substrates protein, fat, carbohydrate, and alcohol. Protein provides 4 kcal per gram, fat provides 9, carbohydrate provides 4, and alcohol provides 7. Foods vary widely in composition, even within the same food group. Food composition tables, nutrition labels, and your own calculations can all be used to determine the energy nutrient content of your diet.

▶ Food energy that is not needed right away is stored in the body, though not always in the same form in which it was consumed. Carbohydrates are broken down to produce intermediate compounds that ultimately form **glucose,** which is either used fairly quickly for energy, stored as **glycogen,** or converted to fat. Proteins are broken down and reassembled into body proteins or are converted to intermediates of glucose and used for energy production. Fats are either used fairly quickly for energy or stored as body fat (the same is true of alcohol). Excess carbohydrate and protein components are also stored as body fat; for the most part they are not converted back to their original form.

▶ The proportions of carbohydrate and fat used for energy production vary, depending on several factors. The amount of oxygen available influences what the source of energy will be. **Anaerobic oxidation** occurs when oxygen is inadequate for the amount of energy production needed; a major form of anaerobic oxidation is **glycolysis,** which is fueled by carbohydrate. **Aerobic oxidation** involves the **citric acid cycle** and **electron transport chain,** requires ample oxygen, and is fueled mainly (though not exclusively) by fat and carbohydrate. A person's state of training and diet composition also influence the proportions of nutrients used for energy.

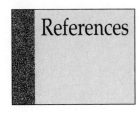
References

Astrand, P.-O. 1988. Whole-body metabolism. In *Exercise, nutrition, and energy metabolism*, eds. E.S. Horton and R.L. Terjung. New York: Macmillan Publishing Company.

Durnin, J.V.G.A. and R. Passmore. 1967. Energy, work, and leisure. In *Energy and protein requirements. FAO/WHO technical report no. 522, 1973.*

Elliott, D.L., L. Goldberg, K.S. Kuehl, and W.M. Bennett. 1989. Sustained depression of the resting metabolic rate after massive weight loss. *American Journal of Clinical Nutrition* 49: 93–96.

Ganong, W.F. 1989. *Review of medical physiology.* San Mateo, CA: Lange Medical Publications.

Heymsfield, S.B. and P.J. Williams. Nutritional assessment by clinical and biochemical methods. In *Modern nutrition in health and disease*, eds. M.E. Shils and V.R. Young. Philadelphia: Lea & Febiger.

Kinney, J.M. 1988. Food as fuel: The development of concepts. In *Modern nutrition in health and disease*, eds. M.E. Shils and V.R. Young. Philadelphia: Lea & Febiger.

McArdle, W.D., F.I. Katch, and V.L. Katch. 1981. *Exercise physiology*. Philadelphia: Lea & Febiger.

Owen, O.E. 1988. Resting metabolic requirements in men and women. *Mayo Clinic Proceedings* 63:503–510.

Passmore, R. and J.V.G.A. Durnin. 1955. Human energy expenditure. *Physiological Reviews* 35:801–840.

Poehlman, E.T. and E.S. Horton. 1989. The impact of food intake and exercise on energy expenditure. *Nutrition Reviews* 47:129–137.

Ravussin, E., S. Lillioja, T.E. Anderson, L. Christin, and C. Bogardus. 1986. Determinants of 24-hour energy expenditure in man. *The Journal of Clinical Investigation* 78:1568–1578.

RDA Subcommittee. 1989. *Recommended dietary allowances.* Washington, DC: The National Academy Press.

Saltin, B. and P.D. Gollnick. 1988. Fuel for muscular exercise: Role of carbohydrate. In *Exercise, nutrition, and energy metabolism*, eds. E.S. Horton and R.L. Terjung. New York: The Macmillan Company.

Smith, E.L., R.L. Hill, I.R. Lehman, R.J. Lefkowitz, P. Handler, and A. White. 1983. *Principles of biochemistry: General aspects*, 7th edition, page 407. New York: McGraw-Hill Book Company.

Taylor, C.M. and G. McLeod. 1949. *Rose's laboratory handbook for dietetics*, 5th edition, p. 18. New York: Macmillan Company.

6

Carbohydrates

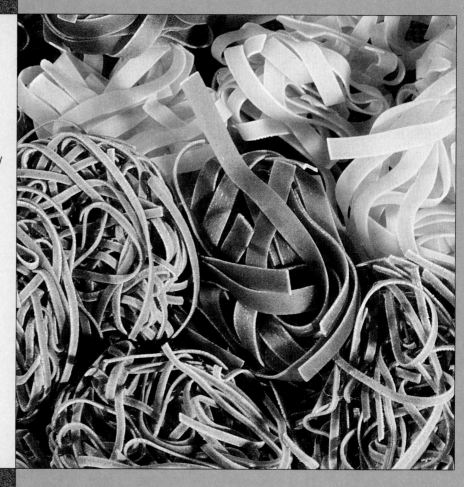

Carbohydrates have an undeservedly bad reputation due, in part, to the commonly held belief that they are fattening; many weight-reduction diets in the popular press include only very limited amounts of high-carbohydrate foods. However, athletes (many of whom are also concerned about controlling body weight) are counseled about the *benefits* of a high-carbohydrate diet.

Part of the confusion may come from the false impression that carbohydrates are especially high in kcalories. Other misconceptions may arise from the fact that there are several types of carbohydrates. Sugars, starches, and fiber are all forms of carbohydrate, and each has somewhat different characteristics and functions. General statements about carbohydrate (as if it were a single substance) are often inaccurate because they may not be true of all forms.

Another source of confusion is that certain kinds of carbohydrates seem to have split personalities. Sugar, maligned as a "poison" by some people, is touted by others as the best source of quick energy. Fiber, long ignored as a nonnutrient, now enjoys such heightened status that it is being deliberately added to foods. However, some experts caution that unusually high fiber intakes may interfere with the body's access to other nutrients.

This chapter provides the background to help you evaluate these claims about carbohydrates. It deals with how the body uses carbohydrates, what foods contain them, and how they relate to various health problems.

Carbohydrates Have Two Major Functions in the Human Body

When you think "carbohydrate," you probably think "energy." That is appropriate, since carbohydrates are the fundamental human fuel. Not all forms of carbohydrate are major energy providers, though. Most sugars and starches are; they are called **available carbohydrates.** Most **dietary fiber,** however, isn't; it is only minimally available for human energy production. Its primary function is to enhance the activities of the GI tract.

available carbohydrates—sugars and starches that can be hydrolyzed by human digestive processes

dietary fiber—plant food components made of linked carbohydrate units that cannot be separated by human digestive secretions

• **Available carbohydrates provide energy.** Sugars and starches furnish 4 kcalories per gram and are metabolized by the body to help meet its energy needs. All cells readily utilize glucose, a major breakdown product of available carbohydrate, but red blood cells and the cells of the central nervous system have a particular preference for it; inadequate dietary carbohydrate can result in impaired functioning of the higher centers of the brain (Macdonald, 1987).

In addition to being a major energy substrate itself, available carbohydrate plays a role in metabolizing fat for energy; a small amount of carbohydrate is needed for the series of reactions involved in fat metabolism. Therefore, even when you are deriving a high proportion of your energy

Carbohydrate sources. Plants are the source of almost all the carbohydrates we eat. The only significant animal sources of carbohydrate are milk and some milk products.

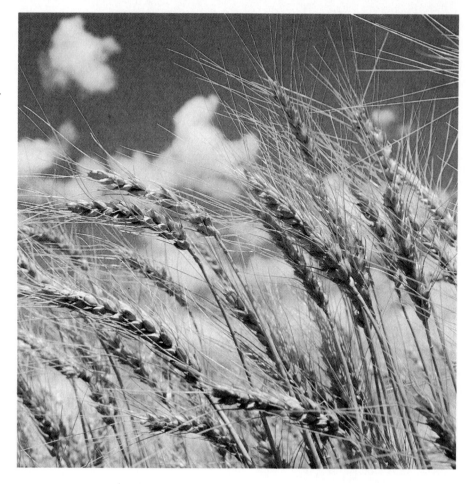

from fat, a small amount of carbohydrate *must* be involved; one of the compounds needed for the operation of the citric acid cycle is derived from carbohydrate.

As was discussed in Chapter 5, if sufficient carbohydrate is not available, protein will be dismantled and used as carbohydrate. This, of course, is not desirable, since protein is needed for functions only it can accomplish. Therefore, when a person consumes at least the recommended level of available carbohydrate, protein that is needed for other purposes is spared from being used for energy. This is referred to as the *protein-sparing effect* of carbohydrate.

• **Dietary fiber (unavailable carbohydrate) enhances the activities of the GI tract.** For the most part, human digestive processes cannot break down dietary fiber; therefore, much of it remains as solid material in the large intestine after other components of food have been absorbed. The bulk it provides (and the water it holds) dilutes the other materials in the colon and gives intestinal muscles the opportunity for healthy muscular work, moving solid waste through the colon more rapidly.

Fiber also serves as a food source for bacteria in the gut. Although

Table 6.1 Major Carbohydrates Occurring in Foods, As Produced by Nature

Source	Major Sugars		Available Polysaccharides	Fiber (polysaccharides not digested by humans)
	Monosaccharides	Disaccharides		
Plants	Glucose Fructose	Sucrose Maltose	Starches Dextrins	Cellulose Hemicellulose Pectins Gums Mucilages
Animals		Lactose		

human digestive processes cannot break fiber apart, bacteria can partially use it. These organisms thrive, multiply, and are eventually excreted, thereby contributing to the mass of solid waste.

In addition, fiber in the gut can have an effect beyond the GI tract itself: some types of fiber are believed to lower blood *cholesterol*, a substance that can increase a person's risk of heart disease if it is in excess. Although the mechanism is not well understood, it appears that certain types of fiber reduce the absorption of cholesterol from the GI tract.

Chapter 7 will provide much more information about cholesterol and the risk of heart disease.

Types and Amounts of Carbohydrates in Foods Vary

The vast majority of the carbohydrates we eat are produced by plants. Milk and some products made from milk are the only significant animal sources.

This section describes the forms of carbohydrate in foods, both as they occur in nature and as they can be made available by processing. Table 6.1 gives an overview of the types of carbohydrate found in nature and their sources.

Sugars

Sugars are the smallest and least complicated of the carbohydrates; they are of varying sweetness and are soluble in water. Their solubility allows them to move readily through the watery systems of plants and animals. Names of sugars are easy to recognize by their *-ose* endings; examples are gluc*ose*, fruct*ose*, sucr*ose*.

Glucose is a good example of a simple sugar. You have already encountered glucose in Chapter 5 (on energy), where it was described as a small carbohydrate molecule found in the blood. Glucose is not only important in the human system, it is also a key substance in all living systems, plant and animal.

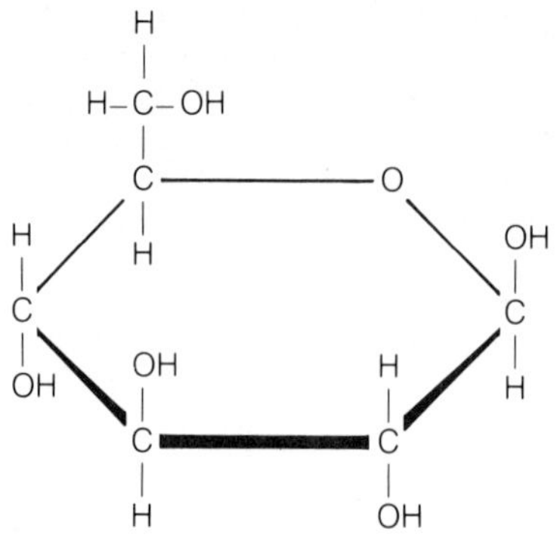

Figure 6.1 The structure of glucose. This structural model of a single molecule of glucose exemplifies the organization of carbohydrates; their units have a carbon skeleton, with oxygen, hydrogen, and hydroxyl groups attached to the carbon.
Key: C = carbon, H = hydrogen, O = oxygen, and OH = hydroxyl group.

The chemist depicts glucose as shown in Figure 6.1. Although you will not see many chemical structures in this book, an occasional one gives you an idea of the composition and relative complexity of various substances. This one illustrates that six carbon atoms (or sometimes five) form the skeleton of the less complex sugar molecules. Hydrogen (H), oxygen (O), and OH groups, called hydroxyl groups, are attached to the carbons in an arrangement that is specific for each type of sugar.

Sugars—in fact, all carbohydrates—contain the equivalent of one water molecule for each carbon in the structure. The term *carbohydrate* reflects the carbon, hydrogen, and oxygen contained in all carbohydrates.

Scientists refer to substances that contain carbon—such as carbohydrates, fats, proteins, and vitamins—as **organic** substances. All living organisms, both plant and animal, use and/or produce organic materials. The public has given a somewhat different meaning to the term *organic*. Many people assume it to mean "grown without use of laboratory-produced chemicals." This popular definition is not scientifically accurate, but a number of states have established some form of the latter definition as having a legal meaning in advertising. Federal regulations have even been considered; however, as we go to press the term *organic* on a food label guarantees very little about the conditions under which the food was grown.

organic—scientifically means carbon-containing substances, whether they originate in nature or in a laboratory; legal but nonscientific definition(s) may be developed.

Sugars in Nature The cells of green plants produce carbohydrate molecules by photosynthesis, a sunlight-requiring process in which carbon dioxide and water are combined to yield glucose and oxygen.

Some of the *glucose* that is synthesized by plants remains in that form, and some of it is converted into another sugar, *fructose,* by rearrangement of the hydrogen, oxygen, and hydroxyl groups. These sugars and a few other less common ones that consist of independent units with 5- or 6-carbon skeletons are called **monosaccharides.**

monosaccharides—the simplest sugars, having 5- or 6-carbon skeletons (examples: glucose, fructose)

Glucose, fructose, and other monosaccharide molecules can be combined into **disaccharides,** which consist of two monosaccharide units linked together. Two molecules of glucose can unite to form a molecule of *maltose* (Figure 6.2), or a molecule of glucose can join a molecule of fructose to form *sucrose.* Several types of sugar usually exist simultaneously in a food of plant origin.

disaccharides—simple sugars consisting of two monosaccharide units linked together (examples: sucrose, lactose)

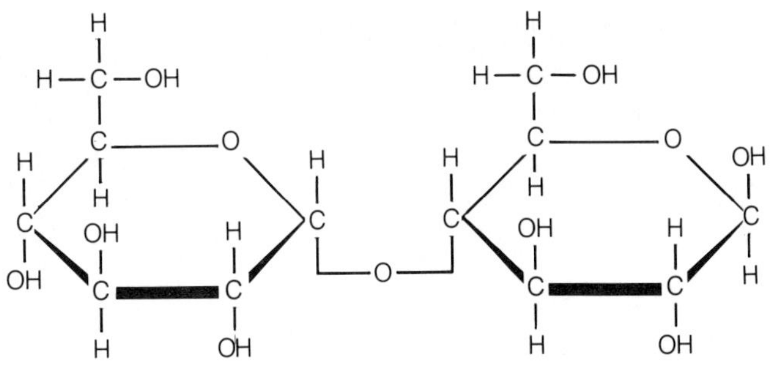

Figure 6.2 The structure of a disaccharide. This model shows how two monosaccharide units (here, two units of glucose) are joined in a disaccharide (here, maltose). In more complex forms of carbohydrates, similar bonds join many monosaccharide units together in either long chains or branched structures. Starches, for example, are composed of many units of glucose.

In which plants are sugars found? Actually, all plants contain some sugar in their juices, although the amounts vary from one part of the plant to another. Fruits usually contain more liberal amounts of sugar; most roots, leaves, stems, and tubers contain less; and seeds have varying amounts. There are a few unusually high nonfruit sources of sugar, though, such as sugar cane (stem) and sugar beet (root).

A major sugar that occurs naturally in animal foods is the disaccharide *lactose,* which is found in animal milks. Lactose consists of a unit of glucose joined to a unit of *galactose,* another 6-carbon sugar molecule.

Sugars and Processing The preceding discussion explains that *nature* produces sugars within foods. However, many foods also contain sugar that people—not nature—have put there. We do this because we are born with a preference for the sweet taste, and although this preference tends to diminish to some degree after childhood, sweetness continues to influence many people's food choices (see Chapter 9). Ever since we learned how to make **concentrated sugars** from naturally sweet sources, sweeteners such as maple syrup, molasses, brown sugar, white sugar (pure sucrose), and honey have been added to food. (Of course, the honey bee gets credit for the production of the last one.)

Food scientists have found ways to produce sweeteners from the starches in grains such as corn, rice, and barley. These are the sources of many of the sweet syrups and much of the glucose (sometimes called *dextrose*) and fructose (sometimes called *levulose*) currently used in processed foods. They are major ingredients in products such as soft drinks, sherbet, ice cream, gelatin desserts, sweet baked goods, and some cereals. Lactose is another sugar commonly added to foods; it is obtained from whey, the watery by-product of cheesemaking.

Other carbohydrate terms you may see are *turbinado sugar* (a steam-cleaned, partially refined sugar) and *total invert sugar* (a modified, liquefied form of sucrose that is used commercially). Sugars that are produced technologically are chemically identical to their counterparts from nature and are metabolized in the same way. The body cannot distinguish between the two.

Read the ingredient list on the labels of foods you eat, and see how many

concentrated sugars—solid or liquid substances consisting largely of sugar that are added to other foods as sweeteners (examples: cane sugar, beet sugar, maple syrup, corn syrup)

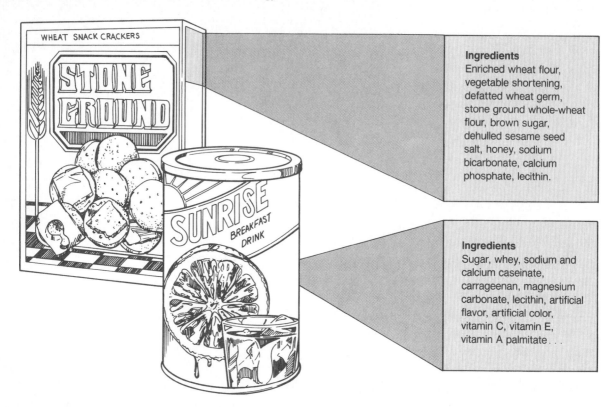

WHEAT SNACK CRACKERS

STONE GROUND

SUNRISE
BREAKFAST DRINK

Ingredients
Enriched wheat flour, vegetable shortening, defatted wheat germ, stone ground whole-wheat flour, brown sugar, dehulled sesame seed salt, honey, sodium bicarbonate, calcium phosphate, lecithin.

Ingredients
Sugar, whey, sodium and calcium caseinate, carrageenan, magnesium carbonate, lecithin, artificial flavor, artificial color, vitamin C, vitamin E, vitamin A palmitate . . .

Figure 6.3 Examples of sugars in two processed foods. You can find out if foods contain sugary components by checking their ingredient lists. It is not possible to tell exactly how much sugar is present, but you can get a rough idea of the relative amount because ingredients must be listed in order from the heaviest to the lightest amount of ingredient in the product.

standards of identity—U.S. regulations that specify the ingredients and their proportions in certain foods with multiple ingredients

sugar substitutes—substances that are sweet but are chemically different from ordinary natural sugars; may or may not have kcaloric value

sugar alcohols—compounds structurally related to sugars and used as sweeteners

sugar sources you can identify. Figure 6.3 shows two examples. You can get a rough idea of how much added sugar a food contains by noting the position of the sugars on the list, since ingredients must be ranked according to their weights in the product, from the greatest to the smallest. (Foods for which there is a federally standardized recipe recorded in the Code of Federal Regulation do not require an ingredient list. Hundreds of common foods such as mayonnaise and macaroni have such **standards of identity**.)

Data collected by the U.S. Department of Agriculture indicate that in 1986, the average per capita intake of refined sugar was 60 pounds for the year, and the intake of sweeteners made from corn was an additional 87 pounds (Bailey et al., 1988).

Some people want to have the sweetness of sugar without experiencing the negative consequences of sugar ingestion. To meet this demand, a number of **sugar substitutes** have been developed for use in food products. Some of these are derivatives of naturally occurring carbohydrates or other natural components of food, and some are new to the food supply.

One negative characteristic of sugars is that they promote tooth decay (discussed in more detail later in the chapter). To circumvent this problem, derivatives of sugars and starches called **sugar alcohols,** which are sweet but do not promote tooth decay, are used in some foods; the sugar alcohols are *maltitol, mannitol, sorbitol,* and *xylitol*. In fact, xylitol has been shown in a number of studies to actually *inhibit* tooth decay (Pepper and Olinger, 1988). The sugar alcohols, because of their close structural relationship to carbohydrates, have the same energy value as carbohydrates: they provide

4 kcalories per gram. (Take a look at a package of chewing gum or candy that contains one of these substances, and you will see that it says "NOT NON-CALORIC"; in other words, it *DOES* HAVE KCALORIES.)

Another aspect of sugar that some people want to avoid is its kcalorie value. Sugar substitutes that are sweet but have few if any kcalories are therefore used in many products. Table 6.2 summarizes information about many sugar substitutes. Some substitutes, such as *aspartame* and *thaumatin*, consist of chemicals similar to those occurring naturally in the food supply but unrelated to sugars. Others are different than substances commonly found in the food supply; examples are *acesulfame-K* and *saccharine*.

Because sugar substitutes vary considerably in their characteristics and effects, you need to be selective to get the feature(s) you want. The safety of some sugar substitutes has been questioned and will be discussed in the appropriate chapters. More information on artificial sweeteners in general is found in Chapter 15 (on food safety issues); discussion of aspartame occurs in Chapter 8 (on proteins).

Starches and Dextrins

Some of the glucose produced in plants is converted into *starches* and *dextrins*, which are the insoluble, nonsweet forms of carbohydrate in which plants store energy. Because they are composed of from ten to hundreds of units of glucose linked together, they are also referred to as available **polysaccharides** or **complex carbohydrates**. Starches have larger molecules (consist of more glucose units) than dextrins.

polysaccharides (complex carbohydrates)—carbohydrates composed of many monosaccharide units linked together (examples: starches, dextrins)

Starches and Dextrins in Nature Starches and dextrins usually concentrate in plant seeds, roots, and tubers. Grains, nuts, legumes, root vegetables, and potatoes are particularly good sources. Fruits have much less of these complex carbohydrates.

Starches, Dextrins, and Processing Processing can alter the nature of starches in food. When starch is exposed to dry heat (as it is in the production of cold cereals or in the baking of bread), some of the large starch molecules are broken down into dextrins. Starches that have been broken down further are called *malted starches*; these are often found in cereals. *Modified starch*, which you find in some processed foods such as puddings, is starch that has been treated to enhance its ability to thicken or gel.

Fiber

Thus far, we have pointed out that fiber in foods of plant origin provides little energy for humans and that it increases the bulk of the intestinal contents. You might think that we can dismiss it quickly as being relatively unimportant. However, recent studies have turned fiber into a prominent and controversial topic on the frontier of nutrition research.

Table 6.2 Sugar Substitutes

Substance	Description	Typical Uses	Comments
Acesulfame-K Sunette® Sweet One®	Chemical not in food supply naturally	Table top sweetener, dry foods and mixes, chewing gum, soft drinks	200 times as sweet as sucrose; no kcalories
Aspartame Nutrasweet® Equal®	Two naturally occurring components of protein linked together	Candy, carbonated beverages, chewing gum, gelatin dessert, puddings	180–200 times as sweet as sucrose; has 4 kcalories/gram, but contributes few kcalories because so little is needed (more on this substance in Chapter 8)
Maltitol Lycasin® Almalty®	Sugar alcohol made from starch	Candy; approval pending for more applications	75% as sweet as sucrose; has 4 kcal/g; does not cause tooth decay
Mannitol	Sugar alcohol	Chewing gum	65% as sweet as sucrose; has 4 kcal/g; does not cause tooth decay
Saccharine	Chemical not in food supply naturally	Primarily being replaced by aspartame but used in some chewing gums	300–400 times as sweet as sucrose; has no kcalories (more on this substance in Chapter 15)
Sorbitol	Sugar alcohol made from glucose	Candy, chewing gum, cough drops, breath mints	50% as sweet as sucrose; causes bloating and diarrhea in some people; has 4 kcal/g; does not cause tooth decay
Thaumatin Talin®	Protein	Chewing gum	400–2,000 times as sweet as sucrose; few kcalories because so little is needed
Xylitol	Sugar alcohol made from substances high in hemicellulose; naturally present in many fruits and vegetables	Special diet candies and chewing gums	Same sweetness as sucrose; has 4 kcal/g; helps prevent tooth decay

References: 1) Institute of Food Technologists (IFT). 1989. Ingredients for sweet success. *Food Technology* 43:94–116. 2) IFT. 1987. Sweeteners: Nutritive and non-nutritive. *Contemporary Nutrition* 12 (no. 9). 3) Jain, N.K., V.P. Patel, and C.S. Pitchumone. 1987. Sorbitol intolerance in adults. *Journal of Clinical Gastroenterology* 9:317–319.

Fiber in Nature   Fiber is often defined as a plant food component that cannot be broken down by human digestive processes. Many forms of fiber are polysaccharides made of sugar units joined together in linkages that human enzymes cannot separate. This is why fiber is largely unavailable for energy production: it cannot be broken into units small enough for absorption.

There are two major types of fiber. One is **insoluble fiber,** the rigid material that gives structure to plants. *Cellulose* and *hemicellulose*, both of which are found in plant cell walls are examples of insoluble fiber. Fruits, vegetables, grains, nuts, and seeds contain both of these types of fiber. They are concentrated in the protective outer layers of whole grains, called the *bran layers,* and in seeds and edible skins and peels.

The other major type of fiber is soluble fiber; examples are *pectins, gums,* and *mucilages.* Apples are a notable source of pectin; other fruits have less. Gums and mucilages are generally found in only small amounts in common plant foods.

insoluble fiber—unavailable carbohydrate that does not dissolve in water; an example is cellulose, a major component of wheat bran.

soluble fiber—unavailable carbohydrate that is soluble in water; an example is pectin, found in apples.

Fiber and Processing   Food processing can change the fiber content of foods. On the one hand, the most fibrous parts of a food are sometimes removed and discarded during processing; apple skins are peeled away while making applesauce, and the bran layers of wheat are removed in the production of white flour (Figure 6.4).

On the other hand, fiber is sometimes added to food by processors in response to the positive public image fiber currently enjoys. For example,

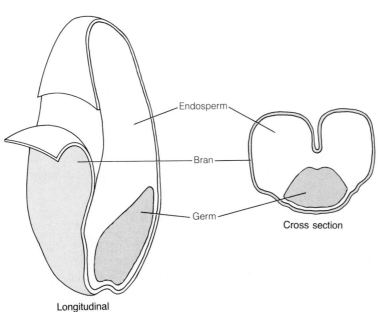

Longitudinal
section

Figure 6.4 A kernel of wheat. The three parts of a wheat kernel have different nutrient characteristics. The endosperm contains most of the starch and protein; the bran and germ contain most of the fiber and micronutrients. When wheat is milled and made into white flour, much of the bran and germ are removed.

the bran of various grains is being added to an increasing number of breakfast cereals. Bran is also marketed by itself so that consumers can add it to other foods. Cellulose that has been refined from wood is added to some breads, both to raise the fiber content and to lower the kcalories by substituting it for some of the available carbohydrates.

Sometimes pectins and gums are refined and used as additives to thicken, gel, or stabilize foods, or to emulsify them so that their different components do not separate. Commercially, pectin is usually refined from citrus peel and apples and is added to jams, jellies, and candies. Gums are extracted from less familiar sources: certain African and Asian shrubs, trees, and seed pods are their natural origins. They are used in ice cream, fruit drinks, and canned meats, to name just a few. You have seen them listed on labels as *guar gum, locust bean gum, gum tragacanth, gum arabic,* and *xanthan gum. Agar, carrageenan,* and *alginates* are extracts of seaweed that also are widely used as stabilizers and thickeners.

In recent years a new fiberlike substance, *polydextrose,* has been developed primarily for use as a bulking and moisture-retaining agent and a texturizer in reduced-kcalorie processed foods. Although this substance does not yield to human digestive processes, it nonetheless provides approximately 1 kcalorie/gram from by-products of colonic bacterial metabolism.

Amounts of Carbohydrates in Various Kinds of Foods

There is substantial variation in carbohydrate content between the four food groups—and even variation within the groups.

Available Carbohydrate   Table 6.3 shows how the total amounts of digestible carbohydrates compare among foods from the basic food groups. The solid parts of the bars represent naturally occurring sugars and starches; the broken parts of the bars indicate added concentrated sugars.

You may be surprised at the total available carbohydrate values of some foods compared to others. For example, did you know that a cup of milk contains almost as much carbohydrate as an average serving of fruit, or that a can of cola beverage has almost as much carbohydrate as three slices of bread?

Appendices E and F give available carbohydrate values for hundreds of foods. Nutrition labels also identify available carbohydrate content per serving.

Unavailable Carbohydrate (Fiber)   It is difficult to determine how much fiber is in food. To measure it, scientists have had to develop special laboratory analyses to approximate human GI processes; various methods have been developed, but some are considerably better than others. A major problem is that the many different substances of which fiber is composed require many different methods of analysis. There is no simple, universally

Table 6.3 Carbohydrate in Standard Servings of Various Foods[a]

Food	Household Measure	Carbohydrate (grams)
Fruits and vegetables		
Many unsugared fruits and fruit juices	½ cup	
Many sugared fruits	½ cup	
Leafy vegetables	1 cup	
Carrots, beets	½ cup	
Peas	½ cup	
Potatoes, corn	½ cup	
Grain products		
Bread	1 slice	
Cake (white with chocolate frosting)	2½ ounces	
Cookies (chocolate chip)	4 medium	
Cereals (plain, cooked)	½ cup	
Cornflakes	1¼ cups	
Pasta or rice, cooked	½ cup	
Milk and milk products		
Cheese (hard types)	1⅓ ounces	
Ice cream	1½ cups	
Milk	1 cup	
Yogurt (plain, low fat)	1 cup	
Yogurt (fruited, low fat)	1 cup	
Meats and meat alternates		
Meat, fish, poultry	3 ounces	
Navy beans	1 cup	
Nuts	½ cup	
Combination foods		
Burrito (bean)	6 ounces	
Chicken chow mein	1 cup	
Macaroni and cheese	1 cup	
Pie (cherry)	⅙ pie	
Pizza (cheese)	⅛ of 15″ pie	
Soup (beef noodle)	1 cup	
Soup (cream of mushroom)	1 cup	
Spaghetti and meatballs	1 cup	
Limited extras		
Butter, oils	1 teaspoon	
Cola beverage	12 ounces	
Gelatin dessert	½ cup	
Sugar, syrup, jelly	1 tablespoon	

(Carbohydrate scale: 0, 10, 20, 30, 40, 50, 60, 70, 80 grams)

[a]Broken sections of bars represent added concentrated sugars.

Data sources: 1) Matthews, R.H., P.R. Pehrsson, and M. Farhat-Sabet. 1987. Sugar Content of Selected Foods. Washington, DC: United States Department of Agriculture.
2) Pennington, J.A. 1989. Food Values of Portions Commonly Used. New York: Harper and Row.
3) Calculation from recipes.

accepted assay (test) (IFT Expert Panel, 1989). Consequently, there can be considerable variation in tables that state the amounts of fiber in a given food (Marlett, 1989). Table 6.4 provides data by David Southgate, from sources thought to be among the most complete and accurate at the time this book went to press. Newer methodology has been developed, but data on only a few foods are available thus far (Marlett et al., 1989).

Table 6.4 Total Dietary Fiber in Some Foods[a]

Food	Household Measure	Total Dietary Fiber (grams)
Fruits and vegetables		
Apple, peeled	1 medium	
Banana, sliced	$\frac{1}{2}$ cup	
Broccoli, cooked	top from 1 stalk	
Carrots	$\frac{1}{2}$ cup	
Cherries	10	
Lettuce, chopped	1 cup	
Onions, raw	1 tablespoon	
Peaches, sliced	$\frac{1}{2}$ cup	
Peas, canned	$\frac{1}{2}$ cup	
Pear, peeled	1 medium	
Plum	1 medium	
Potatoes, french fried	10 strips	
Potatoes, canned	$\frac{3}{5}$ cup	
Strawberries	$\frac{1}{2}$ cup	
Tomatoes, canned	$\frac{2}{5}$ cup	
Grain products		
Bread	1 slice	
White		
Whole wheat		
Rye		
Cake, iced chocolate	3 ounce piece	
Cereals, ready to eat	1 ounce	
All-Bran	$\frac{1}{3}$ cup	
Cornflakes	$1\frac{1}{4}$ cup	
Grapenuts	$\frac{1}{4}$ cup	
Rice Krispies	1 cup	
Shredded Wheat	$\frac{2}{3}$ cup	
Special K	$1\frac{1}{3}$ cup	
Flour, white	$\frac{1}{4}$ cup	
Flour, whole wheat	$\frac{1}{4}$ cup	
Muffin, bran	1	

Total Dietary Fiber (grams) scale: 0 5 10 15 20

Table 6.4 continued

Food	Household Measure	Total Dietary Fiber (grams) 0 5 10 15 20
Spaghetti, boiled	$\frac{1}{2}$ cup	
White		
Whole wheat		
Tortilla, flour	1	
Meat alternates		
Beans, baked	1 cup	
Brazil nuts	1 ounce	
Peanuts	$\frac{1}{2}$ cup	
Peanut butter	$\frac{1}{4}$ cup	
Combination foods		
Fruit pie, 2-crust	$\frac{1}{8}$ pie	
Macaroni and cheese, canned	1 cup	
Pizza, frozen	$\frac{1}{4}$	
Ravioli in tomato sauce, canned	1 cup	

aData sources: 1) Southgate, D.A. 1986. Dietary fiber content of selected foods by the Southgate methods. In *CRC Handbook of Dietary Fiber in Human Nutrition*, G.A. Spiller, ed. Boca Raton, FL: CRC Press, Inc. 2) Holland, B., I.D. Unwin, and D.H. Buss. 1988. *McCance and Widdowson's The Composition of Foods: Cereals and Cereal Products* (Southgate data). Old Woking, Surrey, UK: Unwin Brothers Limited.

The Body Deals with Different Carbohydrates in Different Ways

What happens to carbohydrates when people eat them? You have some idea from Chapter 3, in which the general process of digestion was described. Here we will relate that information specifically to carbohydrates, and then go on to see what the body does with the end-products of digestion.

Digestion and Absorption of Carbohydrates

Carbohydrate digestion begins with chewing. Chewing makes food particles smaller and mechanically breaks apart some cell walls that may have digestible carbohydrates trapped within them. The biochemical processes that carbohydrates go through in the digestive tract vary depending on how complex their molecular structures are.

Monosaccharides Monosaccharides, the smallest carbohydrate units, are able to be absorbed intact through the small intestine.

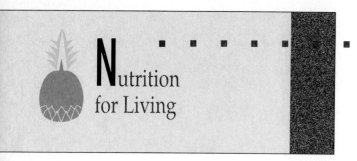

Nutrition for Living

Adding Available Carbohydrate and Fiber to Your Diet

Current dietary recommendations advise Americans to eat *more* of certain types of carbohydrates. This surprises many people who for years have thought that the right thing to do was to *limit* carbohydrate intake.

Here are some dietary changes you can make that will increase your intake of available carbohydrates and fiber, as is promoted in current dietary guidelines:

- Gradually add more fruits and vegetables to your diet. Eat more whole items (in preference to juice) and eat the edible peels.
- Gradually increase your consumption of breads, especially coarse whole-grain types. *Whole-wheat* bread has more fiber than bread simply described as *wheat* bread. (By law, bread that is labeled "whole wheat" must be made from 100% whole-wheat flour, whereas "wheat bread" may be made from varying proportions of white flour and whole-wheat flour.)
- For variety, try cracked-wheat bread, bran muffins, cornbread from whole cornmeal, graham crackers, oatmeal bread, pumpernickel bread, rye bread, and corn tortillas.
- Gradually increase your consumption of grains, cereals, and pasta products; emphasize whole-grain varieties. Choose brown rice instead of white rice, and try whole-wheat noodles or macaroni for a change. Cereals vary widely in their fiber content; many now list values on the label. (If you choose cereals with fiber as a major ingredient or use concentrated bran, limit your

consumption to one serving of this food per day.) You may find that traditional hot cereals (such as oatmeal) are cheaper than new special cold cereals.
- When you use flour in a recipe, substitute whole-grain flour for $\frac{1}{4}$ to $\frac{1}{2}$ of the regular all-purpose type.
- Gradually increase your consumption of cooked dry beans or peas (legumes). These provide generous amounts of both starch and fiber and are good sources of protein and certain micronutrients. They are very versatile: they work well in soups (lentil soup, black-bean soup); salads (kidney-bean salad, Italian salad with garbanzo beans); dips (hummus dipped with pita bread); and main dishes (lima-bean and ham casserole, chili con carne).

Many of these suggestions encourage you to try one type of food *in place of* another. Other suggestions involve *increasing* your intake of certain kinds of foods. Of course, if you increase your overall food intake, you will also increase your energy intake, which results in body fat gain—a result that most people do not want. The way to avoid fat gain is to gradually decrease your intake of some other energy sources as you increase your carbohydrate intake.

You may do this automatically, since foods that are high in available carbohydrates and fiber are satisfying. But if you want to be deliberate about decreasing your intake of other foods, cut down on the limited extras and also those foods within the basic food groups that are high in fat or added sugar.

Disaccharides Disaccharides need to be separated by hydrolysis into their monosaccharide components before they can be absorbed. The small intestine is the primary location along the tract that produces enzymes for this purpose; they are called **disaccharidases.** Once hydrolysis has taken place, the resulting monosaccharides are quickly absorbed.

disaccharidases—enzymes that divide disaccharides into monosaccharide units

Starches and Dextrins Starches and dextrins are more complex and are processed primarily in two regions of the alimentary canal: the mouth and the small intestine. In the mouth, starch-splitting enzymes called **amylases,** which are present in saliva, begin the process of hydrolyzing the many bonds that hold starches and dextrins together. As a result of this initial action, shorter-length dextrins and some maltose are formed. Since food does not remain in the mouth for long, however, there is not much time for hydrolysis to occur; much work remains to be done to these carbohydrates after food is swallowed.

amylases—enzymes that break the bonds that hold starches and dextrins together

Little progress is made in the stomach, since the hydrochloric acid there destroys most of the amylase. Digestion actively resumes in the small intestine, where pancreatic amylases and intestinal disaccharidases complete the job on most carbohydrates present. Those that are reduced to monosaccharides are quickly absorbed; the others move along through the tract.

Rate of Digestion and Absorption of Carbohydrates It does not take long for digestion and absorption of carbohydrates to begin. If sucrose is consumed alone, it starts to show up as blood glucose (blood sugar) in 1 to 5 minutes. Even from a mixed meal, blood glucose begins to rise in 30 to 60 minutes. The timing, extent, and duration of changes in blood sugar are affected by many factors. Different starchy foods consumed as part of a meal can have different effects on blood sugar (Mourot et al., 1988; Thompson, 1988), and the other constituents of the meal have an effect as well. The form of the starchy food can also make a difference: the blenderized versions of some foods cause a greater rise in blood sugar than their whole forms do (Crapo and Henry, 1988). And surprisingly, the body's response to the carbohydrate in one meal can linger to affect its response to the carbohydrate in the next meal (Wolever et al., 1988).

A portion of starches escapes digestion, but it is not a constant percentage from all foods; the amount varies considerably from one food to another (Southgate and Johnson, 1987). For example, in one study, less than 1% of available carbohydrates from rice remained undigested and therefore arrived in the colon, but 7–10% of the carbohydrates from wheat, oats, potatoes, and corn reached the large intestine.

Fiber Most fiber and undigested starch simply moves from one part of the digestive tract to the next with few changes due to human enzymes.

The amount and type of ingested fiber influence the rate of transit in various regions of the GI tract; soluble fiber tends to delay gastric emptying, whereas insoluble fiber speeds transit through the lower part of the tract (Anderson and Clark, 1986).

In the large intestine, bacteria are able to digest the undigested starch and a portion of the fiber. Some of these bacterial end-products are absorbed and used for energy.

Table 6.5 summarizes the phases of carbohydrate digestion.

Table 6.5 Summary of Phases of Carbohydrate Digestion and Absorption

	Mono-saccharides	Disaccharides	Starches and Dextrins	Fiber
Mouth	—	—	Enzymatic hydrolysis to maltose and dextrins	—
Stomach	—	—	(Amylase inactivated by stomach acid)	—
Small intestine	Absorption	Enzymatic hydrolysis to monosaccharides by intestinal enzymes; absorption	Completion of digestion by pancreatic and intestinal enzymes; absorption	—
Large intestine	—	—		Bacterial degradation of some fiber; limited absorption

Failure to Digest and/or Absorb Carbohydrates

There is an important sequel to this chronicle of events: what happens to the carbohydrates that aren't digested and absorbed?

When carbohydrates get to the colon, two consequences may occur. One is that the bacteria there will use some of the carbohydrates to meet their own energy needs. Colonic bacteria are able to digest a wide variety of carbohydrates, even some that are indigestible to humans, producing gas in the process. This is why people are likely to feel "gassy" after eating beans or members of the onion family: those foods contain some carbohydrates that people cannot digest but that bacteria can use readily.

The other possibility is that these carbohydrates will hold water in the colon, or even draw water from surrounding tissues into the lumen. The greater the amounts of carbohydrate and water involved, the faster the transit of the intestinal contents probably will be.

Usually, the amounts of fiber and available carbohydrates consumed result in normal transit times and in such minimal gas production that it goes unnoticed. However, there are several circumstances in which more exaggerated reactions may occur.

lactose intolerance—reduced ability to digest lactose, resulting from unusually low lactase production

Lactose Intolerance **Lactose intolerance** (related terms: *lactase deficiency, lactase nonpersistence, lactose malabsorption, lactose maldigestion*) is a condition in which a person is unable to digest much lactose because his or her body produces only a low level of lactase, the enzyme that splits this disaccharide.

If a severely lactose-intolerant person eats foods that contain a large amount of lactose, most of it will not be digested but will move along to the colon. There, bacteria will metabolize some of the lactose, and the remaining lactose and unabsorbed components will draw water into the lumen. As a consequence, the person will experience intestinal cramping, sometimes followed by an explosive, watery diarrhea. Symptoms can begin anywhere from 30 minutes to two hours after eating (National Dairy Council, 1989).

Lactose intolerance of some degree is common among adults, especially those of African, Asian, Mediterranean, or Native American heritage (Scrimshaw and Murray, 1988). Approximately 70% of the world's population has it; those who are not affected are mainly people of Northern European ancestry, although approximately 20% of North American Caucasians also have it.

Lactose intolerance is a condition that usually develops gradually. People who have it as adults probably did not have it as infants or young children. Most people are born with the ability to produce lactase, but starting as early as two years of age, their bodies begin to produce less and less of it. Nevertheless, even most lactose-intolerant people produce at least a small amount of lactase. Therefore, the amount of lactose a person can tolerate is a very individual matter; each person with lactose intolerance has to find that out independently. Most of these people will not develop symptoms from consuming a single 8-ounce serving of milk, especially if it is consumed with other foods (Savaiano and Kotz, 1988), but at some level above that, problems will occur.

The levels of lactose in various dairy foods are shown in Table 6.6, but it is found in other consumables as well. It is the predominant ingredient of nondairy creamer, for example, and is used in a wide variety of food products and medications. People who are extremely lactose intolerant need to become careful label readers.

Table 6.6 Lactose Content of Some Dairy Products

Measure	Food	Grams Lactose per Serving
1 cup	Human milk	17
1 cup	Cow's milk (milk solids added)	14
1½ cups	Ice cream	13
1 cup	Cow's milk (no solids added)	12
1 cup	Buttermilk	12
2 cups	Cottage cheese	12
1 cup	Yogurt	9
1⅓ ounces	Cheddar cheese	trace

The lactose content of the diet is not the only determinant of the body's response, however. The rate of gastric emptying also makes a difference: the more rapidly chyme empties into the small intestine, the more likely it is that a given load of lactose will lead to distress. Conversely, the factors that slow gastric emptying—such as the presence of solid food in the stomach or the inclusion of fat and/or protein—reduce the likelihood of problems. People with lactose intolerance can use this knowledge to their advantage; they may be able to avoid problems if they consume a moderate amount of milk *with meals* (National Dairy Council, 1989).

Many people with lactase insufficiency tolerate yogurt that contains live cultures, even though yogurt has a relatively high lactose content (Kolars et al., 1984). This tolerance may be possible because the bacteria used in the production of yogurt from milk—a process that results in the metabolism of some of the milk's lactose—become more active again when they are warmed by body temperature. The enzymes in the bacteria then digest an additional amount of lactose before the yogurt arrives at the small intestine.

There are other ways of coping with lactose intolerance. Lactase enzyme powders are available; when added to milk, they digest 90% of its lactose during 24 hours in the refrigerator. Lactase tablets or capsules that can be taken with a lactose-containing meal have also been tested and found helpful. And an increasing number of special products with little or no lactose are being developed (Houts, 1988), which means that special milk, ice cream, and various look-alikes can now be consumed quite freely by those who have exercised caution before. Most hard cheeses also contain little lactose but provide other nutrients found in milk.

Despite the fact that *lactose* intolerance is common among adults, this condition does not explain all instances of *milk* intolerance; some people experience GI distress and other symptoms because they are allergic to the *protein* in milk. A *protein* allergy is distinctly different from lactose intolerance. (Allergies are discussed in Chapter 8.) This is most likely to occur in very young infants, but less than 1 percent of babies have this condition (Scrimshaw and Murray, 1988). People allergic to milk protein will not be helped by avoiding lactose.

Ingestion of Sugar Alcohols Sugar alcohols, which do not require digestion, are absorbed relatively slowly because of the mechanism by which they are transported through the villi of the small intestine. Therefore, a portion of ingested sugar alcohols usually fails to be absorbed and moves on to the colon. If large amounts of them have been consumed, some people may experience symptoms similar to those of lactose intolerance. The amounts that are present in chewing gum are not usually large enough to cause this effect, but eating large amounts of sugar alcohol-sweetened candies could cause symptoms. Sorbitol also occurs naturally in many fruits; prunes have the most (Tuft's Letter, 1986).

Athletic Activity Sometimes athletes consume sugary foods or drinks before or during athletic activity, thinking that the sugars will provide extra energy; generally they do, but in some situations this practice may be counterproductive.

One problem with a very high sugar intake during exercise is its negative effect on hydration. A high concentration of sugar delays stomach emptying and hence absorption of water; concentrations in excess of 100 grams of fructose and/or glucose per liter of beverage cause some interference (American Dietetic Association, 1987). Some fruit juices, fruit drinks, and other sugar-sweetened beverages have more than this amount; if the sugar content exceeds 24 grams per 8 ounces of beverage, it should probably be diluted.

Another problem involves the lower GI tract. If a person's intestines react to activity (or the nervousness that may accompany competition) by moving material through the small intestine more rapidly than usual, undigested disaccharides and/or unabsorbed monosaccharides will reach the colon, which could result in a very inopportune bout of diarrhea.

Influences on Transport and Regulation of Carbohydrates

Most sugars travel via the bloodstream to the liver, where the majority are converted to glucose. What happens to the glucose after this? Ultimately, of course, it is used by the body's cells for energy production, but it is not all needed at once. As you learned in Chapter 5 (on energy), only a small amount of glucose is metabolized for energy right away. Another small portion stays conveniently available in the bloodstream. The largest amounts are converted to energy-storage materials.

Several factors work together to affect how and when the glucose is handled. They are the activity of the liver, several hormones, muscles, and enzymes.

The Liver After every meal, your body puts most of the glucose you have absorbed into energy-storage forms: the liver converts much of it into materials that will later make up glycogen and fat molecules. This helps keep the level of glucose in your blood within a normal range, even after a substantial carbohydrate intake. (A condition in which the body does not respond normally to carbohydrate intake—called reactive hypoglycemia—will be discussed shortly.)

In the opposite situation—if you have not eaten anything for several hours—your blood glucose gradually drifts to a low level within the normal range. This prompts your liver to break glycogen apart into glucose and release it into the blood, raising the glucose level back up. You can often sense when these events are occurring. When your blood glucose drops to low-normal, you initially feel hungry and possibly tired; but after a while, even if you do not eat anything, the hunger and tiredness seem less pronounced as glycogen is converted into blood glucose. This sequence of events is totally normal and desirable.

Hormones Several hormones also cooperate in regulating the blood sugar level. **Insulin,** a hormone produced by the pancreas, is one that has a major

insulin—hormone produced by the pancreas; helps to regulate the blood sugar level by promoting glucose utilization, protein synthesis, and formation and storage of lipids

influence. Part of its function is to help glucose be transported into body cells.

When the blood glucose level rises, the pancreas produces more than the maintenance level of insulin and releases it into the bloodstream. The insulin acts on body cells, causing them to remove the excess glucose from the blood. It promotes the production of glycogen in both liver and skeletal muscle cells, and it promotes the formation of fat in both liver and fat cells. At the same time, it discourages the breakdown of fat for energy, which causes the body to rely more heavily on the recently acquired carbohydrate load for energy production.

When the blood sugar level falls, the pancreas increases its production of a different hormone, **glucagon,** which has the opposite effect of insulin. Glucagon encourages the liver to break glycogen back down into glucose. Glucagon also promotes the utilization of fat. Some other hormones have this same effect, particularly *epinephrine,* which is produced by the adrenal glands when the body has a sudden, high demand for energy.

Figure 6.5 shows the effects of various levels of blood glucose on the production of insulin and glucagon.

glucagon—hormone produced by the pancreas; has the opposite effect of insulin, helping to regulate the blood sugar level by promoting the breakdown of glycogen and fat

Muscles   Exercise depresses insulin production. Although it seems as though this would interfere with energy production, exercise has another effect that compensates: exercise prompts skeletal muscle cells to take in more glucose from the bloodstream than usual, resulting in more energy being available to the muscles for continued work.

Figure 6.5 Relative blood levels of glucose, insulin, and glucagon. When the blood glucose level rises (b), as it does after a meal, the pancreas produces more insulin, which helps to lower the blood glucose level. When blood glucose falls too low (as in a and e), the pancreas produces more glucagon, which causes blood glucose to rise. (Reference: Barrington, E.J.W. 1975. *An introduction to general and comparative endocrinology.* Oxford: Clarendon Press.)

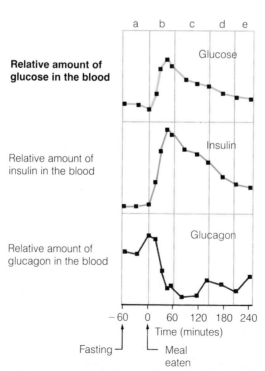

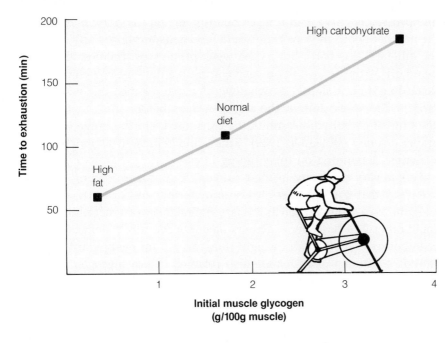

Figure 6.6 The relationship between diet, muscle glycogen, and endurance. When subjects were fed high-fat/high-protein diets for several days, leg muscle glycogen was low, and endurance for pedaling an exercise bicycle was lower than normal. When fed a high-carbohydrate diet (approximately 80% of kcalories) for several days, both muscle glycogen and work increased dramatically. (From McArdle, W.D., Katch, F.I., and Katch, V.L.: *Exercise physiology: energy, nutrition and human performance.* Lea & Febiger, Philadelphia, 1981. [Adapted from Bergstrom, J., et al.: Diet, muscle glycogen and physical performance. *Acta Physiol. Scand.,* 71:140, 1967.])

Enzymes As a person's reserves of glycogen in the liver and muscles are used up, the body produces a greater supply of enzymes for synthesizing glycogen. In this way, as soon as more carbohydrate becomes available, more glycogen can be synthesized and deposited in the liver and/or muscles.

Applications for Athletes

Athletes who are involved in endurance activities—sports in which they are continuously active for more than an hour—can perform longer by having the largest possible amount of glycogen in their liver and muscles before they begin. Classic studies have demonstrated that the amount of glycogen in muscles at the start of a bout of exercise is directly proportional to the amount of time until exhaustion occurs (Figure 6.6).

People who exercise heavily day after day need to consume a high carbohydrate diet to restore glycogen after exercise. Whereas the average nonathlete is advised to get at least half his or her kcalories from carbohydrate, the endurance athlete is advised to consume 70% of kcalories as carbohydrate routinely (Sherman, 1989). Athletes do not always achieve this. A group of marathon runners averaged 52% of kcalories as carbohydrate (Nieman et al., 1989), but a group of triathletes seemed more aware of their increased need for carbohydrate and consumed approximately 67% of kcalories as carbohydrate (Green et al., 1989).

If they do not routinely consume the recommended 70% of kcalories from carbohydrate, athletes preparing for an endurance event can increase muscle and liver glycogen through **glycogen loading** or **carbohydrate loading**.

glycogen loading—controlling both exercise and food consumption in such a way as to maximize body stores of glycogen

The process begins about a week before the event and involves modifying the nature of both their workouts and food consumption. Early in the week, the athlete trains hard; but as the week progresses, training should be tapered off, with just rest or an easy warm-up a day or two before the event. Regarding diet, it should be whatever is usual for the athlete at the beginning of the week; but in the last few days before the event, very high amounts of carbohydrate should be consumed—in the range of 500 to 600 grams per day (Williams, 1989). This could represent as much as 80% of kcalories, depending on total energy intake.

People vary markedly in their reaction to glycogen loading. Those who like it say that it allows them to continue farther and/or faster at the end of an endurance activity (such as the last several miles of a marathon) than they could otherwise have done. Others have not felt this benefit but may have been bothered by the extra weight they carried: for every gram of glycogen stored, 2.7 grams of water are also retained. Since glycogen loading can increase muscle glycogen by two or more times the normal amount (normal is about 400 grams in a 150-pound man), some people may carry several pounds of extra water-weight in the major muscles used. This may make the muscles feel heavy and stiff. Therefore, if you want to try carbohydrate loading, do not do it for the first time just before an event that is important to you.

In the past, despite the known benefits of carbohydrate consumption, athletes were often warned against taking in much carbohydrate 30 to 60 minutes before the start of an event. That was because experiments had revealed changes in muscle glycogen and blood glucose levels that were *presumed* to negatively affect endurance; however, more recent *actual tests of endurance* found no such penalty. Therefore, this is the current advice: "A carbohydrate meal or beverage can be consumed from 4 hours before exercise up to minutes before exercise without a detrimental effect on performance in most athletes" (Sherman, 1989). (However, remember the effects of *very large* intakes of carbohydrate on body water. Also, the advice given in Chapter 3 about not eating too large a meal and not eating much fat or protein before competition still holds.)

During endurance exercise, it has been found helpful to take in some carbohydrate intermittently as exercise continues; 15–20 grams of carbohydrate every 15–20 minutes is recommended. If you are consuming it as a fluid, a 5–10% solution (that is, up to 12 grams of carbohydrate per half cup of fluid) is recommended (Williams, 1989). This does not affect performance at the beginning of activity, but can extend endurance at the end of a very long event.

Carbohydrate consumption *after exercise* is an interesting area of current research. It appears that glycogen restoration in liver and muscles is influenced by when and in what form carbohydrate is consumed (Ivy, 1989). Consuming carbohydrate immediately after exercise (rather than waiting for several hours) favors greater glycogen deposition. Solutions of specially formulated sugars called *glucose polymers* have been used in some of these studies.

Abnormalities in Insulin Production and Function

Some people's bodies do not handle carbohydrate in the ways just described because of an abnormality in the amount of insulin the body produces or how body cells react to the insulin. Approximately 11 million Americans are estimated to have these conditions (Surgeon General's Report, 1988).

It is possible that a person's pancreas may not produce enough insulin to accomplish its usual tasks. In such instances, sugar builds up in the blood; without sufficient insulin it cannot be taken into body cells for energy production or converted to glycogen or fat. This condition is called **insulin-dependent (or type I) diabetes:** people with this disease need to inject insulin to make up for their lack of it.

insulin-dependent (or type I) diabetes—condition in which the pancreas does not produce enough insulin to regulate blood sugar adequately

In the past, insulin-dependent diabetics have been advised to rigidly restrict their carbohydrate intake. But in recent years, studies with insulin-dependent diabetics have shown that blood sugar levels are influenced not only by the total amount of carbohydrate eaten, but also by the type of carbohydrate and/or the food(s) in which it was consumed. In general, diabetics achieve better blood sugar control on diets that are high in complex carbohydrates and soluble fiber (Anderson et al., 1987). Research in the years ahead should add to our understanding of the best diet for the insulin-dependent diabetic.

Do not assume that consumption of sugar or other carbohydrates causes diabetes; epidemiological evidence indicates that it does not. Rather, researchers theorize that diabetes may result from a hereditary tendency of a person's body to destroy insulin-producing cells, a process that may be hastened by such stress as a viral infection.

Another possible abnormality occurs when a person (usually an adult) produces plenty of insulin, but for some reason the insulin cannot perform its role of carrying glucose into body cells. This is a form of diabetes quite different from and approximately ten times more prevalent than the one just mentioned; it is called **non-insulin-dependent (or type II) diabetes.** Since people who get it are often overweight, it is primarily treated with a weight-reduction program, which may in itself bring the condition under control; sometimes a diet that is high in soluble fiber or an oral drug that helps lower blood glucose is also part of the treatment. There is probably also a hereditary influence on this condition.

non-insulin-dependent (or type II) diabetes—condition in which adequate amounts of insulin are produced but not used normally

Yet another unusual metabolic dysfunction occurs when insulin is *overproduced* in response to carbohydrate ingestion. In this case, a small rise in blood glucose from a normal diet causes an abnormally large outpouring of insulin from the pancreas, and blood sugar drops sharply below the normal range two to four hours after a meal. At the same time, sweating, palpitations, hunger, weakness, and anxiety occur. The condition is called **reactive hypoglycemia. Hypoglycemia** simply refers to blood sugar that has fallen below the normal range. This can be caused by various abnormalities. The adjective *reactive* specifies that the hypoglycemia occurs *in reaction to* normal ingestion of carbohydrate.

hypoglycemia—condition in which blood sugar falls below the normal range

reactive hypoglycemia—condition in which abnormally low blood sugar results from overproduction of insulin despite ordinary levels of carbohydrate intake

Although reactive hypoglycemia has received substantial popular press coverage, very few people have it. Scientists now suspect that in many people what seem to be symptoms of reactive hypoglycemia are actually the result of stress and anxiety (Mayo Clinic Nutrition Letter, 1989). Stress causes the release of the hormone epinephrine, which ultimately brings about some of the same symptoms as excessive insulin. Dealing directly with the causes of the stress and anxiety may be more productive in the long run than changing the diet; however, people with these symptoms may also benefit from eating evenly spaced meals with lots of variety, avoiding highly sugared snacks, and exercising regularly.

Carbohydrates Affect Certain Health Conditions

Carbohydrates have been accused, sometimes unjustly, of damaging health. Here we take a look at various salvos that have been fired at carbohydrates and also acknowledge the conditions in which carbohydrates can be helpful.

Excess Weight

Do carbohydrates make people fat? No, carbohydrates are not inherently fattening. Neither sugars nor starches are fattening per se. What makes people overly fat is excess kcalories from *any* source. The kcalories from carbohydrates are no more fattening than surplus kcalories from proteins, fats, or alcohol.

Sometimes fiber is credited with being a weight loss aid, but studies designed to test this have yielded mixed results (Stevens, 1988). There is little doubt that eating more high-fiber foods *in place of* some high-kcalorie foods will reduce overall energy intake and result in weight loss.

Chapter 10 is devoted to a thorough discussion of body weight and methods for changing it.

Dental Caries

Carbohydrate—or at least one type of it—bears more guilt when it comes to the matter of tooth decay.

dental caries (cavities)—tooth enamel destruction caused by acid by-products of bacterial metabolism of certain carbohydrates

In essence, **dental caries,** or **cavities,** occur when susceptible teeth are exposed over time to acids, which are produced when bacteria metabolize any fermentable carbohydrates (but especially common sugars) in the mouth. Fortunately, there are counterbalancing factors that can discourage decay.

Factors That Promote Acid Production and Decay   Some people's teeth are more prone to decay than others. *Susceptibility* can be inherited, but diet can also be involved. If a child has had access to a sufficient amount of the mineral fluoride during the tooth-forming years, the tooth surface (enamel) will be harder and less likely to decay throughout life than if the child has not. As a result, susceptibility is an individual variable.

A factor that almost everybody is subject to is *mouth bacteria*. The organism most often implicated is *Streptococcus mutans,* a common mouth resident that metabolizes fermentable sugars. The bacteria produce acid by-products that slowly dissolve the minerals from the enamel on the outside of the tooth; this makes the softer structures inside the tooth more vulnerable to decay. Other bacteria are thought to play a less important role.

The common sugars sucrose, glucose, fructose, maltose, and lactose are all highly fermentable and are almost equally **cariogenic** on a gram-for-gram basis (National Dairy Council, 1986). This is true whether the sugars occur naturally in food or are added to it. Sugar alcohols, on the other hand, are not as easily metabolized by mouth bacteria; that is why they are commonly used in "sugarless" chewing gum and candy. Another factor in dental caries is a food's *stickiness.* Sticky-sweet foods cling to tooth surfaces, making sugar available to mouth bacteria for an extended period. Foods such as caramels and raisins are more cariogenic than less sticky items.

cariogenic—likely to cause cavity production

Frequency of eating is important as well, since acid production continues for approximately 30 minutes after the last mouthful is swallowed (National Research Council, 1989). That means it is less damaging to consume a popsicle that is eaten quickly than to eat hard candy (with an equivalent amount of sugar) at intervals throughout the day. Even apples, once thought of as "nature's toothbrush," can contribute to tooth decay if consumed very frequently: Farm workers who ate at least 8 apples per day during the harvest season had substantially more decayed, missing, and filled teeth than controls (Grobler and Blignaut, 1989).

Timing of eating also plays a role: fermentable carbohydrates consumed *between meals rather than with meals* are more likely to result in tooth decay. For example, it has been found that drinking soft drinks with meals was not associated with high incidence of decay, but drinking sodas three times or more between meals daily was associated with almost twice the likelihood of having a high incidence of decay (Nutrition Reviews, 1987).

Deterrents to Decay Besides changing diet and eating habits, there are other ways to discourage tooth decay.

Saliva helps deter decay in a number of ways: it washes sugars away from teeth, and it contains materials that actually promote remineralization of eroded tooth enamel to a certain extent (Featherstone, 1987). As a result, any practice that stimulates saliva production is helpful. For example, eating fibrous foods stimulates saliva flow, and eating sugary foods with meals— when saliva flow is more copious—results in fewer cavities than eating sugary foods between meals.

Some scientists think that *certain food components* are protective. Fats may provide a coating for teeth, and high-phosphorus foods may be protective as well. These experts think that ending a meal with cheese or nuts may help prevent dental caries.

Xylitol, as mentioned earlier, has been found to discourage the formation of dental caries. In a study funded by the World Health Organization, xylitol was substituted for some of the sugar in the diets of children living on two islands, while the children on another island (with dietary habits originally similar to the other two) continued their usual diets. After almost three years, the children who were ingesting xylitol as part of their diet had significantly fewer dental caries than those who were not (Kandelman and Hefti, 1988). A number of other studies have had similar findings (Pepper and Olinger, 1988).

Of course, *good dental hygiene* immediately after eating reduces the amount of time that sugars are in the mouth and is also helpful.

The American Dental Association incorporates these suggestions into its decay-prevention program: it recommends a nutritious diet, limited snacking (especially on sweets), careful hygiene, and regular dental checkups.

Figure 6.7 summarizes factors that increase the risk of decay.

Decrease in Micronutrient Status

Both available and unavailable carbohydrates have been criticized for interfering with micronutrient status. Dietary recommendations also advise against eating too much concentrated sugar on the grounds that foods that contain a lot of sugar tend to be low in nutrient density. If sugary foods represent a large share of a person's diet, vitamin and mineral intake could be inadequate overall. Experts in the United States have not set any particular limit on intake, because they do not believe that a specific limit is supported by the data (Diet and Health, 1989). However, the general dietary recommendations of some other countries suggest that added sugars should not constitute more than 10–12% of kcaloric intake.

High levels of fiber in the diet dilute nutrient density too. In addition, fiber and/or substances found along with it in plants decrease the absorption of some essential minerals and vitamins. For example, some studies done in the United States found that adding a total of 6 tablespoons of wheat bran to the day's meals decreased apparent calcium absorption by about 50% (Balasubramanian et al., 1987). Different nutrients are not affected in the same way; the type of fiber is another variable.

The dilution of nutrient density and interference with absorption of minerals by fiber have been found to have substantial practical significance in the developing countries. Some groups of people in Egypt and Iran, whose typical diets are extremely high in fiber and related compounds but marginal in minerals, have developed mineral deficiency syndromes. Much remains to be learned about the bioavailability (usability) of minerals when they are consumed with various kinds of fiber and about how much fiber is too much. (More on this in Chapter 13 on minerals.) Therefore, despite the

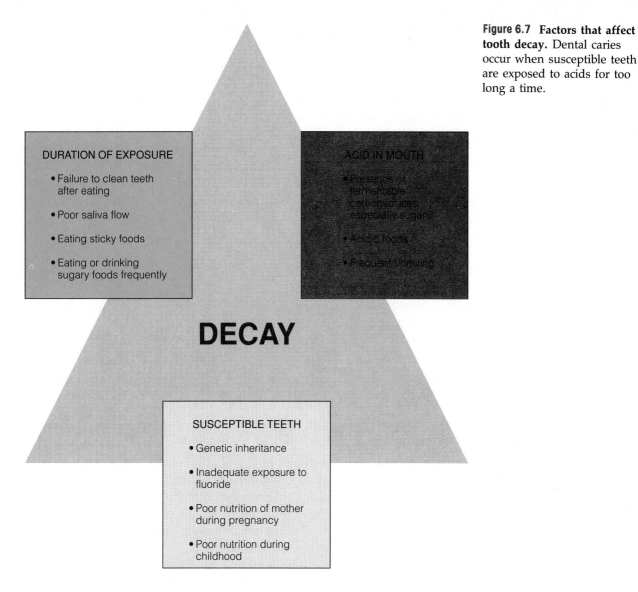

Figure 6.7 Factors that affect tooth decay. Dental caries occur when susceptible teeth are exposed to acids for too long a time.

benefits we can get from dietary fiber, like any other ingested substance, it should not be overused.

Constipation

Adequate fiber in the diet relieves constipation. Fiber and the water it absorbs make the feces bulkier. Carrot fiber, for example, can hold 20 to 30 times its weight in water, and wheat bran can hold about 5 times its weight. Bulk is also influenced by the size of fiber particles. Whole-wheat flour that is coarsely ground results in more fecal bulk than finely ground whole-wheat flour (IFT Expert Panel, 1989).

Bulky feces cause the colonic muscles to exercise more, which makes them stronger and able to function better. In addition, the fecal mass moves through the tract more easily because it is softer. When a diet contains the recommended amount of fiber, transit time is typically between 24 and 72 hours; if fiber intake is very low, transit time may be longer.

Vegetarians who rely largely on plant foods and therefore have high fiber intakes rarely experience constipation.

Diverticular Disease

diverticular disease—condition in which pressure in the lumen of the colon causes outpouchings called diverticula to occur in its walls

Diverticular disease is a condition in which pressure in the lumen of the colon causes outpouchings (diverticula) to occur in its wall (Figure 6.8). An estimated 30–40% of people aged 50 and over in the United States are thought to have this condition, although they may not be aware of it (National Research Council, 1989). Diverticula will not cause any pain unless waste collects in them and causes irritation, resulting in *diverticulitis*. (The suffix *-itis* means *inflammation*.)

A diet generous in fiber has been found to help relieve the symptoms of uncomplicated diverticular disease. Some epidemiologists further believe that a high-fiber diet may help prevent the condition, since another effect of increased fecal bulk and decreased transit time is decreased colonic pressure.

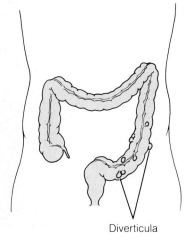

Diverticula

Figure 6.8 Diverticular disease. In diverticular disease, a common condition in the elderly, outpouchings form in the wall of the colon.

Colon Cancer

Cancer is a disease in which body cells multiply out of control. Research over the past several decades suggests that there may be over 100 different clinical conditions with this characteristic, all of which are called cancer. Certain components in the diet have been linked to cancer, which puts this topic on the leading edge of nutrition research.

Epidemiological studies suggest that dietary fiber may provide protection against colon cancer; populations that consume a high-fiber diet tend to have less colon cancer than populations that eat low-fiber diets (Bright-See, 1988). Note, however, that high-fiber diets often have the coexisting characteristic of being lower in fat and kcalories than low-fiber diets. Consequently, it may be just as valid to suggest that the low-fat and/or low-energy features of the diet are protective—it may even be that none of the three is involved. Other possibilities are that some types of fiber may be protective whereas others are not or that another substance associated with fiber in food is a helpful factor. Animal studies have been done to try to clarify the relationship between fiber and colon cancer, but they have not produced consistent results (National Research Council, 1989).

Despite these uncertainties, the National Cancer Institute and many other health organizations recommend that Americans eat a variety of fiber and a large number of fiber-containing foods. They believe that it may help; in any event, it won't hurt. The fiber intakes of many populations are double those of average Americans and have not caused detrimental effects (Greenwald and Lanza, 1986).

Cardiovascular Disease

The effect of diet on cardiovascular (heart and blood vessel) disease is a topic that has been on the nutrition frontier for decades. Dietary fats are believed to be more influential in the development of cardiovascular (CV) disease than carbohydrates are, so we will devote a major section in Chapter 7 (on fat) to this health concern, including the definition of many important terms.

Suffice it to say here that different forms of carbohydrates seem to have different effects on CV disease because of their influence on blood cholesterol, a fatty substance in blood. The higher your total blood cholesterol is, the greater statistical likelihood you have of developing CV disease.

Studies of both animals and humans have indicated that the bran of grains such as oats, corn, and rice can lower blood cholesterol levels in some individuals, whereas wheat bran does not. Legumes and some fruits and vegetables also lower blood lipid levels. These effects are generally attributed to the soluble fibers present (Anderson and Gustafson, 1988; National Research Council, 1989). In addition, a water-soluble fiber found in psyllium seed, originally marketed as a bulking agent, has also been found to reduce blood cholesterol (Abraham and Mehta, 1988; Anderson et al., 1988).

It may not take dramatic levels of fiber to achieve some benefit; moderately increasing the intake of fibrous foods may lead to small, persistent decreases in blood cholesterol levels that may significantly lessen risk over a long period. The debate about the benefits of fiber in reducing the incidence of CV disease continues.

The effect of other carbohydrates on CV disease is less clear-cut. Studies attempting to determine if sugars or starches increase blood cholesterol have yielded mixed results; future work may provide more definitive answers.

Interestingly enough, epidemiological studies show that groups of Seventh Day Adventist vegetarians—whose diets are likely to be high in fiber and starch—have considerably less heart disease than the general population (Trowell and Burkitt, 1986). However, such studies have not ascertained which dietary constituent (if any) is responsible for the decreased risk. It is also possible that the effect may be due to differences in other lifestyle factors such as less smoking and little alcohol consumption.

Assess Your Own Carbohydrate Intake Compared to Recommendations

Now we will deal with the matter of how much available and unavailable carbohydrate is the right amount to consume, and how to determine whether you are getting it.

Recommended Minimal Intake for Total Available Carbohydrate

Even though it is a biochemically important substance, there is no RDA for carbohydrate, since it can be produced from protein. However, if body proteins were used heavily for carbohydrate production, physiological damage would eventually result. Therefore, estimates have been made of how much carbohydrate is needed to provide for important functions and to preserve body protein.

Experts in the United States recommend that *at the very least*, a person should take in 50 to 100 grams of carbohydrate daily (RDA Subcommittee, 1989). The United Nations Food and Agriculture Organization and the World Health Organization suggest a more generous *minimum* of 180 grams daily (720 kcalories from carbohydrate). If you add up the carbohydrate in the minimal amount of foods recommended by the Basic Food Guide, you will find that it ranges anywhere from about 110 to 200 grams, depending on which foods are selected—especially on whether legumes are used as meat alternates.

Interestingly, the traditional diets of many of the world's cultures emphasize high-carbohydrate foods. For example, rice is a staple food in much of China, Japan, and southeast Asia; for many people in Ireland and in the Andes Mountains, potatoes are a very important food; and bread is basic to many Eastern Europeans. Such dietary practices make it probable that recommended intakes for carbohydrate will be achieved with no difficulty.

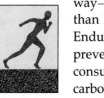

Carbohydrate recommendations are sometimes expressed in another way—as a proportion of kcalories. The 1989 RDA recommends that more than half of a person's energy requirement be provided by carbohydrates. Endurance athletes who train daily are advised to consume even more to prevent becoming progressively glycogen-depleted. Of course, individuals consuming 50% or more of their kcalories as carbohydrate will get far more carbohydrate than the minimum recommendations given above.

Suggested Intake for Fiber

It is difficult to recommend a specific fiber intake because the amounts of fiber in foods are not known with certainty and the consequences of taking in different kinds and amounts of fiber are not entirely understood. Yet, people want and need some guidance regarding how much is enough without being too much. While most groups have avoided recommending any specific level of intake because of the many uncertainties about fiber, some health organizations have offered suggestions in light of what is currently known. (Surgeon General, 1988; National Research Council, 1989; AMA Council of Scientific Affairs, 1989).

In 1984, the National Institutes of Health suggested that Americans should eat foods that provide a total of 25–35 grams of fiber per day; the American Dietetic Association recommended 20–35 grams (1988). Another fiber researcher points out that many vegetarians in our population consume 40–50 grams of dietary fiber daily without ill effect (Slavin, 1987); in fact, many studies show better health among adult vegetarians than among the general population. Nonetheless, all groups agree that the intake of fiber should be increased above the 10–20 grams per day that is currently consumed by Americans, and that the fiber should come from food rather than from supplements.

These reports reflect the spirit of the 1985 *Dietary Guidelines*, which suggested, "Select foods that are good sources of fiber and starch, such as whole-grain breads and cereals, fruits and vegetables, beans, peas and nuts. . . . There is no reason to add fiber to foods. . . ."

Assessment 6.1 shows how you can estimate your fiber intake. Then, Critical Thinking 6.1 helps you consider how to increase your fiber intake if it is warranted.

Estimating Your Total Fiber Intake for One Day

1. Keep a record of your food intake for 24 hours.
2. Write down the fiber content for each food from Table 6.4. If foods you have eaten are not on the table, use a value for a food that is similar. If you have eaten a high-fiber cereal that is not on Table 6.4, check the label for specific data for that product, since there can be a tremendous difference between products.
3. Total the fiber column.
4. How does your fiber intake compare with the average American intake of 10–20 grams per day? Check whether it is:

_____ less than average

_____ within the average range

_____ above the average range

5. If your intake for this day was less than 20 grams, in the far column suggest some additions or substitutions you could have made to increase it to at least 20 grams. Be sure they are changes that would be acceptable to you.

Assessment 6.1

Sample Assessment 6.1 Estimating your total fiber intake for one day

Food or Beverage	Amount Eaten	Fiber (Grams)	Changes to Reach 20 Grams for the Day
Orange juice	1 cup	(est) 0.1	
Special K	1⅓ cup	1.5	try shredded wheat (2 grams more fiber)
Milk, 2%	¾ cup	0	
Sugar	1 teaspoon	0	
Submarine sandwich:			
Roll (est.) like	4 slices white bread	2.4	
Meat	2 ounces	0	
Cheese	2 ounces	0	
Lettuce, chopped	½ cup	0.4	substitute shredded carrot salad or sticks (2.5 g more fiber)
Mayonnaise	3 tablespoons	0	
Tomato, fresh	3 thin slices	(est) 0.3	
Cola	12 ounces	0	
Apple (with peel)	1 medium	(est) 2.4	
Baked chicken	4 ounces	0	
Baked potato	1 medium	(est) 1.6	
Sour cream	3 tablespoons	0	
Lettuce, shredded	1 cup	0.8	
French dressing	1 ounce	0	
Peas, frozen, cooked	½ cup	canned value: 5.3	
Chocolate sandwich cookies	4	(est) 1.0	
Milk, 2%	1½ cup	0	
Snack crackers, refined	10 small	(est) 1.0	
Apple juice	1 cup	(est) 0	
TOTAL DIETARY FIBER		16.8	

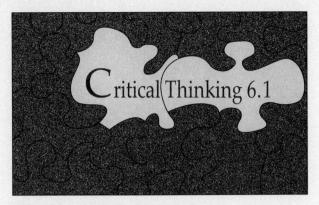

Fiber, Fiber Everywhere— So What?

The situation

You are watching your favorite TV morning news show as you eat breakfast, and now they are showing another breakfast cereal commercial. The last one was for a cereal that had oat bran added to it—they said it is supposed to keep your blood cholesterol down. This one is for a wheat bran cereal, and they're claiming it can reduce your risk of colon cancer.

You take a bite of your English muffin, and you eye it somewhat critically. No bran here, from the looks of things. You wonder whether you ought to start eating a fiber-enriched cereal for breakfast, as everybody seems to be recommending, instead of your usual muffin or bagel.

Is the information accurate and relevant?

■ It is true that oat bran has been found to lower blood cholesterol; a human metabolic study showed that eating either two ounces of oat bran or oatmeal daily along with a low fat, low cholesterol diet reduced blood cholesterol. The fat-modified diet initially lowered blood cholesterol by about 5%; later, when the oat products were added, blood cholesterol went down by an additional 3% (Van Horn et al., 1986).

■ There is epidemiological evidence that diets higher in whole grains reduce the risk of colon cancer. Animal studies using grain fiber have yielded mixed results, but wheat bran has had the most consistent beneficial effect in this regard (National Research Council, 1989).
■ The recommendation to include sources of fiber in the diet has been one of the most consistent pieces of dietary advice given to Americans since the early part of this century. Recent recommendations have suggested increasing these intakes beyond what is typically consumed.

What else needs to be considered?

Fiber and its relationship to health is a hot research topic at present, and that means there is much yet to be learned. We need to know a great deal more about the types and amounts of fiber in foods and how they affect the body before very specific recommendations can be made.

Although in general it appears that diets higher in fiber offer some protection against heart disease and cancer, it is not always clear whether it is the *presence of the fiber per se*, or *the presence of a particular type or amount of fiber*, or *either the presence or absence of something else in high fiber foods* that has the beneficial effect. More research on both laboratory animals and humans is needed.

For these reasons, many scientists and scientific groups are hesitant to make very specific recommendations for fiber intake. Most do not recommend fiber supplements but are willing to recommend that we should eat a variety of foods that are naturally high in fiber.

There are some possible negative effects of high fiber intake. A few individuals who have taken fiber supplements without adequate fluid have produced compacted feces that were difficult to eliminate. Of more general concern is that at some level of intake, certain types of fiber reduce absorption of minerals such as calcium and iron—which are already in short supply in the diets of many Americans.

Many products now being promoted as fiber-enriched vary not only in the types of fiber they contain, but also in the amounts included. You can get a general idea of how much fiber is present by the location of the fiber source on the ingredient list: the closer it is to the top of the list, the more fiber is there.

Some "fiber-enriched" foods contain so little that their fiber content is lower than that of an ordinary whole-grain product; nonetheless, a premium price is often charged for the "extra fiber." On the other hand, products that have bran or cellulose listed as one of the first few ingredients are essentially fiber supplements, since the fiber is present in amounts much higher than is naturally found in food.

What do you think?

You are left with the question of whether you should increase your fiber intake; and if so, what's the best way to get the benefits of fiber without the possible penalties?

Here are some options you may consider:

- ■ Option 1   You decide that since there is quite a bit that is unknown about fiber, there's no point in changing your fiber intake.
- ■ Option 2   You decide not to worry about fiber intake at present but to increase your overall carbohydrate intake and lower your fat intake. You'll ask your physician's advice at your next checkup.
- ■ Option 3   You evaluate your diet for its current fiber content on a typical day using Assessment 6.1. If you find that you usually consume over 20 grams of dietary fiber per day, you decide there is no need to increase your fiber intake at this time. If you find your fiber intake is less than 20 grams, you consider options 4 and 5.
- ■ Option 4   You decide to use more foods with their natural fiber intact: more whole-grain products instead of refined and more fruits and vegetables with edible peels.
- ■ Option 5   You decide to try one of the fiber-enriched cereals.

Do you see other options? Which approach makes most sense to you and why?

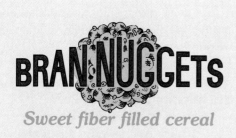

BRAN NUGGETS

Sweet fiber filled cereal

Ingredients: Oat bran, wheat bran, brown sugar, partially hydrogenated soybean oil, sugar, corn syrup, walnuts, wheat starch, salt.

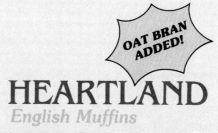

OAT BRAN ADDED!

HEARTLAND
English Muffins

Ingredients: Enriched flour, malted barley flour, water, whole blueberries, sugar, yeast, oat bran, salt, corn meal, baking powder, lactic acid.

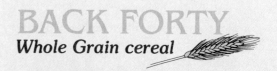

BACK FORTY
Whole Grain cereal

Ingredients: Cracked wheat, cracked rye, whole flax.

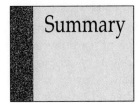
Summary

▶ Sugars, starches, and fiber are all forms of carbohydrate that differ somewhat in their characteristics and functions. As a group, they have two major functions in the body: they provide energy, and they enhance GI functioning.

▶ The types and amounts of carbohydrates in foods vary. All are **organic** substances regardless of their origin. Sugars are the smallest and simplest carbohydrates; glucose is a typical and important example. **Mono-** and **disaccharides** are found in all plant foods; the disaccharide lactose occurs in animal milks. Sugar can also be added to foods during processing; you can get a general idea of how much added sugar a food contains from the food label. Starches and dextrins **(polysaccharides)** are also commonly found in plant foods, and can be altered in or added to processed foods. Sugars and starches are available for human energy production and are thus considered **available carbohydrates.**

▶ **Fiber** cannot be digested by human processes, but it is nevertheless important to the healthy functioning of the digestive tract. Fiber is a plant food component that exists in both **soluble** and **insoluble** forms, and can be removed from or added to foods during processing. The fiber content of specific foods is difficult to quantify.

▶ A healthy person digests and absorbs carbohydrates quickly and efficiently. Disaccharides are **hydrolyzed** in the small intestine, where all monosaccharides are then absorbed. Starch digestion begins in the mouth with the activity of **amylases,** and then resumes in the small intestine. Fiber progresses along the upper tract without modification. Carbohydrates that are not digested (including fiber) and move along to the colon are used by bacteria and draw water from surrounding tissues into the lumen; normally neither event causes problems. However, under conditions of **lactose intolerance,** unusually high ingestion of sugar alcohols, or the stress of athletic activity, carbohydrates are sometimes not digested or absorbed properly and the consequences cause discomfort.

▶ Several factors determine what happens to glucose, the ultimate product of carbohydrate digestion. Some is used right away for energy production and some remains in the bloodstream, but most is converted to glycogen or fat for storage. The hormones **insulin** and **glucagon,** both produced by the pancreas, help to regulate the blood glucose level. The activities of the liver, muscles, and enzymes also affect blood glucose.

▶ Athletes, in some cases, can maximize their muscle glycogen using a diet and exercise regimen called **glycogen loading.** A successful alternative is for an endurance athlete to consume a high carbohydrate diet every day.

▶ Various abnormalities in carbohydrate metabolism can be traced to problems in **insulin** production or function. These include **insulin-dependent (type I) diabetes, non-insulin-dependent (type II) diabetes,** and **reactive hypoglycemia.**

▶ Carbohydrates affect certain aspects of health in various ways. Sugars can be metabolized by bacteria in the mouth and, over time, the resulting acid can cause decay in susceptible teeth; thus, the common food sugars are **cariogenic. Sugar alcohols,** which are not as likely to be metabolized in the mouth, are not. Fiber can relieve constipation and help prevent **diverticular disease,** but if it is ingested in large amounts it can interfere with the bioavailability of certain minerals. Fiber may or may not provide some protection against certain types of cancer and cardiovascular disease; these are active areas of research and debate.

▶ Americans are encouraged to consume carbohydrates in amounts that represent at least 50% of their kcalorie intake. Such intakes should provide more than the minimum of 50–100 grams of carbohydrate needed by the body.

▶ Recommendations for fiber intake suggest that most Americans should increase their consumption of fiber-containing foods.

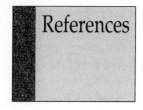
References

Abraham, Z.D. and T. Mehta. 1988. Three-week psyllium-husk supplementation: Effect on plasma cholesterol concentrations, fecal steroid excretion, and carbohydrate absorption in men. *American Journal of Clinical Nutrition* 47:67–74.

American Dietetic Association, House of Delegates. 1987. Position of the American Dietetic Association: Nutrition for physical fitness and athletic performance in adults. *Journal of the American Dietetic Association* 87:933–939.

American Dietetic Association, House of Delegates. 1988. Position of the American Dietetic Association: Health implications of dietary fiber. *Journal of the American Dietetic Association* 88:216–221.

American Medical Association (AMA), Council on Scientific Affairs. 1989. Dietary fiber and health. *Journal of the American Medical Association* 262:542–546.

Anderson, J.W. and N.J. Gustafson. 1988. Hypocholesterolemic effects of oat and bean products. *American Journal of Clinical Nutrition* 48:749–753.

Anderson, J.W., N.J. Gustafson, C.A. Bryant, and J. Tietyen-Clark. 1987. Dietary fiber and diabetes: A comprehensive review and practical application. *Journal of the American Dietetic Association* 87:1189–1197.

Anderson, J.W., N. Zettwoch, T. Feldman, J. Tietyen-Clark, P. Oeltgen, and C.W. Bishop. 1988. Cholesterol-lowering effects of psyllium hydrophilic mucilloid for hypercholesterolemic men. *Archives of Internal Medicine* 148:292–296.

Bailey, L., L. Duewer, F. Gray, R. Hoskin, J. Putnam, and S. Short. 1988. Food consumption. *National Food Review* 11(No. 2):1–11.

Balasubramanian, R., E.J. Johnson, and J.A. Marlett. 1987. Effect of wheat bran on bowel function and fecal calcium in older adults. *Journal of the American College of Nutrition* 6:199–208.

Bantle, J.P., D.C. Laine, G.W. Castle, J.W. Thomas, B.J. Hoogwerf, and F.C. Goetz. 1983. Postprandial glucose and insulin responses to meals containing different carbohydrates in normal and diabetic subjects. *New England Journal of Medicine* 309:7–12.

Bright-See, E. 1988. Dietary fiber and cancer. *Nutrition Today* 23(No. 4):4–10.

Crapo, P.A. and R.R. Henry. 1988. Postprandial metabolic responses to the influence of food form. *American Journal of Clinical Nutrition* 48:560–564.

Featherstone, J.D. 1987. The mechanism of dental decay. *Nutrition Today* May/June, 1987:10–16.

Green, D.R., C. Gibbons, M. O'Toole, and W.B. Hiller. 1989. An evaluation of dietary intakes of triathletes: Are RDAs being met? *Journal of the American Dietetic Association* 89:1653–1654.

Grobler, S.R. and J.B. Blignaut. 1989. The effect of a high consumption of apples or grapes on dental caries and periodontal disease in humans. *Clinical Preventive Dentistry* 11:8–12.

Houts, S.S. 1988. Lactose intolerance. *Food Technology* 42:110–113.

Institute of Food Technologists. 1989. Ingredients for sweet success. *Food Technology* 43:94–116.

Institute of Food Technologists (IFT), Expert Panel on Food Safety and Nutrition. 1989. Dietary fiber. *Food Technology* 43:133–139.

Ivy, J.L. 1989. Carbohydrate supplementation for rapid muscle glycogen storage in the hours immediately after exercise. In *The theory and practice of athletic nutrition: Bridging the gap*, A.M. Cameron, ed. Columbus, Ohio: Ross Laboratories.

Jain, N.K., V.P. Patel, and C.S. Pitchumoni. 1987. Sorbitol intolerance in adults. *Journal of Clinical Gastroenterology* 9:317–319.

Kandelman, A.B. and A. Hefti. 1988. Collaborative WHO xylitol field study in French Polynesia. *Caries Research* 22(No. 1):55–62.

Kolars, J.C., M.D. Levitt, M. Aouji, and D.A. Savaiano. 1984. Yogurt—an autodigesting source of lactose. *New England Journal of Medicine* 310:1–3.

Macdonald, I. 1987. Metabolic requirements for

dietary carbohydrate. *American Journal of Clinical Nutrition* 45:1193–1196.

Marlett, J.A. 1989. Measuring dietary fiber. *Animal Feed Science and Technology* 23:1–13.

Marlett, J.A., J.G. Chesters, M.J. Longacre, and J.J. Bogdanske. 1989. Recovery of soluble dietary fiber is dependent on the method of analysis. *American Journal of Clinical Nutrition* 50:479–485.

Mayo Clinic Nutrition Letter. 1989. Hypoglycemia: Low blood sugar rarely explains why you feel lousy. *Mayo Clinic Nutrition Letter* 2:4–5.

Mourot, J., P. Thouvenot, C. Couet, J.M. Antoine, A. Krobicka, and G. Debry. 1988. Relationship between the rate of gastric emptying and glucose and insulin responses to starchy foods in young healthy adults. *American Journal of Clinical Nutrition* 48:1035–1040.

National Dairy Council. 1986. The role of diet and nutrition in oral health. *Dairy Council Digest* 57:13–18.

National Dairy Council. 1989. Food sensitivity and dairy products. *Dairy Council Digest* 60(No. 5): 25–30.

National Research Council. 1989. *Diet and health: Implications for reducing chronic disease risk.* Washington, DC: National Academy Press.

Nieman, D.C., J.V. Butler, L.M. Pollett, S.J. Dietrich, and R.D. Lutz. 1989. Nutrient intake of marathon runners. *Journal of the American Dietetic Association* 89:1273–1278.

Nutrition Reviews. 1987. Diet and dental health as measured by NHANES I data. *Nutrition Reviews* 45:302–304.

Pepper, T. and P.M. Olinger. 1988. Xylitol in sugar-free confections. *Food Technology* 42:98–106.

RDA Subcommittee. 1989. *Recommended dietary allowances.* Washington, DC: National Academy Press.

Savaiano, D.A. and C. Kotz. 1988. Recent advances in the management of lactose intolerance. *Contemporary Nutrition* 13(No. 9, 10). Minneapolis, MN: General Mills, Inc.

Scrimshaw, N.S. and E.B. Murray. 1988. Lactose tolerance and milk consumption. *American Journal of Clinical Nutrition* 48:1059–1083.

Sherman, W.M. and D.A. Wright. 1989. Preevent nutrition for prolonged exercise. In *The theory and practice of athletic nutrition: Bridging the gap,* A.M. Cameron, ed. Columbus, Ohio: Ross Laboratories.

Slavin, J.L. 1987. Dietary fiber: Classification, chemical analysis, and food sources. *Journal of the American Dietetic Association* 87:1164–1171.

Southgate, D.A. and I.T. Johnson. 1987. New thoughts on carbohydrate digestion. *Contemporary Nutrition* 12(No. 10).

Stevens, J. 1988. Does dietary fiber affect food intake and body weight? *Journal of the American Dietetic Association* 88:939–942.

Surgeon General's Report. 1988. *Surgeon General's report on nutrition and health.* Washington, DC: United States Department of Health and Human Services.

Thompson, L.U. 1988. Antinutrients and blood glucose. *Food Technology* 42:123–132.

Tuft's Letter. 1986. Sorbitol is not for all. *Tuft's University Diet and Nutrition Letter* 4(No. 7) September, 1986.

Van Horn, L.V., K. Liu, D. Parker, L. Emidy, Y. Liao, W.H. Pan, D. Giumetti, J. Hewitt, and J. Stamler. 1986. Serum lipid response to oat product intake with a fat-modified diet. *Journal of the American Dietetic Association* 86:759–764.

Williams, M.H. 1989. Nutritional ergogenic aids and athletic performance. *Nutrition Today* January/February 1989:7–14.

Wolever, T.M., D.J. Jenkins, A.M. Ocana, V.A. Rau, and G.R. Collier. 1988. Second-meal effect: Low-glycemic-index foods eaten at dinner improve subsequent breakfast glycemic response. *American Journal of Clinical Nutrition* 48:1041–1047.

7

Lipids

In This Chapter

- Lipids Have Six Important Functions
- Different Types of Lipids Are Found in Foods
- The Amounts of Lipids in Different Foods Vary Considerably
- Different Lipids Are Digested and Absorbed at Different Rates
- Your Body Produces Lipids from Various Materials
- Lipoproteins Have a Special Role in Transporting Lipids
- Lipids Are Involved in Major Health Problems
- Assess Your Own Lipid Intake Compared with Recommendations

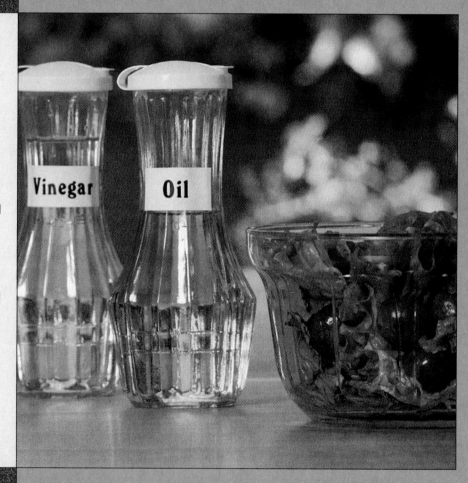

ave you ever noticed on the ingredient list of a food product label the terms *monoglycerides* and *diglycerides?* Or *lecithin?* Or have you ever had a laboratory test done to determine the level of your *blood cholesterol?* These substances are all examples of lipids.

Lipids are fatty substances that usually do not dissolve in water but that do dissolve in ether. **Fats** are lipids that are solid at room temperature; **oils** are pourable at room temperature.

Fats, oils, and their chemical relatives have had a bad reputation among the general public in recent years. One reason is cosmetic; our society has come to think that body fat is ugly. Other reasons are health-related. Over the years, we have learned to be concerned about limiting our overall fat intakes to 30% of total kcalories. We are also concerned about our levels of blood cholesterol, knowing that this form of lipid has been implicated in the development of atherosclerosis, a type of cardiovascular disease.

We think negatively about lipids; nonetheless, we enjoy eating them and find ourselves repeatedly tempted by them. Lipids often contribute to the tantalizing aromas of foods; lipids also largely account for the sense of satiety (hunger satisfaction) that is experienced from eating rich foods. Magazines that place an article about new, buttery desserts alongside a feature on how to slim down exemplify these conflicting attitudes about fat.

This chapter will help give a balanced perspective on the topic. It starts by emphasizing the positive values of lipids: they have important functions besides those you have already read about in previous chapters. We will discuss the many forms of lipids found in foods, both as nature produces them and as food technology modifies them; how the body handles lipids; how much fat a person needs; and how health can be affected by consuming various amounts of lipids for long periods of time.

lipids—fatty substances that usually do not dissolve in water because of their chemical structure

fats—lipids that are solid at room temperature

oils—lipids that are liquid at room temperature

Lipids Have Six Important Functions

Fats are important contributors to our health and well-being. As dietary constituents, they perform all three of the general functions of nutrients—providing energy, supplying materials for physiological structures, and serving as regulators of body processes. Although excess body fat is a real problem for some people, a certain amount of fat serves us well as a thermal insulator and as a cushion for internal organs.

1. *Providing energy.* Lipids are the most potent providers of energy. At 9 kcalories per gram, they provide more than twice as much energy as the 4 kcalories per gram that carbohydrates and proteins furnish. Because fat is such a concentrated source of energy, high-fat diets are more likely to result in high energy intakes and body fat gain than are low-fat diets.

A large share of the body's lipids are stored in **adipose tissue** (body fat) (Figure 7.1). It is fortunate that we can store energy in such a compact

adipose tissue—an aggregation of cells specialized in fat storage

Figure 7.1 An adipose cell. (a) Although every cell can hold some fat, cells of adipose tissue are designed for storage of large amounts of fat. Other normal cell components—the nucleus and other bodies—are compressed into a small portion of the adipose cell. (b) Pictured here are adipose cells. Note the large droplets of lipid in each adipose cell.

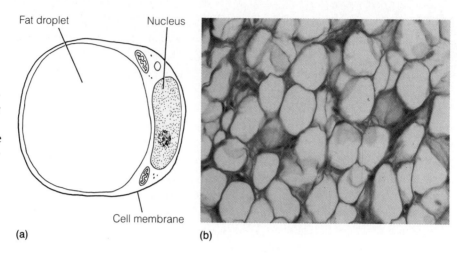

Fat droplet   Nucleus

Cell membrane

(a)   (b)

form: we would be very much larger and heavier than we are now if the kcalories carried as fat were stored as glycogen instead. For example, if the energy contained in 25 pounds of fat were stored in your body as glycogen, the glycogen would weigh about 55 pounds, and the water associated with it would weigh over 150 pounds, making you more than 180 pounds heavier than the 25 pounds of fat would.

2. *Providing essential nutrients.* There is an essential nutrient in lipids called **linoleic acid.** Although a deficiency of linoleic acid is rarely seen in humans, if it were absent from the diet for a long time, it would result in skin that is scaly and rough; tendency to bleeding; abnormal kidney function; and diminished reproductive capacity (Kinsella, 1988). If a child does not get enough linoleic acid, growth is impaired. Fortunately, it is widespread enough in the food supply that most people who eat a varied diet are likely to fulfill their need for this nutrient.

linoleic acid—essential fatty acid present in lipids

Some research indicates that **linolenic acid,** another widely available fatty acid, may also be essential. Both of these fatty acids are abundant in plant oils.

linolenic acid—fatty acid that may be essential (different from linoleic acid)

3. *Carrying fat-soluble vitamins into the body.* Some vitamins—A, D, E, and K—are absorbed into the body much more easily if they are dissolved in fat. (This is a good example of how nutrients influence each other in the body.)

4. *Providing components for many body materials.* Besides being the stuff of which adipose tissue is largely made, lipids are also necessary components of cell membranes, some hormones and **prostaglandins** (hormone-like substances), nerve coverings, vitamin D, and some digestive secretions.

prostaglandins—certain naturally occurring lipid substances with hormone-like activity; they have important effects on various body systems and functions

Cholesterol is one lipid that performs many of these functions. It is important for you to know that cholesterol, which has had so much bad press, is a necessary body substance. It is so important that people's bodies actually *produce* it, usually in larger amounts than people consume in their diets.

5. *Providing thermal insulation.* If you are of average weight, roughly half of the adipose tissue in your body is just under the skin and is called **subcutaneous fat.** Located there, it constitutes an internal blanket that helps hold in your body heat. Whether this is an advantage or a disadvantage depends on how much subcutaneous fat you have and what the usual temperature of your environment is.

6. *Protecting vital organs.* The rest of your adipose tissue surrounds your internal organs, where it cushions them from shocks and bruises.

subcutaneous fat—adipose tissue located just under the skin

Different Types of Lipids Are Found in Foods

Lipids are categorized according to their structural similarities. We will deal here with glycerides, phospholipids, and sterols. They are of major importance because of their prevalence in the diet and the body and because of their implications for health. We will begin by discussing them as they occur in nature, and then we will discuss various technological modifications developed for use in food.

Glycerides in Nature

Glycerides are the most common forms of lipids. By definition, glycerides consist of a molecule of the 3-carbon compound **glycerol** to which one, two, or three **fatty acids** are attached (*mono-, di-, or triglycerides*).

Triglycerides (called *triacylglycerols* by some biochemists) account for about 90% of the weight of lipids in foods; fats and oils are both largely triglycerides. Mono- and diglycerides also occur in nature, as do some unattached or "free" fatty acids.

Even though the name of these compounds draws attention to the glycerol portion of the lipid molecule, the attached fatty acids are the components responsible for giving different glycerides their characteristics. Fatty acids differ from each other in several ways.

One such difference is their *chain length;* this refers to the number of linked carbon atoms in the fatty acid skeleton. Chain length is significant because, generally speaking, the shorter the fatty acid chains, the more likely a glyceride is to be liquid at room temperature. (Milk fat has many short-chain fatty acids.) Triglycerides with long saturated fatty acids, such as those found in red meats, tend to be solid at room temperature. Fatty acids may have anywhere from 4 to 22 carbons; oleic acid, the most common fatty acid in nature, has 18 carbons in its chain.

Another important characteristic of a fatty acid is its *degree of saturation.* **Saturation** refers to the number of hydrogen atoms attached to the carbons in the fatty acid skeletons. If the fatty acid chain can accommodate more

glycerides—the most common lipids, consisting of one, two, or three fatty acids attached to a molecule of glycerol; triglycerides have three fatty acids

glycerol—the 3-carbon compound that is the backbone of glycerides

fatty acids—units attached to glycerol in glycerides

saturation—the degree to which hydrogen atoms fill all available positions along the fatty acid skeleton; a saturated fatty acid is holding as many hydrogens as it has room for, whereas an unsaturated fatty acid is not

hydrogen than it currently does, the fatty acid is said to be *unsaturated*, and the unsaturated carbons will be connected by double bonds.

A fatty acid with no double bonds between carbons is a *saturated fatty acid (SFA)*; a fatty acid with one double bond is a *monounsaturated fatty acid (MUFA)*; and a fatty acid with two or more double bonds is a *polyunsaturated fatty acid (PUFA)*.

Figure 7.2 shows a theoretical example of a triglyceride containing fatty acids of varying chain lengths and saturation.

Triglycerides containing large amounts of SFAs are usually solid at room temperature and are generally found in animal products, such as beef fat and butter. Triglycerides high in MUFAs are usually liquid at room temperature and are generally found in plant products, such as olive oil and nuts. Triglycerides containing mostly PUFAs are also usually liquid at room temperature and are generally found in plant products, such as cottonseed oil and corn oil. Notable exceptions to these generalizations are coconut and palm oils, often referred to as *tropical oils*. The tropical oils, which have been commonly used in processed foods, contain a high proportion of SFAs. Another exception is fish oils, which might be expected to contain primarily SFAs but, in fact, contain many PUFAs. Table 7.1 shows the proportions of saturated, monounsaturated, and polyunsaturated fatty acids in various lipids.

Scientists have learned that there is another important variable in unsaturated fatty acids: the *position* of the last unsaturated bond. This, along with the other distinguishing characteristics of fatty acids, will be discussed further in the section on lipids and health.

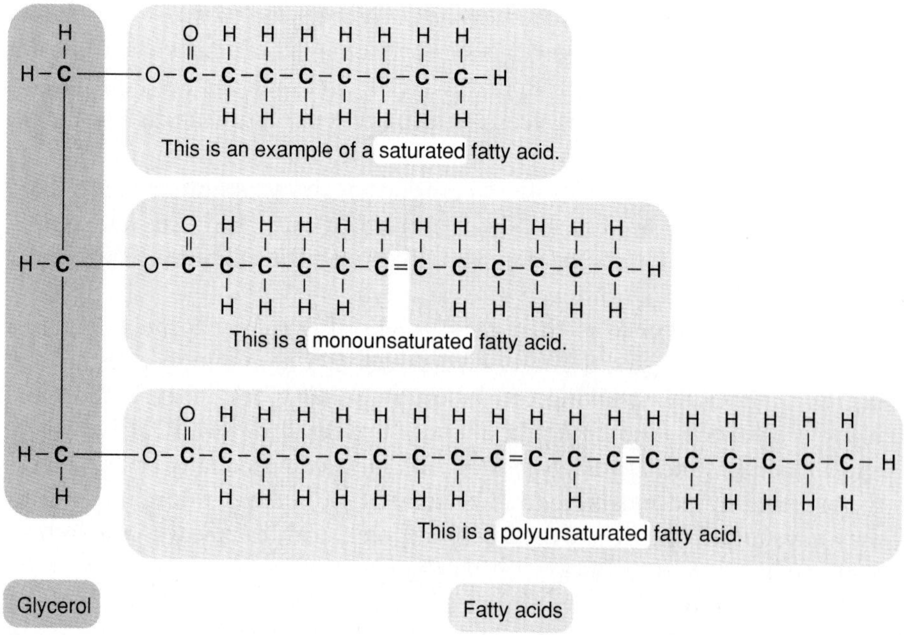

Figure 7.2 Theoretical example of a triglyceride. Triglycerides, which consist of a molecule of glycerol with three fatty acids attached, are the most common forms of lipids found in foods and in the body. Fatty acids can be saturated (no double bonds between carbon atoms); monounsaturated (one double bond); or polyunsaturated (two or more double bonds). Fatty acids can also differ in the position of their double bonds and the length of their carbon chains.

Phospholipids in Nature

Phospholipids are compounds that resemble triglycerides except that a phosphorus-containing unit is substituted for one of the fatty acids. **Lecithins,** a common and important group of phospholipids found in cell membranes, have the biologically useful characteristic of mixing well with both watery and oily substances, which is an unusual trait that a few types of lipids have. This property classifies them as **emulsifiers.**

Sterols in Nature

Sterols are unlike triglycerides in the organization of their carbon, hydrogen, and oxygen components. Nonetheless, they qualify as lipids because they are organic substances with insolubility in water and solubility in ether.

Undoubtedly the most well-known sterol is **cholesterol,** a compound produced by animals, including humans. Cholesterol is particularly abundant in egg yolks and organ meats such as liver. Although cholesterol and satu-

phospholipids—compounds similar to triglycerides but having a phosphorus-containing unit in place of one of the fatty acids

lecithin—type of phospholipid that mixes well with both watery and oily substances

emulsifiers—substances that mix with both fat-soluble and water-soluble materials to help create and maintain suspensions

sterols—class of lipids that includes certain hormones and vitamin D

cholesterol—important sterol that is produced by the body and ingested in foods of animal origin

Table 7.1 Comparison of Dietary Fats

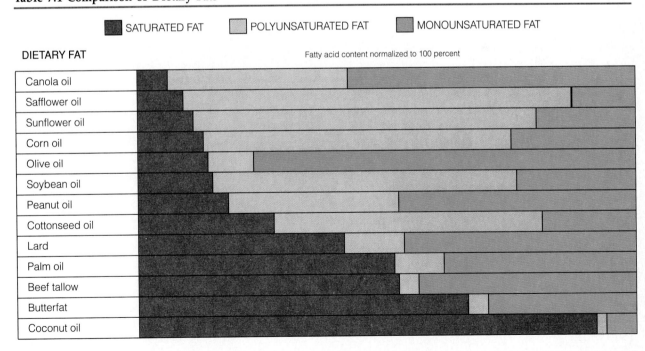

rated fats are both lipids typically found in animal products, they are distinctly different from each other. Other sterols in food include vitamin D and **precursors** of vitamin D; they will be discussed in Chapter 12 (on vitamins).

precursor—a substance from which another substance is formed

Lipids and Processing

Food scientists have developed ways to modify food fats, just as they have modified carbohydrates. For example, it is possible to separate fats and oils (such as butter and lard, and soybean, peanut, and safflower oils) from their natural sources so they can be used as ingredients or as frying agents. Food technology can also prolong the shelf life and sensory appeal of fats and oils through techniques such as refining, bleaching, and deodorizing.

The food industry has also utilized other properties of some of the naturally occurring lipids. Mono- and diglycerides are good emulsifiers, for example, so they are often used as additives to prevent the separation of watery and fatty fractions of products such as salad dressings, margarines, and baking batters. Lecithin can also serve that purpose.

Another application of food science to lipid modification is the **hydrogenation** of oils. This process forces hydrogen into oils with a high PUFA content, thereby increasing their degree of saturation, firming them, and lengthening their shelf life. Hydrogenation can be controlled so as to be partial or complete. A whole range of margarines and shortenings on the market have been hydrogenated to varying degrees; to some extent, you can

hydrogenation—The forcing of hydrogen into unsaturated oils to make them firmer and prolong shelf life

Figure 7.3 Examples of lipids in three processed foods.

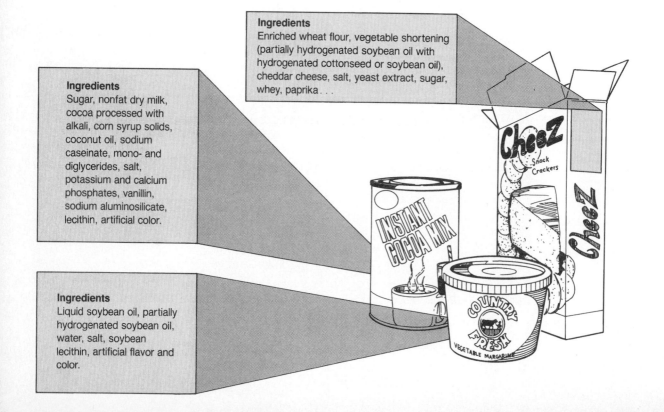

Ingredients
Enriched wheat flour, vegetable shortening (partially hydrogenated soybean oil with hydrogenated cottonseed or soybean oil), cheddar cheese, salt, yeast extract, sugar, whey, paprika . . .

Ingredients
Sugar, nonfat dry milk, cocoa processed with alkali, corn syrup solids, coconut oil, sodium caseinate, mono- and diglycerides, salt, potassium and calcium phosphates, vanillin, sodium aluminosilicate, lecithin, artificial color.

Ingredients
Liquid soybean oil, partially hydrogenated soybean oil, water, salt, soybean lecithin, artificial flavor and color.

judge the level of hydrogenation by how firm or soft they are. Figure 7.3 shows examples of lipids listed on food labels.

In recent years, food technologists have been developing **fat substitutes** that have some of the sensory characteristics (such as look, taste, or mouth feel) of common dietary fats without the same high kcaloric value. One promising fat substitute is **sucrose polyester** (a proposed brand name is *Olestra*), an indigestible compound of fat components and sucrose units. Another is *Simplesse,* made from proteins found in egg white and milk. Of the substitutes just mentioned, only *Simplesse* had been approved for retail purposes by the Food and Drug Administration as of mid-1990—and only for use in frozen desserts. Various carbohydrate-derived products such as *maltodextrin* and *polydextrose* have been in use as partial fat replacements for more than a decade.

Although the idea of having substances that seem like fat without the kcaloric value is appealing, there are problems in the use of most fat substitutes. One problem is defining safe levels of intake, which is important when advising consumers how to avoid excessive use of these products.

fat substitutes—substances that have the sensory properties of fat without the high-kcalorie value of fat

sucrose polyester—a laboratory-produced fat substitute made from a union of carbohydrate and lipid components.

Table 7.2 Fat Substitutes

Substance	Description	Typical Uses	Comments
Maltodextrin Maltrin®	Hydrolyzed corn-starch; water can be added	Used commercially in salad dressings, table spreads, frozen desserts	1–4 kcal/g, depending on water content; can partially replace fat
Nutrifat C®	Hydrolyzed dextrins from wheat, potato, corn, tapioca	Used commercially in cakes, ice cream, mayonnaise, salad dressings	1.2 kcal/g; can partially replace fat
Polydextrose	Water-soluble fiber made from dextrose	Used commercially in baked goods, frostings, frozen desserts, puddings, dry cake and cookie mixes	1 kcal/g due to partial metabolism; serves as a bulking agent and partial replacement for fat and sugar
Shortening replacer N-Flate®	Mixture of emulsifiers, modified food starch, guar gum, non-fat dry milk	Used commercially in baked goods	Can reduce kcal content of cakes by one-third
Simplesse®	Physically modified milk protein and/or egg white protein; water added	Approval limited to frozen desserts; suitable only for unheated foods	1–2 kcalories/gram, depending on formulation; breaks down if heated
Sucrose polyester Olestra®	Chemical union of sucrose and lipid components	Pending approval; suitable for frying; potentially wide variety of uses	0 kcalories; indigestible; will only partially replace fat
Tapioca dextrin N-Oil ®	Hydrolyzed tapioca starch; water can be added	Used commercially in salad dressings, table spreads, frozen desserts	1–4 kcal/g, depending on water content
Trailblazer®	Similar to Simplesse® but by different manufacturer	Pending approval	See comments for Simplesse®

References: 1) Anon. 1989. Fats, oils, and fat substitutes. *Food Technology* 43:66–74. 2) Anon. 1990. Fat substitute update. *Food Technology* 44:92–97. 3) Waring, S. 1988. Shortening replacement in cakes. *Food Technology* 42:114–117. 4) Anon. 1988. Nutrifat. *Food Engineering,* November, 1988.

Another concern is whether these "fake fats" will affect the body's use of other food components. For example, preliminary data indicate that sucrose polyester interferes with absorption of vitamin E from the diet (Toma et al., 1988). Table 7.2 describes various fat substitutes and their characteristics and uses. Several are in use; others are awaiting approval by the FDA or are being developed.

The Amounts of Lipids in Different Foods Vary Considerably

Although you can sometimes see how much lipid is in a food simply by looking at it (such as the fat on meat, or butter on bread), fats are often hidden in food (such as shortening in pie crust or fat in avocado). Therefore, it is hard for most people to estimate their fat intake. In the United States, people consume a higher proportion of "hidden" fats than visible ones (National Research Council, 1989). Table 7.3 compares the approximate amounts of lipids that are present in various foods and food groups.

Table 7.3 Amounts of Lipids in Standard Servings of Various Foods

Food	Household Measure	Lipids (g)
Fruits and vegetables		
Most plain, fresh, frozen, canned fruits and vegetables	½ cup	tr
Potato chips	1 ounce	
Avocado	½ medium	
Grain products		
Quick bread	1 slice	
Plain bread	1 slice	
Cake, frosted chocolate	2 ounces	
Cookies, oatmeal	4 small	
Corn chips	1 ounce	
Plain rice, pasta, most cereal	½ cup	
Milk and milk products		
Milk, whole	1 cup	
Milk, 2%	1 cup	
Milk, skim	1 cup	tr
Cheese, cheddar	1⅓ ounces	
Cheese, processed	2 ounces	
Ice cream	1½ cups	

Table 7.3 continued

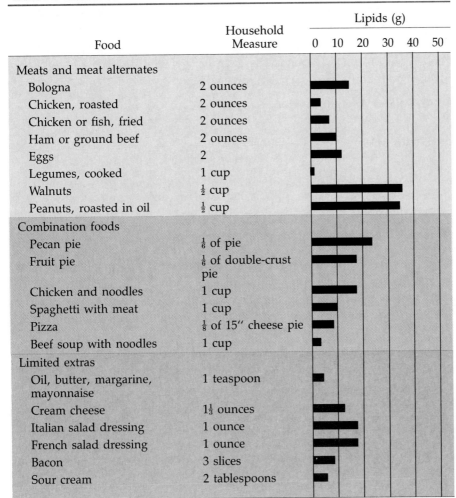

Food	Household Measure	Lipids (g) 0 10 20 30 40 50
Meats and meat alternates		
Bologna	2 ounces	
Chicken, roasted	2 ounces	
Chicken or fish, fried	2 ounces	
Ham or ground beef	2 ounces	
Eggs	2	
Legumes, cooked	1 cup	
Walnuts	½ cup	
Peanuts, roasted in oil	½ cup	
Combination foods		
Pecan pie	⅙ of pie	
Fruit pie	⅙ of double-crust pie	
Chicken and noodles	1 cup	
Spaghetti with meat	1 cup	
Pizza	⅛ of 15″ cheese pie	
Beef soup with noodles	1 cup	
Limited extras		
Oil, butter, margarine, mayonnaise	1 teaspoon	
Cream cheese	1⅓ ounces	
Italian salad dressing	1 ounce	
French salad dressing	1 ounce	
Bacon	3 slices	
Sour cream	2 tablespoons	

Glycerides

As found in nature, fruits, vegetables, and grains have little fat. Fats added during processing or home cooking, however, can substantially raise the lipid level of a product. Look at what happens when plain, fresh vegetables such as potatoes are processed into potato chips, and notice the difference in lipid levels between bread and cake (Table 7.3).

The foods that are naturally high in fat include some dairy products, many meats, and nuts. In the case of dairy products, food technology has developed ways of removing fat to provide some lower fat options: skim milk is almost devoid of fat, for example, as are products made from it, such as yogurt cultured from skim milk. Several cheeses that can be made from partly skimmed milk, such as mozzarella, ricotta, and low-fat cottage cheese, have less fat than their full-fat counterparts. Read the label to be sure. Now, thanks to food processing techniques, cheeses that taste like traditional Swiss and cheddar are produced with reduced fat content.

Many meats and meat products are also being trimmed of their traditionally higher fat values. Both the methods of raising the animals and of processing the meat contribute to this decrease in fat (see Chapter 14).

Critical Thinking 7.1 will help you understand the labeling of some of these new products. Appendices E and F give the lipid levels for many foods. Foods containing fat substitutes will have variable levels; check product nutrition labels.

Cholesterol

Compared to glycerides, cholesterol occurs in only minute amounts in foods. An average serving of food may contain many *grams* of triglycerides, but it will contain only *milligrams* of cholesterol. Your own body produces more cholesterol than your diet provides. This will be discussed in more detail later.

As we mentioned earlier, cholesterol is found only in products of animal origin. Table 7.4 on page 191 compares the amounts of cholesterol in standard serving sizes of certain foods. Notice that there are not many concentrated sources of cholesterol; egg yolk and liver are the only commonly eaten foods that stand out.

Different Lipids Are Digested and Absorbed at Different Rates

In this section we will discuss the digestion and absorption of just two important types of dietary lipids: triglycerides (since they represent the overwhelming majority of lipids we consume) and cholesterol (because it not only is an important structural material but also is associated with heart disease).

Digestion and Absorption of Triglycerides

When triglycerides are consumed, they encounter a small amount of lipase in the stomach, but the vast majority of lipid digestion takes place in the small intestine. There, two types of substances—bile and lipases—play vital roles in preparing lipids for absorption.

bile—substance produced by the liver that maintains emulsions in the small intestine

bile acids—derivatives of cholesterol that are components of bile

lipases—enzymes that digest lipids

Bile is a greenish liquid that is synthesized in the liver and released into the small intestine when fat is present. It contains cholesterol, lecithin, and **bile acids,** which are emulsifiers. Bile salts help keep the triglycerides in small droplets, which makes them more readily available to digestive enzymes.

Lipases, the enzymes that digest lipids, are produced primarily in the pancreas and in the small intestine. They break down triglycerides into monoglycerides, glycerol, and fatty acids, all of which are then incorporated

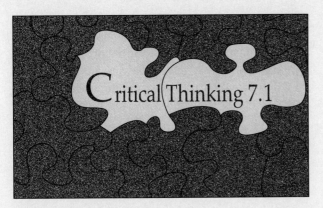

Critical Thinking 7.1

Interpreting Fat Claims on Meat Labels

The situation

You are shopping for groceries, and because you know that your typical daily intake of fat substantially exceeds the recommended 30% of kcalories (you did Assessment 5.2 for several days), you are trying to find foods with less fat. Looking in the lunchmeat and sausage case, you see a number of products with claims on the labels suggesting that the products don't contain much fat.

One type of lunchmeat is labeled "95% fat free," another is labeled "lean," and a package of turkey frankfurters carries a large banner across it reading "lower in fat." With a touch of skepticism, you wonder whether the "95% fat free" claim could possibly be accurate, and you wonder just how much fat is present in the "lean" and "lower in fat" products. You like meat sandwiches and hot dogs, and you hope that these products can help you achieve the lower fat intake you are shooting for.

Is the information accurate and relevant?

Producers of meat and poultry products are required to submit all labels to the United States Department of Agriculture (USDA) for approval before they can be used. This makes it likely that the nutritional claims on these products are technically accurate.

What else needs to be considered?

You pick up the "95% fat free" lunchmeat, assuming that this means only 5% of the kcalories come from fat, but when you look at the nutrition label, you realize that this is not the case. The nutrition label says that each slice contains 1 gram of fat and 25 kcalories. Since 1 gram of fat provides 9 kcalories, fat accounts for 36% of the kcalories.

Then how can the processor claim that this lunchmeat is "95% fat free"? The explanation is that, unless stated otherwise, the percentage of fat on a label *represents the percent of the weight of the product*, not the percent of the kcalorie value. That's true for milk as well: "2% milk" is 2% *fat by weight* but approximately 37% *fat based on kcalories*.

Surely, this can cause a great deal of confusion, but it is not intentional. The problem has historical roots: in the past, many food products such as milk were *valued* for their fat content, and percentage of fat by weight was a convenient measure used by agricultural producers and the food industry to indicate quality; it is the traditional way to express fat content. It is a relatively recent development that nutritional scientists and others concerned about health have suggested limiting fat intake *based on % of kcalories*. Both ways of describing fat content are valid for their purposes, but they are not interchangeable.

Now back to the lunchmeat department. When you check the label of the "lower fat" hot dogs, you find that each hot dog has 9 grams of fat and 110 kcalories. That means that 81 of the 110 kcalories (74%) come from fat! It may seem odd that something can be called "lower in fat" and can have 74% of its kcalories as fat, but this product was appropriately labeled too; in this case, it helps to know the USDA definitions of these terms.

USDA policy memos that went into effect in 1987 state that "lean" and "low fat" can be used only on meat products containing no more than 10% fat, and "lower fat" (also "light," "lite," or "leaner") can be used only on products that contain at least 25% less fat than the majority of their traditional counterparts in the marketplace (Committee on Technological Options, 1988). That means that regular hot dogs have even more fat (i.e., 12 grams or more per hot dog).

What do you think?

Can you include these products in your diet if you want to get no more than 30% of your kcalories for the day from fat? Which of the following options do you think has the most merit? Would you decide differently regarding the lunchmeat and hot dogs?

- Option 1   Give up processed meats, because more than 30% of their kcalories come from fat, even in the lower-fat varieties.
- Option 2   Avoid the regular processed meats, but allow yourself the reduced-fat products a couple of days a week, ignoring your fat intake on those days. You don't have time to do "fancy" calculations.
- Option 3   Decide that a total diet with 30% of kcalories from fat can tolerate some items that

have (on an individual basis) more than 30% of their kcalories from fat, because many other foods have less. Keep food records on several days when you use these products, and see whether you can avoid fat in other foods to come out within the 30% overall limit.

- Option 4   Use Assessment 7.1 (on page 218) to determine a "daily fat budget" for yourself—that is, the number of grams of fat that represents 30% of your usual daily kcalorie intake. Then choose foods with a variety of fat levels, noting the number of grams of fat per serving on the nutrition label, as long as your total intake stays within your daily fat budget.

Do you see other options or combinations that would work?

What makes the most sense to you? Your decision may be influenced by how much time you are willing to spend planning your diet and how important it is to you to reduce your fat intake.

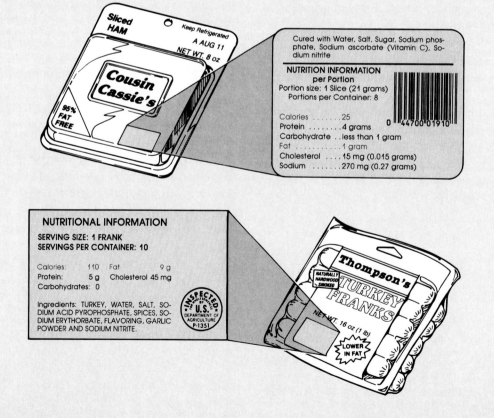

Sliced HAM   Keep Refrigerated
A AUG 11
NET WT. 8 OZ

Cousin Cassie's

95% FAT FREE

Cured with Water, Salt, Sugar, Sodium phosphate, Sodium ascorbate (Vitamin C), Sodium nitrite

NUTRITION INFORMATION
per Portion
Portion size: 1 Slice (21 grams)
Portions per Container: 8

Calories 25
Protein . . . . 4 grams
Carbohydrate . . less than 1 gram
Fat . . . . 1 gram
Cholesterol . . . . 15 mg (0.015 grams)
Sodium . . . . 270 mg (0.27 grams)

0 44700 01910

NUTRITIONAL INFORMATION

SERVING SIZE: 1 FRANK
SERVINGS PER CONTAINER: 10

Calories: 110   Fat   9 g
Protein: 5 g   Cholesterol 45 mg
Carbohydrates: 0

Ingredients: TURKEY, WATER, SALT, SODIUM ACID PYROPHOSPHATE, SPICES, SODIUM ERYTHORBATE, FLAVORING, GARLIC POWDER AND SODIUM NITRITE.

INSPECTED U.S. DEPARTMENT OF AGRICULTURE P-1351

Thompson's TURKEY FRANKS

NATURALLY HARDWOOD SMOKED

NET WT. 16 oz (1 lb)

LOWER IN FAT

Table 7.4 Cholesterol in Some Foods

Food	Household Measure	Cholesterol (mg)
Fruits and vegetables		
All types	½ cup	
Grain products		
Bread, plain	1 slice	
Cake (most plain mix or commercial)	1 piece	tr
Cereal, pasta, grains	½ cup	
Milk and milk products		
Milk, whole	1 cup	~20
Milk, 2%	1 cup	~18
Milk, skim	1 cup	~5
Cheese, cheddar	1⅓ ounces	~30
Ice cream	1½ cups	~100
Meats and meat alternates		
Beef, ground, baked	2 ounces	~55
Chicken, baked, with skin	2 ounces	~55
Fish (cod), baked	2 ounces	~55
Shrimp, boiled	2 ounces	~130
Eggs	2 large	~425
Legumes, nuts	½ cup	
Liver, beef	2 ounces	~270
Limited extras		
Alcoholic beverages	1 serving	
Butter	1 tablespoon	~35
Cream cheese	1¼ ounces	~35
Mayonnaise	1 tablespoon	~10
Vegetable oils	1 tablespoon	

Data sources: 1) United States Department of Agriculture. 1976–1990. *Revised agricultural handbook no. 8 series.* Washington, DC: USDA. 2) Human Nutrition Information Service. 1989. *Agricultural handbook, no. 8, 1989 supplement.* Washington DC: USDA. 3) Pennington, J.A.T. 1989. *Food values of portions commonly used.* New York: Harper & Row.

along with bile salts into conglomerations called *micelles.* Micelles ferry the lipid fragments to the intestinal wall cells for absorption, after which most of the remaining components are recycled to continue the process.

Normally, this system works very effectively. If there is an abundance of bile salts present, over 95% of all fats are usually digested and absorbed by the healthy small intestine (RDA Subcommittee, 1989).

Digestion and Absorption of Cholesterol

Cholesterol in food is often found with a fatty acid attached to it; this is called a **cholesterol ester.** The fatty acid must be removed before cholesterol

cholesterol esters—derivatives of cholesterol and fatty acids

can be absorbed; this is accomplished by enzymes in the small intestine. Cholesterol is best absorbed when micelles are available to ferry it to the intestinal wall cells. In contrast to the thorough digestion and absorption of triglycerides, dietary cholesterol is only partially absorbed; estimates range from 25–75% (Kantor, 1989b), with the average at about 55% (McNamara, 1987). Table 7.5 summarizes the phases of digestion of both triglycerides and cholesterol.

Table 7.5 Summary of Phases of Digestion and Absorption of Two Types of Lipids

	Triglycerides	Cholesterol and Cholesterol Esters
Mouth	—	—
Stomach	Very small amount of enzymatic hydrolysis	—
Small intestine	Emulsification by bile acids; enzymatic hydrolysis to glycerol, fatty acids, and monoglycerides by pancreatic and intestinal enzymes; ferrying by micelles to intestinal wall cells; absorption	Enzymatic hydrolysis of cholesterol esters to free cholesterol and fatty acids; secretion of bile acids (containing cholesterol); ferrying by micelles to intestinal wall cells; absorption
Large intestine	—	—

Your Body Produces Lipids from Various Materials

The products of lipid digestion are largely made into body lipids; however, dietary lipids are not the only source of the fats in our bodies. Here we will discuss the production of triglycerides and cholesterol.

Triglycerides

Once inside your body, many absorbed fragments from dietary triglycerides are reassembled into other triglycerides right in the cells of the intestines; but triglycerides can be synthesized from other materials as well. Remember from Chapter 5 that a surplus of kcalories from any source—that means carbohydrates, proteins, and alcohol as well as lipids—can be converted by the body into body fat. This metabolic thriftiness has served humans through the ages as an important survival mechanism. But if food supplies are seldom scarce and you consistently take in more than you need, you will gradually accumulate an excessive amount of body fat.

Cholesterol

The cholesterol you absorb from food is not the only cholesterol you have in your body; the body, especially the liver, readily produces cholesterol so that there is always enough for its many important functions.

The liver can produce cholesterol from fragments of any of the energy nutrients. In most people, the liver adjusts the amount of cholesterol it produces according to the amount absorbed from the diet. In general, the more cholesterol there is in the diet, the less the liver produces; the less the diet contains, the more the body produces. This *feedback mechanism* works effectively for most people to keep the total amount of cholesterol in their blood quite stable under ordinary circumstances (McNamara et al., 1987). On the other hand, some people's bodies do not compensate as successfully for the cholesterol absorbed from the diet; at least one-third of the population experiences an increase in blood cholesterol when they consume dietary cholesterol (Food and Nutrition Board, 1989). In any event, for most people, the amount of cholesterol produced by the body (primarily in the liver) is substantially larger than the amount absorbed from the diet. Figure 7.4 reinforces this point.

Why is it that the body is so intent on making sure it has enough cholesterol? It is because, as we have mentioned, cholesterol is a very important biological substance. The major use of cholesterol in the body is to be part of bile acids. Additionally, it is an important structural element in cell membranes; it comprises the protective covering on nerves; and it is the material

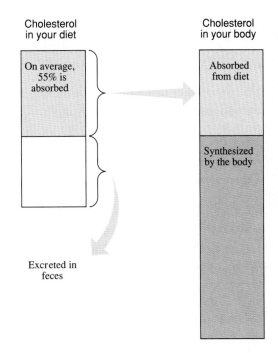

Cholesterol in your diet

On average, 55% is absorbed

Excreted in feces

Cholesterol in your body

Absorbed from diet

Synthesized by the body

Figure 7.4 Where the cholesterol in your body comes from. Only part of the cholesterol in your body is absorbed from food. On average, we absorb 55% of the cholesterol present in the small intestine; therefore, the typical North American 70-kg man, who consumes approximately 450 mg of cholesterol per day, absorbs approximately 250 mg of it. The body of that same man synthesizes approximately 840 mg of cholesterol per day, largely in his liver (From McNamara, D.M. 1987. Effects of fat modified diets on cholesterol and lipoprotein metabolism. *Annual Review of Nutrition* 7:273–290).

from which steroid hormones, vitamin D, and various other body substances are derived. Unfortunately, it can also accumulate in blood vessel walls; this is the one characteristic of cholesterol that is not healthy, because it can cause narrowing of the affected vessels and could ultimately result in blockage. This is how the most common form of cardiovascular disease develops.

We'll say much more about this shortly. In preparation, let's become familiar with how lipids are transported in the body.

Lipoproteins Have a Special Role in Transporting Lipids

As you read above, many of the absorbed lipid breakdown products are quickly reassembled inside the cells of the small intestine into glycerides and cholesterol esters. Other components are not; for example, short- and medium-chain fatty acids, which are water-soluble, can be absorbed directly into the bloodstream and are transported via the portal vein to the liver. But the reassembled triglycerides and cholesterol esters are not soluble in water; they must be put into a water-soluble form, or they would clump together and possibly clog up the vessels. The body makes them soluble by combining them into conglomerates with phospholipids and encasing them in a surface coat that includes protein. The resulting soluble compounds are called **lipoproteins** (Figure 7.5). Lipoproteins can be made not only in the small intestine, but also in the liver. The various types of lipoproteins differ from one another in the amounts of triglyceride, phospholipid, and cholesterol they contain. They also differ in their amounts and types of protein.

lipoproteins—water-soluble aggregates of triglycerides, phospholipids, cholesterol, and protein that can be transported in the bloodstream

Lipoprotein Formed in the Intestine

The principal type of lipoprotein formed in the intestinal wall cell is the **chylomicron.** It contains more triglyceride than any other type of lipoprotein. Chylomicrons move from the intestinal wall cells into the lacteals of the lymphatic system and eventually join the bloodstream. As these and other lipoproteins move through the body, many of them give up their triglycerides to muscle and fat cells along the way.

chylomicron—principal type of lipoprotein formed in the intestinal wall cells; consists mostly of triglyceride

Chylomicrons are short-lived: several hours after an average meal, chylomicrons have been broken apart and their components used for energy and for making other lipids. If you have a blood sample drawn an hour or two after a meal, the level of chylomicrons will be much higher than if you have a sample drawn after many hours without food (Linscheer and Vergroesen, 1988).

On the other hand, the levels of lipoproteins that are synthesized by the liver tend to be present in the blood at more consistent levels throughout the day because they are regulated by the feedback mechanism described earlier.

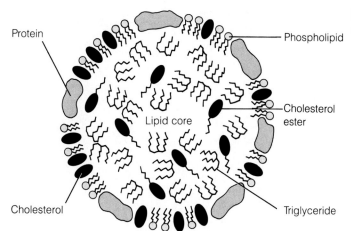

Figure 7.5 General structure
of lipoproteins.

Lipoproteins Formed in the Liver

The lipoproteins formed by the liver are named according to their relative *density* (mass per unit volume). The substances within lipoproteins that are the most dense are the proteins; therefore the lipoproteins containing the most protein are called **high density lipoproteins (HDL).** Other lipoproteins produced by the liver are **very low density lipoproteins (VLDL)** and **low density lipoproteins (LDL).** All of these lipoproteins are released from the liver into the bloodstream, where they undergo considerable change: components of various lipoproteins are plucked off and traded back and forth, sometimes even changing them into different types. For example, much of the VLDL eventually is converted into LDL. Table 7.6 indicates the relative size of these lipoproteins and proportions of various components they contain.

From here on, we will deal primarily with HDL and LDL, the two types of lipoproteins that assume particular importance in the upcoming discussion of cardiovascular disease.

In all individuals, there is much more LDL than HDL present in the blood; this is normal. But there is considerable individual variation in the absolute amounts of LDL and HDL.

Statistics show that individuals who have elevated total cholesterol or elevated LDL cholesterol are statistically at greater risk of coronary heart disease (CHD). On the other hand, high blood HDL levels are *inversely* correlated to CHD. This is why the popular press often refers to LDL as "bad cholesterol" and to HDL as "good cholesterol."

But what is it that *makes* "bad cholesterol" bad and "good cholesterol" good? Scientists are working hard to find an answer. It appears that HDL is likely to take cholesterol *away* from the tissues (i.e., from the linings of blood vessels) and carry it back to the liver. This takes it out of harm's way, at least for a while.

Researchers Michael Brown and Joseph Goldstein shed light on another factor that can affect levels of blood cholesterol (1986). They discovered that

high density lipoprotein (HDL)—lipoprotein containing a high proportion of protein

very low density lipoprotein (VLDL)—lipoprotein containing about half its substance as triglyceride

low density lipoprotein (LDL)—lipoprotein containing a high proportion of cholesterol

Table 7.6 Some Important Lipoproteins in the Bloodstream

Type of Lipoprotein	Major Site of Synthesis	Relative Size and Composition	Comments
Chylomicrons	Small intestine	Triglyceride — Phospholipid — Cholesterol and derivatives — Protein	Present in blood for a few hours after meals; are processed into other forms
Very low density lipoproteins (VLDL)	Small intestine Liver	Triglyceride — Cholesterol and derivatives — Phospholipid — Protein	Most gets converted to LDL
Low density lipoproteins (LDL)	Liver	Cholesterol and derivatives — Phospholipid — Protein — Triglyceride	Some used for bile production; the rest circulates in blood for use in other body materials. Some may accumulate in the walls of blood vessels
High density lipoproteins (HDL)	Liver	Protein — Phospholipid — Triglyceride — Cholesterol and derivatives	Some used for bile production; the rest circulates in blood for other uses

Data source: Linscheer, W.G. and A.J. Vergroesen. 1988. Lipids. In *Modern nutrition in health and disease*, M.E. Shils and V.R. Young, eds. Philadelphia: Lea & Febiger.

there are special structures *(lipoprotein receptors)* on the membranes of liver cells that enable the cells to take in lipoprotein cholesterol, thereby removing cholesterol from the blood and inhibiting cholesterol synthesis by liver cells. If a person's liver cells have fewer of these receptors than normal, the level of cholesterol in the blood is likely to be higher. The relative number of cholesterol receptors a person has appears to be an inherited trait. This discovery was deemed so important that Brown and Goldstein received a Nobel Prize for their work.

Additional research suggests that the receptors recognize lipoproteins based in part on the type of *protein* they contain (Linscheer and Vergroesen, 1988). They especially seem to respond to the proteins prominent in LDL and HDL.

Cholesterol that enters liver cells can be used in various ways. It may be recycled into different lipoproteins, or it may be used to make bile acids. As was mentioned earlier, cholesterol is more likely to become a part of bile than to be used for anything else. Approximately 1000 mg of biliary cholesterol enters a person's intestinal tract each day. Of that, about half is reabsorbed and the other half is excreted (McNamara, 1987). This is the major way in which the body rids itself of cholesterol. Figure 7.6 summarizes the various ways in which the body uses cholesterol and recaptures part of what is in bile.

Lipids Are Involved in Major Health Problems

The previous sections have focused on how food lipids are digested and rebuilt into body lipids and how they contribute to the body's healthy functioning. Now let's take a look at the darker side of lipids—the health problems they may cause or partially affect. Lipids have been implicated to varying degrees in the development of diseases of the heart and blood vessels, in the promotion of cancer, and in the accumulation of excess body fat.

Atherosclerosis and Coronary Heart Disease

Atherosclerosis is the major disease affecting the heart and blood vessels. Heart and blood vessel diseases account for more deaths in the United States

atherosclerosis—disease in which certain materials gradually accumulate in the lining of blood vessels, interfering with their function

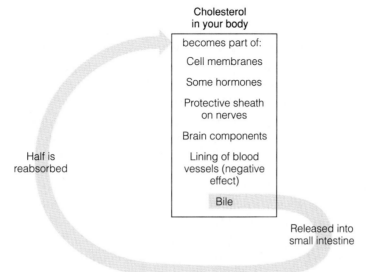

Cholesterol
in your body

becomes part of:

Cell membranes

Some hormones

Protective sheath
on nerves

Brain components

Lining of blood
vessels (negative
effect)

Bile

Half is
reabsorbed

Released into
small intestine

Half is excreted

Figure 7.6 Cholesterol is needed by the body. Many important body substances contain cholesterol. More goes into bile than into anything else, and about half of the cholesterol from bile is reabsorbed (McNamara, 1987 *Annual Review of Nutrition* 7:273–290). The one negative characteristic of cholesterol is that sometimes it is deposited in the linings of blood vessels where it may eventually interfere with blood flow.

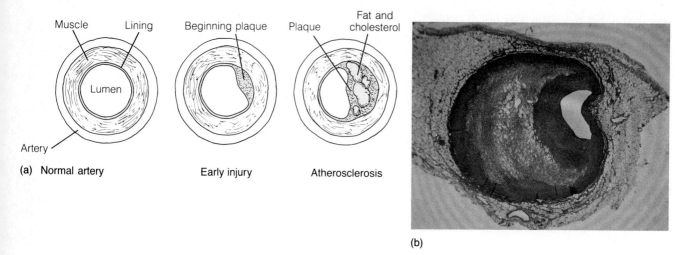

(b)

Figure 7.7 The development of atherosclerosis. (a) This figure shows the progression of atherosclerosis in the cross-section of an artery. The lumen of the vessel becomes progressively smaller as the disease advances, restricting blood flow. (b) This micrograph shows a human artery that is almost completely blocked.

plaque—patches of material that form in the lining of blood vessels in a person with atherosclerosis; consists of cells of the blood vessel lining, cholesterol, calcium, blood cells, and various other materials

stroke, cerebrovascular accident (CVA)—result of interruption of blood flow to the brain

heart attack, myocardial infarction (MI), coronary occlusion—result of interruption of blood flow to the heart

and other developed countries than any other cause. Although the number of these deaths has been declining steadily in the United States since the 1960s, heart and blood vessel diseases still account for almost half of the deaths in this country (Surgeon General, 1988).

Although atherosclerosis has been the subject of thousands of studies of various kinds, *there is currently no absolute proof as to what causes it.* There are two major theories, however (Addis and Park, 1989). One theory proposes that a minor injury to a blood vessel lining—caused by high blood pressure, for instance—prompts certain blood cells, lipoproteins, and other substances in the blood to attach to the injured site, which in turn stimulates the blood vessel to produce more cells to cover over the area. Another theory suggests that the presence of high levels of blood cholesterol or cholesterol metabolites initiate the process by its unusually close contact with the blood vessel linings. In any event, the material that forms inside the blood vessel, which is called **plaque,** progressively narrows the opening (lumen) of the blood vessel and causes it to lose its flexibility (Figure 7.7).

As plaque builds up in a blood vessel, the chances for damage increase: a bit of loose plaque or blood clot could clog the narrowed vessel, a spasm could block it, or a rise in blood pressure could become severe enough to cause the vessel to rupture. Any of these occurrences interrupts the delivery of oxygen and nutrients to the body cells served by the vessel, causing these cells to die within a couple of hours. If the group of cells that die is very important and/or very extensive, the person dies. With less damage, varying degrees of recovery are possible.

Although atherosclerosis can occur in various regions of the body (Figure 7.8), two areas in which the effects of atherosclerosis are most critical are the brain and the heart. If atherosclerosis interrupts blood flow to the brain, a **stroke** or **cerebrovascular accident (CVA)** occurs. If atherosclerosis causes interference with blood flow to the heart muscle, a **heart attack, myocardial infarction (MI),** or **coronary occlusion** will result. The development of atherosclerosis in any of the body's blood vessels, including those of the heart, is

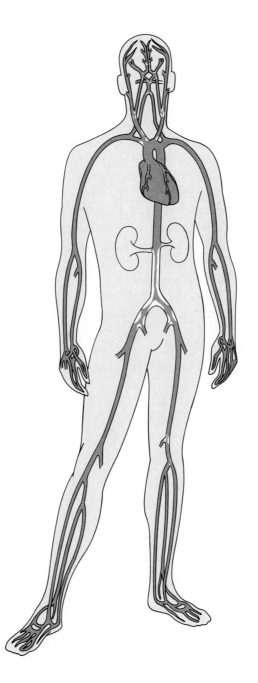

Figure 7.8 More common locations of atherosclerosis. Typical sites of atherosclerosis are shown in this diagram of the major arteries. Plaque tends to collect at points where an artery branches.

known as **cardiovascular (CV) disease;** when it occurs in the heart, it is usually called **coronary heart disease (CHD).**

Although both heart attacks and strokes can result in death, they are not always fatal; important determining factors are the extent of damage and the promptness and quality of care. One third of heart attack victims die within hours of the attack. Here we will look mainly at what is known about CHD, since it is a common type of atherosclerosis and has been the subject of much research.

cardiovascular (CV) disease—gradual impairment of the body's blood vessel function; **coronary heart disease (CHD)** refers specifically to impairment of the heart's blood vessels

risk factors—factors associated with an increased chance of developing a given health problem

Risk Factors for CHD We are not certain of the cause(s) of CHD, but epidemiological and animal studies have shown that it occurs with greater frequency in association with certain characteristics called **risk factors.** Data on risk factors have been collected in many important studies. One such epidemiological research study began in the late 1940s in the town of Framingham, Massachusetts, and data are still being collected and analyzed today on the more than 5000 original participants. Another long-term study involves the community of Tecumseh, Michigan; and the Seven Countries Study provides useful information with a broad geographical sweep. Studies of cardiovascular risk factors in children are being conducted in Bogalusa, Louisiana and Muscatine, Iowa. These and thousands of other studies have identified over 20 risk factors for CHD.

Some risk factors have higher correlations with CHD than others. Some of the high risk factors cannot be changed; being male, growing older, and having a family history of atherosclerosis are *uncontrollable risk factors.* Certain *clinical measurements* can determine other risks; these include such factors as high blood pressure (hypertension), obesity, high blood cholesterol, abnormal electrocardiogram (test of electrical activity of the heart), and diabetes. In addition, particular *lifestyle habits,* such as smoking, consuming too many kcalories and/or fats, being physically inactive, and taking certain medications, correlate with risk. Figure 7.9 shows many of these factors and some of their relationships.

High blood cholesterol, high blood pressure, and smoking emerge as the major modifiable risk factors; they have the strongest statistical association with heart attacks in white American males, a population segment prone to

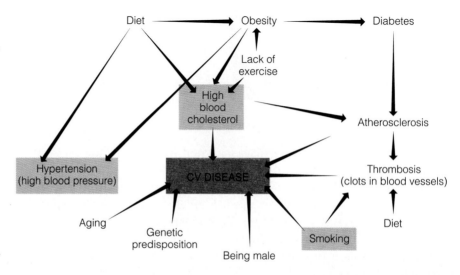

Figure 7.9 Some known contributors to cardiovascular (CV) disease. This model represents some of the risk factors for CV disease that have been identified and some ways they are interrelated. The three most influential *modifiable* risk factors are smoking, hypertension, and high blood cholesterol. Diet influences several risk factors. (Modified from Zilversmit, D.B. and C. Stark. 1984. Diet and cardiovascular disease. *Professional Perspectives.* June, 1984. Ithaca, NY: Cornell University Extension.)

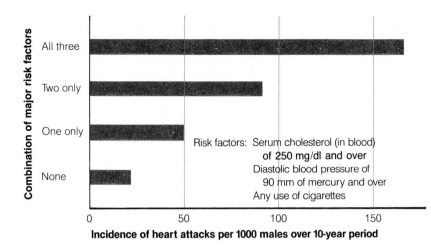

Figure 7.10 The effect of three major risk factors on the incidence of heart attacks in white American males. When the data from many studies were assembled in the National Cooperative Pooling Project, the impact of having one, two, or all three of the risk factors was evaluated. Each additional risk factor almost doubled the risk. (Adapted from Farrand, M.E., and L. Mojonnier. 1980. Nutrition in the multiple risk factor intervention trial [MRFIT]. *Journal of the American Dietetic Association* 76:347–351.) Diastolic blood pressure is the lower number in a blood pressure value, such as 125/72. The 72 indicates the pressure in the arteries when the heart is relaxing. The upper number is the systolic pressure, the pressure in arteries when the heart is contracting.

CHD. Figure 7.10 shows how these factors affected the occurrence of first heart attacks during a ten-year period. Several important points are made by this figure: (1) the more of these risk factors the men had, the more likely they were to have a heart attack; (2) even if they had none of these three risk factors, 20 out of 1000 had heart attacks anyway; and (3) even if they had *all three* of these risk factors, 830 out of 1000 did not have heart attacks during the ten years. It is obvious that although these factors are influential, they do not explain all occurrences of heart disease. Nonetheless, their relative importance has made them the target of major efforts to reduce the incidence of heart disease.

Blood Cholesterol As a Risk Factor for CHD   A high total blood cholesterol level, as indicated above, is one of the three major modifiable risk factors for CHD. Figure 7.11 shows the relationship between serum cholesterol levels and the likelihood of developing CHD. As we saw in Figure 7.10, however, the statistical relationship between blood cholesterol and CHD does not explain all cases of heart disease: *a number of people who have heart attacks do not have excessive levels of total blood cholesterol.*

Many researchers and medical professionals, therefore, are reluctant to rely too heavily on blood cholesterol tests for assessment of risk. Furthermore, it is difficult to pinpoint what a person's blood cholesterol is (Roberts, 1987); different samples from the same person can yield different cholesterol values, and there can be variability between test results that use different laboratory methods (Koch et al., 1988). Methods of standardizing these tests have been suggested for improving their reliability (Laboratory Standardization Panel, 1988). Blood cholesterol values can also vary with the season of the year and even with a person's level of anxiety. For all of these reasons, more than one blood cholesterol test should be done before a diagnosis is made or treatment is initiated.

Figure 7.11 Relationship of serum cholesterol to CHD death. These data were collected on over 350,000 men ages 35 to 57 who were followed for an average of 6 years. Each point represents the median for 5% of the men. (From National Research Council. 1989. *Diet and health*. Washington, DC: National Academy Press.)

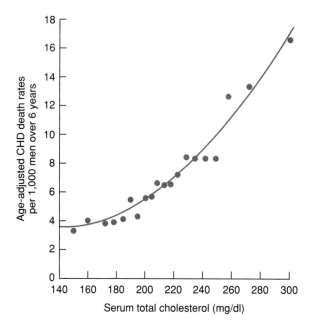

Despite the shortcomings of blood cholesterol data, many experts believe that it is best to keep blood cholesterol levels below 200 mg/dl (that is, 200 mg per deciliter or 100 ml of blood) while also taking steps to reduce other risk factors. Forty-one percent of U.S. adults are estimated to have blood cholesterol values in excess of 200 mg/dl (Sempos et al., 1989). The National Cholesterol Education Program, a public health education campaign involving 20 major health organizations, regards blood cholesterol levels of 200–239 mg/dl as "borderline," and 240 mg/dl or more as high. If a person in the borderline range has two or more of various other risk factors, their risk of CHD is also regarded as high. Table 7.7 lists these factors; note that simply being male is one of them.

Although total cholesterol is a recognized risk factor, we can predict an individual's susceptibility to CHD more accurately by analyzing blood for *the amounts of different types of lipoprotein cholesterol* it contains. That is, risk of

Table 7.7 Other Risk Factors for CHD

According to the National Cholesterol Education Program, if your blood cholesterol level is "borderline high" (200–239 mg/dl) and you have two of the following additional risk factors, then you are considered to be at high risk:

- Male sex
- Family history of premature CHD (heart attack before age 55 in a parent or sibling)
- Cigarette smoking (currently more than 10 cigarettes per day)
- Hypertension
- Low HDL-cholesterol concentration (below 35 mg/dl)
- Diabetes mellitus
- History of other vascular disease
- Severe obesity (more than 30% overweight)

CHD increases *when LDL is high* (such as above 160 mg/dl) or *when HDL is low* (less than 35 mg/dl). HDL values are especially predictive for women, for some unknown reason (Abbott et al., 1988).

You might wonder, then, why HDL and LDL analyses aren't done automatically instead of determining total cholesterol. Total cholesterol is regarded by many health care providers as a reasonable starting point. If the test for total cholesterol indicates risk, then the more expensive, more time-intensive tests for HDL and calculations for LDL are done.

In the future, other measurements involving lipoproteins may be used for predicting risk. Researchers are investigating whether the types of *proteins* in the lipoproteins may be even more sensitive indicators of risk than the lipid components are (Kantor, 1989a). Some people with low blood cholesterol levels who have had heart attacks have been found to have elevated levels of these proteins. More research is needed. Until we have clearer evidence, it seems likely that clinicians will continue to focus on cholesterol values rather than on the protein fraction of the lipoproteins.

Ways to Lower Blood Cholesterol   From what they have learned about how the body handles cholesterol, scientists have identified several possible ways to reduce excessive blood cholesterol. One way is to interfere with the amount of cholesterol that is absorbed and reabsorbed from the gut; another is to reduce the liver's production of cholesterol and/or to increase cholesterol uptake by the liver and increase its excretion of cholesterol. There is also an advantage when your body channels more cholesterol into HDL rather than LDL.

Different types of interventions have been tried with varying rates of success. Exercise has a beneficial effect, primarily by raising HDL levels. Some medications have been found to lower blood cholesterol, but they always have undesirable side effects and are usually expensive. For those who smoke, quitting smoking helps; not only does it lower total cholesterol, but it improves circulation and reduces the likelihood of blood clotting in the blood vessels. Also, dietary modifications have been found to help change cholesterol levels. As noted in Chapter 6, for example, soluble fiber (as in oat and rice bran) can lower blood cholesterol; this occurs because the soluble fiber probably interferes with cholesterol absorption.

With the enormous amount of research that has been done on other effects of diet on blood cholesterol, one might expect that we should know exactly how diet affects blood cholesterol. Unfortunately, many questions remain. One thing we have learned with certainty from these studies is that there is tremendous *individual variation* in how people's blood cholesterol levels change with modifications in diet. By changing just the diet, an occasional person might reduce blood cholesterol by about 20%; more often, the decrease is in the range of 10–15% (Kwiterovich, 1989); in some people there may be no change at all.

The extent of change appears to be affected by genetics, weight fluctuation, initial blood cholesterol levels, and the nature and aggressiveness of the dietary measures used. Therefore, some people with high blood cholesterol levels who faithfully follow the recommended diet may not be able to lower their cholesterol at all, while others may have moderate success. Even with some success, the lowered blood cholesterol level may still be too high. In this chapter our discussion focuses on the factors that involve lipids; other factors are discussed in relevant chapters.

As we discuss dietary measures to reduce risk of CHD, we will give the recommendations of the National Cholesterol Education Program (NCEP) for reducing blood cholesterol in people who have elevated levels (Expert Panel, 1988). The NCEP makes the same recommendations for the general public (1990), and so does the American Heart Association (1988). Be aware, though, that some aspects of these recommendations are controversial, and physicians do not unanimously follow them (Roberts, 1987). We will discuss this at the end of the section on heart disease. Anybody who is at high risk for heart disease should seek the advice of a qualified health care professional for planning a comprehensive risk reduction program. The following are diet-related factors that influence blood cholesterol levels:

- **Excessive body fat.** People who are obese are likely to have higher levels of blood lipids in general. Losing excess fat often helps reduce blood lipids.
- **Total amount of dietary fat.** Reducing total fat in the diet can lower total blood cholesterol; however, some studies show that both HDL and LDL are lowered in the process. Nonetheless, the National Cholesterol Education Program recommends limiting fat intake to 30% of kcalories. This can be helpful both for controlling body weight and for reducing saturated fat, the importance of which is discussed next.
- **Saturated fatty acids in the diet.** Saturated fatty acids (SFAs) are known to be strong promoters of higher LDL cholesterol levels. For this reason, people have been advised for many years to reduce their intake of saturated fats, which are primarily found in animal products (meats and full-fat dairy products) and tropical oils (coconut, palm, and palm kernel oils).

Research within the last several years calls into question whether this effect is uniform for all SFAs. For example, one study showed that a liquid diet high in stearic acid, an 18-carbon SFA found primarily in animal products, did not maintain the higher blood cholesterol levels produced by a liquid diet high in palmitic acid (a 16-carbon SFA found in palm oil) (Bonanome and Grundy, 1988). On the other hand, in several other studies, palm oil had less effect on blood cholesterol than butterfat (Nutrition Reviews, 1987).

The results of these studies suggest that the biological effects of a particular fatty acid cannot be predicted from its degree of saturation alone; among others, the length of the fatty acid chain may also be a factor. It is even more difficult to predict the effect of a *food* that contains a mixture of different kinds of fatty acids. For example, palm oil, which contains almost equal amounts of saturated and unsaturated fatty acids, may behave very differently from coconut oil, which is over 90% SFAs.

The National Cholesterol Education Program recommends that people consume less than 10% of kcalories from saturated fats. More research is needed to determine whether certain saturated fatty acids may be excluded from this suggested limit.

• **Polyunsaturated fatty acids in the diet.**   It is well established that polyunsaturated fatty acids (PUFAs) lower blood cholesterol. PUFAs are prominent in plant products such as vegetable oils, and they are also found in the oils of cold-water fish; but not all of the PUFAs these foods act in the same way. This probably has to do with the structure of the polyunsaturated fatty acid.

Scientists have noted that *the location of the last double bond in the fatty acid chain* makes a difference in the physiological activity of the fatty acid and determines what other substances it can become. Its location is described relative to the carbon farthest from where the fatty acid attaches to glycerol; this last carbon is called the "omega" carbon. Using this system, an omega-6 fatty acid (found in vegetable oils) has its last double bond between the sixth and seventh carbon atoms from the end of the chain. Although omega-6 fatty acids have been found to depress total blood cholesterol, both LDL and HDL seem to be lowered in the process (Grundy, 1989), and prolonged high intakes of omega-6 fatty acids may increase blood pressure over time (Berry and Hirsch, 1986). Further, in some (but not all) studies on laboratory animals, very high intakes of PUFAs have increased the incidence of cancer.

Fish oils are rich in *omega-3 fatty acids*. Depending on the dosage of omega-3 fatty acids and the level of saturated fat in the diet, fish oils can either increase or decrease levels of various blood lipoproteins (Harris, 1989). However, omega-3 fatty acids promote the production of certain prostaglandins that improve the flexibility and reduce the stickiness of red blood cells; these are beneficial because they reduce the likelihood of blood clot formation in blood vessels, which could cause a heart attack (Ney, 1990).

Several epidemiological studies that compared the incidence of CHD in fish-eating populations with that of non-fish-eating populations showed that fish-eaters were less likely to die from CHD; on the other hand, they were more likely to die from strokes (Bjerregaard and Dyerberg, 1988). In a study done in the Netherlands, there were only half as many cardiac deaths among men who ate at least 1 ounce of fish per day as among those who ate none (Kromhout et al., 1985). On the other hand, a study in Canada did not reinforce this finding; the death rate from CHD was higher along the Atlantic coast where fish were commonly eaten than it was in the prairie provinces (Hunter et al., 1988). Many other variables could have affected the outcome of that study.

In an attempt to more closely define the effects of fish oils on cardiovascular health, highly purified fish oil is being used in carefully conducted studies with high-risk patients. Only after much more is known about the short-term and long-term effects of taking fish oil will scientists be able to advise who can benefit from it and how much should be consumed. Some day, specific recommendations may be made as to what proportion of PUFAs should come from omega-3 and omega-6 fatty acids (Simopoulos, 1988). The 1990 *Nutrition Recommendations* for Canadians already do this (Appendix B).

Currently, every responsible organization knowledgeable about heart health advises the public *not* to experiment on themselves with fish oil *supplements*, even though they are available over the counter (see this chapter's Slice of Life). They do recommend *eating fish* a couple of times per week, though. Table 7.8 gives the levels of two of the most common omega-3 fatty acids in a variety of seafoods.

The National Cholesterol Education Program recommends that PUFAs

Table 7.8 Omega-3 Fatty Acids in Selected Seafoods

A number of fatty acids can be classified as omega-3. Two of the most common[a] are very long (20 or 22 carbons) and very unsaturated (5 or 6 unsaturated bonds). This table lists the amount of these two fatty acids that are thought to lower the risk of CVD. In general, the best sources (in bold type) are fatty fish that live in extremely cold water.

Food Item	Mg of certain omega-3 fatty acids[a] per 2 oz. of fish
Finfish	
Anchovy, European	0.8
Bass, striped	0.5
Bluefish	0.7
Catfish	0.2
Dogfish, spiny	1.1
Halibut, Greenland	0.5
Herring	1.0
Mackerel, Atlantic	1.5
Pike, walleye	0.2
Pompano, Florida	0.4
Salmon, different varieties	0.5–0.8
Trout, lake	1.0
Tuna	0.3
Whitefish, lake	0.8
Crustaceans and mollusks	
Clams, softshell	0.2
Shrimp, different varieties	0.2–0.3
Oysters	0.2–0.4
Squid	0.2

[a]Omega-3 fatty acids are considered here to be equal to the content of eicosapentaenoic acid (EPA) and docosahexaenoic acid (DHA).

Data source: Hepburn, R.N., J. Exler, and J.L. Weihrauch. 1986. Provisional tables on the content of omega-3 fatty acids and other fat components of selected foods. *Journal of the American Dietetic Association* 86:788–793.

should comprise up to 10% of the kcalories in the diet; within this 10%, they recommend a couple of fish meals per week.

• **Monounsaturated fatty acids in the diet.** Scientists used to think that monounsaturated fatty acids (MUFAs) were neutral in their effect on blood cholesterol. Epidemiological studies have shown, however, that people in the Mediterranean countries, where monounsaturated olive oil

Slice of Life

Don't Get Hooked on Fishy Sales Pitches

While reading his favorite news magazine, Don noticed an ad picturing an Eskimo fishing. The prominent message was "Scientists share the Eskimos' health secret." The product was fish-oil capsules; the ad stated that fish oils lower the risk of heart disease and possibly also relieve high blood pressure, arthritis, psoriasis, migraine headaches, and the risk of cancer. It suggested that taking a daily capsule of their product could help avoid these problems.

Don's dad had a high blood cholesterol level and was working hard to lower it by exercising more and eating differently. Don had been annoyed when his father had mentioned that it might be good for Don to make similar changes in case he had inherited a tendency toward high cholesterol himself. That's why this fish-oil ad appealed to him—it seemed like an easier way to reduce risk of heart disease than changing his exercise habits and the way he ate.

Don was not unique in being attracted to this idea. We would all be glad to find a simple solution to the complex problem of heart disease. But although data from several studies that compare the health of fish-eaters and non-fish-eaters are impressive, they do not automatically mean we can reap the same benefits from taking concentrated

fish-oil supplements. When people *eat fish* as a significant component of their diets, there are other foods they are *not* eating as much of, such as fatty meats and gravies. One must question whether fish oils would be as beneficial when consumed *in addition to* a high intake of other fats. Also it is uncertain whether other substances in fish need to be present along with the fish oil to produce the benefits.

Other questions need to be answered. What is the safe and adequate range of intake; or, as one respected researcher put it, "When does enough become more than enough?" (Lands, 1986). Also consider the fact that Eskimos eating a diet rich in seafood are known to bruise and bleed more easily and have more strokes; these are likely effects of the fatty acids in fish oils. Are there other undesirable consequences of fish oils? Do fish oils contain toxicants? We know that if people take fish *liver* oils, the high amounts of vitamins A and D they contain can accumulate to toxic levels. Are there other toxic substances present as well? Does fish oil increase the need for some other nutrients?

Obviously, then, this "simple solution" is not so simple after all, given our current knowledge.

This explains why experts in nutrition are careful to advocate eating more *fish as part of meals* rather than taking fish-oil supplements. Furthermore, they suggest that the fish be prepared and eaten without the addition of fat; frying the fish or adding rich sauces could negate the benefits of the natural fish oils. ▼

is liberally used in food, have a lower incidence of heart disease than would have been predicted from their total intake of fat; such evidence called for metabolic studies to be done.

To try to identify the effects of the MUFAs, scientists studied the effects of liquid diets containing more extreme levels of fatty acids than are found in ordinary foods. These studies supported the hypothesis that MUFAs could lower blood cholesterol levels when substituted for SFAs. Now studies using ordinary foods are adding further support, but the number of such studies is still small. MUFAs appear to lower total blood cholesterol largely by lowering LDL levels (Mensink and Katan, 1989; Mattson, 1989); they do not seem to lower HDL as omega-6 fatty acids do.

Currently, recommendations for fat intake do not suggest specific levels of MUFAs but allow MUFAs to make up the remainder of the 30% of kcalories budgeted for fat but not consumed as SFAs and PUFAs.

• **Cholesterol in the diet.**   Reducing cholesterol in the diet can lower total blood cholesterol, but again the extent of the change varies greatly among individuals. *For most people, changing the amount of dietary cholesterol appears to be the least important influence on their level of blood cholesterol* (Kris-Etherton et al., 1988). Even so, the National Cholesterol Education Program recommends that the daily intake of dietary cholesterol should not exceed 300 mg. Since egg yolk and liver are the only common foods that contain much cholesterol, this limit is fairly easy to achieve if you restrict those two foods. It's easy to see that advertisers for high-fat foods (such as margarines) who promote products because they have "no cholesterol" are missing the point: to decrease blood cholesterol, it is more productive to reduce *fat* intake than to reduce *dietary cholesterol* intake. That is why in 1990 the FDA proposed that only food with less than a certain amount of fat could make claims regarding cholesterol content.

Several researchers have hypothesized that cholesterol in the *oxidized* form, a conversion that can occur during food processing or even in blood vessels, may be more damaging to blood vessels than unoxidized cholesterol (Addis, 1986). This idea requires further study.

• **Other dietary factors.**   Sucrose polyester, a fat substitute mentioned earlier, has been found to lower LDL cholesterol without affecting HDL levels (Toma et al., 1988). Preliminary studies are promising, but more research is needed.

Another promising development in biotechnology is the ability to change the nature of fatty acids in common foods. In the future, we may have access to fats and oils that contain types and proportions of fatty acids more favorable to health than the foods currently available (Hammond, 1988).

After All, Is Dietary Change Worthwhile?

In addition to all the aforementioned studies involving how various components of the diet affect biochemical functions, large clinical trials have also attempted to determine whether lowering CHD risk factors actually lowers the incidence of CHD and/or prolongs life. It is difficult to conduct such studies. Often they are flawed or their results are difficult to interpret. For example, one large clinical study showed that lowering cholesterol levels in high risk men *did* reduce their chance of CHD—but their blood cholesterol levels were reduced through the use of *both* drugs *and* a modified diet (Lipid Research Clinics Program, 1984). From this study, it was not possible to tell how effective diet alone would have been.

Effectiveness of Lowering Blood Cholesterol   Evidence accumulated from epidemiologic and clinical studies and data collected in animal studies have convinced many experts that lowering serum cholesterol, especially LDL, reduces the incidence of CHD—at least in middle-aged men with high serum cholesterol (Food and Nutrition Board, 1989). This occurs whether blood cholesterol has been reduced by diet, drugs, or a combination of the two.

Lowering serum cholesterol is not as helpful for women or for people over the age of 50. Some studies have actually found that in older people, lower blood cholesterol is statistically related to greater likelihood of death— but some scientists believe that this occurs because certain terminal diseases (other than cardiovascular disease) cause blood cholesterol levels to drop as disease progresses (Anderson et al., 1987).

One group of researchers developed a mathematical model for predicting to what extent lowering blood cholesterol by dietary means would prolong life. They estimated that the greatest benefits could be achieved by those at highest risk. They calculated that high-risk men might be able to gain 1 to $1\frac{1}{2}$ years with a 20% reduction in blood cholesterol; others (of lower risk to begin with, or who lowered cholesterol by less than 20%) would benefit less (Taylor et al., 1987). These figures, of course, cannot be taken too literally because they are based on calculations and not on experience, but they were developed to give patients an estimate of how much payoff in longevity they might expect for making dietary changes. Note, too, that this study addressed only *quantity* of life—it did not estimate the improved *quality* of life that may occur if a modified diet delays or reduces the symptoms of the disease.

Effectiveness of Lowering Other Risk Factors   Some health experts think that too much emphasis has been put on lowering blood cholesterol. They believe that people could benefit more from making other changes such as quitting smoking or eating more fish—which, as mentioned earlier, reduces the likelihood of blood clotting. The mathematical model mentioned above indicated that a high-risk man in his 20s could add almost 6 years to his life if he stopped smoking. And in a study done in Great Britain, a group of post-heart-attack patients was advised to increase their intake of fatty fish while another group of patients was advised to decrease their fat intake or increase their fiber intake. The study reported 29% fewer deaths among the fish-eating group (Burr et al., 1989). This lower death rate was achieved although the men who increased their intake of fatty fish did not experience a decrease in blood cholesterol.

Should Everybody Change Their Diet?   Nutrition and health experts are divided about who should be encouraged to make dietary changes in an attempt to avoid or delay CHD. The experts are likely to fall into one of two groups.

One group believes that the entire population should make dietary changes without delay. Health agencies and professional societies in many countries have already made specific recommendations to their populations. In the United States, the American Heart Association, the National Institutes of Health, and the Food and Nutrition Board suggest limiting fat intake to 30% of kcalories, reducing saturated fat intake, and limiting dietary cholesterol.

The other group believes we should wait for more conclusive evidence that specific dietary changes do cause reductions in CHD before recommending such changes to the general population. Some scientists are generally skeptical about the relationship between diet and CHD (Harper, 1988). They point out that although dietary intakes vary widely from one developed country to another, average ages at the time of death in those countries are remarkably similar; therefore diet cannot be very important. However, lifestyle practices, the environment, or the quality of the health care system also are likely to affect mortality data, making it difficult to identify the effect of an individual factor.

Another critic of broadscale approaches—this one a science writer—is Thomas Moore. In his 1989 book *Heart Failure,* Moore questioned the potential effectiveness of a program such as the National Cholesterol Education Program and expressed concern about its considerable costs and even its safety.

Even these skeptics believe, however, that we should identify and treat high-risk individuals and their families because if one person in a family is at risk, there are likely to be other family members also at risk (Council on Scientific Affairs, 1983). The American Academy of Pediatrics has taken the position that children in high-risk families should be tested to determine whether they have elevated blood cholesterol; if they do, a cholesterol-lowering diet should be part of the treatment (Committee on Nutrition, American Academy of Pediatrics, 1986; 1989). Care must be taken to ensure that such a diet meets the child's needs for growth. For the general public, the Academy advises that children up to the age of two years should not restrict fat intake but that moderate fat restriction is reasonable after age two and throughout the rest of childhood and adolescence (1986).

The upshot of the debate is that if you want to follow the advice of world experts on this matter, you are in a tough spot since even the experts can't agree on all points. All would probably agree, however, that moderation in fat intake is a good goal for everyone. For more personalized advice in determining what your own risk factors are, see your physician. Now you have some understanding of what affects the development of CHD—as well as an awareness of the limitations of our knowledge.

Cancer

Cancer accounts for the second largest number of deaths per year in the United States. Statistical projections suggest that one person out of four will develop cancer during his or her lifetime, and one in eight to ten will die of the disease. As with atherosclerosis, a great deal of evidence links cancer with dietary lipids.

Many experts believe that the term *cancer* encompasses over 100 separate diseases that afflict different body organs by different mechanisms. The most common sites affected are the lungs, colon, breast, pancreas, prostate, stomach, and blood. Figure 7.12 shows the rates of death from some major types of cancer in men and women in the United States.

Cancer occurs when normal body cells, whose growth and division are carefully regulated in healthy individuals, undergo genetic changes *(initiation)* that allow them to ignore the usual controls. If the body's processes for recognizing and destroying such cells are not functioning normally, the abnormal cells can compete with healthy ones for oxygen and nutrients and eventually spread throughout the body if conditions encourage their growth *(promotion* and *progression)*. This process often takes place over a period of several decades (although there are exceptions). Figure 7.13 illustrates the stages in cancer development.

Possible Causes of Cancer   Although there seems to be a genetic aspect to cancer development, epidemiological data suggest that most human cancers are influenced by one or more environmental factors called **carcinogens.** Certain dietary constituents are among the environmental carcinogens; several leading epidemiologists estimate that about one-third of all cancer deaths may be linked to diet (National Research Council, 1989).

Lipids are thought to be among the most important of the dietary factors

cancer—general term for what are probably many diseases, all characterized by uncontrolled cell growth

carcinogen—environmental factor thought to influence the development of cancer

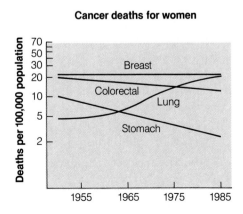

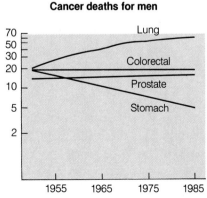

Figure 7.12 **Death rates from cancer for men and women, then and now.** These graphs show age-adjusted death rates for certain cancers in the United States, 1950–1985. [Source: National Center for Health Statistics, 1985. *Health, United States, 1985.* DHHS Pub. no. (PHS) 86-1232. Public Health Service, Washington, DC: U.S. Government Printing Office.]

anticarcinogen—environmental factor thought to interfere with the development of cancer

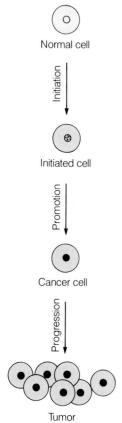

Normal cell

Initiation

Initiated cell

Promotion

Cancer cell

Progression

Tumor

Figure 7.13 Stages in cancer development. Body cells undergo a series of changes in becoming cancerous. Usually initiation occurs in response to certain environmental conditions, including various dietary factors. It is not inevitable that initiated cells will become cancerous; if levels of cancer-promoting factors are low or if cancer-inhibiting factors are high enough, promotion and progression will not occur. It may take 20 or more years for cancer to develop even when conditions that encourage it exist.

related to cancer development; both epidemiological evidence and animal studies support this. Others include excessive amounts of alcohol and toxins produced by molds (see the topic capsule on cancer in the front of the book for others). Examples of nondietary factors are tobacco, radiation (such as ultraviolet and x-ray radiation), viruses, hormones, and various industrial chemicals.

Just as some substances *encourage* cancer, others—called **anticarcinogens**—*prevent* its development. Examples of substances thought to be anticarcinogens are nutrients such as carotenoids and vitamin E (see Chapter 12); others are non-nutrients in food, such as fiber (see Chapter 6). The important point here is that food should not be viewed darkly as only a potential *cause* of cancer; diet can play an important role in cancer *prevention*.

Dietary Lipids As a Risk Factor for Cancer   According to the comprehensive report of the National Academy of Sciences' Committee on Diet, Nutrition, and Cancer, lipids seem to be more closely associated with the development of cancer than any other dietary constituent (1982); this was also the prevailing opinion of the National Research Council in its report *Diet and Health* (National Research Council, 1989). Although some scientists are not convinced, several kinds of data support the hypothesis that lipids are associated with cancer. Epidemiological data from many countries show a correlation between the average daily dietary fat intake of a population and the incidence of cancer of the breast, colon, and prostate (National Research Council, 1989). The data become more convincing when you note what happens to people who leave their homeland and its diet and adopt a new country and its diet; in a generation or two, the incidence of cancer among those people resembles that in the adopted country rather than that in the homeland.

Certain vegetarian groups have been found to have considerably lower rates of cancer than the general population. Although it may be tempting to attribute this finding to the fact that vegetarian diets are often lower in fat, other aspects of diet and lifestyle could influence the incidence of cancer in these population groups. For example, Seventh Day Adventists, approximately 50% of whom avoid meat, experience lower rates of cancer. They generally do not smoke or consume alcohol either, which could also lessen their incidence of certain types of cancer. Mortality rates among Seventh Day Adventists are only 50–70% of the general population rates for cancer in body sites *other* than those related to smoking and drinking. They are also lower for sites *unrelated to fat consumption*. More research is obviously needed to explain the reasons—which are likely to be multifactorial—for the impressively lower rates of cancer among Seventh Day Adventists.

Animal tests strengthen the relationship between dietary fat and cancer (National Research Council, 1989). Animals fed a high-fat diet generally develop more tumors than those fed low-fat diets. This effect may be partially due to the fact that a low-fat diet may also be a low-kcalorie diet, which is known to discourage cancer growth in animals.

Some scientists have been exploring this idea more thoroughly and have become convinced that it is not fat per se that is carcinogenic, but rather *excess kcalories* (Kritchevsky et al., 1986; Pariza, 1986). They point to research that supports their theory. For example, a rat study tested the carcinogenic effect of diets that differed in fat and kcalorie values. Surprisingly, the animals receiving the *most fat* had the *lowest* incidence of breast cancer, but their diet was *lower in total kcalories* by 20% than the other test diets (Boissonneault et al., 1986).

Some human studies have also called into question a link between fat intake and breast cancer in women. One study done in the United States involved almost 90,000 registered nurses from 34 to 59 years of age. They completed a dietary questionnaire designed to measure consumption of fat as well as other nutrients. During the next four years, about 600 cases of breast cancer were diagnosed in these women. When the data were analyzed as to how their intake of fat related to their incidence of cancer, it was found that *the women consuming the* **highest** *proportion of their kcalories as fat (44%) had* **less** *cancer than those consuming the least fat (32%)* (Willett et al., 1987). Other U.S. studies have failed to show a relationship between fat intake and breast cancer (Jones et al., 1987; Mills et al., 1989). A study done in Australia also failed to find an association (Rohan et al., 1988).

How can such conflicting evidence be explained? There are many possibilities. First of all, factors other than diet come to bear on the incidence of breast cancer. One of these is reproductive history: women who have had a full-term pregnancy early in life or who have had more than one pregnancy have a lower risk of breast cancer (Love, 1988). Genetic differences also may have confounded the dietary effects. In addition, when doing studies within a country, the intakes of fat among the women studied may not have occupied a broad enough range of fat quantities to show significant effects; furthermore, even the lowest fat intakes may not have been low enough to affect the incidence. Some experts believe that fat intake earlier in life may be more important than fat intake during adulthood, and studies that assess current diet may not reflect earlier eating habits. Finally, it is possible that total energy intake and body weight, as in the animal study above, were important factors. Until such issues have been addressed, it is impossible to say with absolute certainty whether there is a cause and effect relationship between dietary fat and breast cancer.

Evidence linking cancer of the colon with dietary fat intake, on the other hand, is stronger (National Research Council, 1989). A study done in western New York state substantiated a correlation between high-fat and/or high-kcalorie diets and incidence of colon cancer. Although the influence of other factors such as obesity and an inherited tendency to colon cancer were also seen, men with the highest intakes of fat and kcalories had an incidence of cancer four times higher than that in men with low intakes. For women with high fat intakes, the risk was two-and-one-half times greater than for those with low intakes (Graham et al., 1988).

Attempts have been made to determine whether certain types of fat—

saturated, unsaturated, or the slightly modified fats that can result from hydrogenation—are more closely associated with cancer development than others. It appears that the effects are not even uniform within a given type. For example, some data suggest that certain polyunsaturated fats (especially those high in linoleic acid) are cancer *promoters*. At the same time, there is some evidence that diets containing fish oils may be *protective* (National Research Council, 1989). More studies are needed. In general, the association between total dietary fat and cancer is stronger than the association between any specific type of fat and cancer. But does that statement also hold true for cholesterol?

Cholesterol As a Risk Factor for Cancer   Although there is a general lack of correlation between intake of *dietary* cholesterol and the incidence of cancer, the link between *blood* cholesterol and cancer incidence may be a different matter. A number of studies involving blood cholesterol levels and incidence of all types of cancer together have suggested that if blood cholesterol is low (e.g., less than 190 mg/dl), the statistical risk of cancer is increased. Other studies show an inverse relationship or no relationship at all (National Research Council, 1989).

It is possible that different body sites respond differently to blood cholesterol levels. For example, some studies show that cancer of the lung is more likely to develop in people with low blood cholesterol levels (less than 195 mg/dl) (Isles et al., 1989), and cancer of the colon and rectum are more common in those with elevated blood cholesterol (above 250 mg/dl or 269 mg/dl) (Törnberg et al., 1986; Mannes et al., 1986). These variations could confound studies looking for a similar effect from blood cholesterol on *all types* of cancer.

When studies have shown an inverse relationship between blood cholesterol and cancer, there has been much debate as to whether the low blood cholesterol levels were the *cause* or the *effect* of the cancer. Some experts believe that since the progression of cancer is often accompanied by falling blood cholesterol levels, some cases of low blood cholesterol in these studies were *a result of* a growing cancer that had not yet been detected (preclinical case) (National Dairy Council, 1986). Other researchers seriously consider the possibility that low levels of blood cholesterol *may contribute to the beginning of cancer*, possibly by interfering with the integrity of cell membranes (Isles et al., 1989).

The conflicting information on blood cholesterol and cancer is not consistent enough to be the basis for dietary advice at present. However, there are other suggestions that are on firmer footing about how to reduce risk of cancer through diet, as the next section suggests.

Guidelines for Reducing the Risk of Cancer Through Diet   In the past decade, many organizations have issued advice to the general public about how to use dietary practices to reduce the likelihood of developing cancer. The Committee on Diet, Nutrition, and Cancer of the National Academy of

Sciences issued its advice in 1982, followed by the National Cancer Institute of the National Institutes of Health and by the American Cancer Society, both in 1984. In 1986, the National Cancer Institute revised its recommendations into a format that was similar to the *Dietary Guidelines for Americans.* All of these cancer prevention guidelines have been quite similar in content. In general, these are their recommendations:

- lower fat intake
- increase the intake of whole-grain products
- increase the intake of fruits and vegetables, especially those that are good sources of vitamins A and C and **cruciferous vegetables**
- reduce the intake of pickled, salt-cured, smoked, and charred foods
- limit consumption of alcoholic beverages

Table 7.9 gives more details from the National Cancer Institute's booklet, *Diet, Nutrition & Cancer Prevention: The Good News* (1986).

cruciferous vegetables— vegetables of the mustard or cabbage family (e.g., cabbage, cauliflower, broccoli); so named because their blossoms, when looked at from the top, have the pattern of a cross

Table 7.9 Reducing Risk of Cancer Through Diet

The following recommendations are summarized from *Diet, Nutrition & Cancer Prevention: The Good News,* which was prepared by the Office of Cancer Communications of the National Cancer Institute (NCI, 1986). These reinforce *Dietary Guidelines for Americans,* with comments particularly relevant to cancer risk.

1. **Eat a variety of foods.**
2. **Maintain a desirable weight.**   Some types of cancer are more common among obese individuals.
3. **Avoid too much fat, saturated fat, and cholesterol.**   A diet low in fat may reduce the risk of cancers of the breast, prostate, colon, and rectum; limiting fat intake to less than 30% of kcalories is recommended.
   Choose lean meats, trim visible fat, eat more fish and lean poultry, use low-fat dairy products, use low-fat salad dressings and spreads. Use cooking methods that reduce fat, but avoid charring food, since possible cancer-causing substances may be produced.
4. **Eat foods with adequate starch and fiber.**   Fruits and vegetables with edible peels, lentils, and whole-grain products are generally high in fiber; a high-fiber diet can reduce the risk of colon and rectal cancer. Intakes of 20–30 grams of dietary fiber, not to exceed 35 grams, are recommended per day.
   Regarding fruits and vegetables, choose foods that are good sources of vitamins A and C; these may reduce the risk of certain types of cancer. Vegetables from the mustard family (commonly called the "cabbage family"; technically called *cruciferous* vegetables) contain anticarcinogens that may reduce the risk of cancer.
5. **Avoid too much sugar.**
6. **Avoid too much sodium.**
7. **If you drink alcoholic beverages, do so in moderation.**   Heavy drinking increases the risk of cancers of the mouth, throat, esophagus, and liver.

In addition to dietary factors, there are other ways of modifying your lifestyle to reduce cancer risk. These include avoiding unnecessary x-rays, protecting yourself against too much sun, avoiding dangerous substances in the workplace by following health and safety rules, taking estrogens (female hormones) only as long as necessary, and avoiding smoking. Tobacco smoke causes more cancer deaths than all the other reliably known cancer-causing agents together.

Some scientists say that not enough is known to make such recommendations. Perhaps the best response to that criticism was made in an early set of guidelines by the Committee on Diet, Nutrition, and Cancer (1982) when it stated:

> It is not now possible, and may never be possible, to specify a diet that would protect everyone against all forms of cancer. Nevertheless, the committee believes that it is possible on the basis of current evidence to formulate interim dietary guildelines that are both consistent with good nutritional practice and likely to reduce the risk of cancer. These guidelines are meant to be applied in their entirety to obtain maximal benefit.

With cancer, as with heart disease, consumers must decide which scientific arguments make the most sense to them and whether their own diets put them at risk.

Excess Weight As Body Fat

Excess body fat, as stated previously, results from surplus kcalories from *any* source. But because lipids are so high in kcalories, it is reasonable to say that a high intake of lipids may result in overweight.

Dietary fat may even be "more fattening" than we have long thought: some researchers suggest that kcalories from fat may be more conservatively handled by the body than energy from other sources. In addition, it is possible that the energy value of fat is closer to 11 kcalories per gram, rather than 9 kcalories per gram, the number that experts attributed to fat for many years (Donato and Hegsted, 1985). Research is increasingly finding an association between a high fat diet and a higher proportion of body fat (Bray, 1987; Dreon et al., 1988; Romieu et al., 1988).

Memory Loss

Because many chemicals that are normal constituents of the brain are lipids, some of these substances have come into the limelight in recent years in possible connection with brain function.

choline—component of the phospholipid lecithin

neurotransmitter—chemical substance that conveys a nerve impulse from one cell to another

acetylcholine—a neurotransmitter; choline is a precursor of this substance

Choline, a component of the phospholipid *lecithin,* is one such compound. It is a precursor of a **neurotransmitter**—a chemical substance that is released from a nerve cell when it fires, conveying the nerve impulse to another cell. **Acetylcholine,** the neurotransmitter of which choline is a part, plays a role in memory performance. Further, it has been found that increasing the intake of lecithin increases the formation of acetylcholine. This has led to the hypothesis that increasing lecithin intake might improve memory. Logical as this seems, *normal adults* who took lecithin in a double-blind study did not perform better on memory tests than the control group who took a placebo, even when the lecithin raised their acetylcholine levels to almost double normal levels (Harris et al., 1983).

Alzheimer's disease is one condition in which acetylcholine levels in the brain have been found to be low. Unfortunately, most controlled studies of patients with this disease have not shown improvement in memory when lecithin intake has been increased (National Research Council, 1989). Nevertheless, research continues in the hope that people with disease conditions that include memory loss might ultimately benefit.

Assess Your Own Lipid Intake Compared with Recommendations

With the effects of lipids on health left unsettled in many ways, it may seem difficult to make any recommendations regarding fat intake. However, scientific organizations that are familiar with the literature on both the need for lipids and the risks associated with them have made recommendations that can serve until more is known.

For linoleic acid, the essential fatty acid, the recommended intake is 1–2% of kcalories (RDA Subcommittee, 1989). Based on USDA data, it is possible that Americans get as much as 5–7% of their kcalories as linoleic acid; therefore there is little risk of your developing essential fatty acid deficiency and little need for you to be deliberate about consuming it.

Regarding total fat in the diet, the Food and Agriculture Organization/World Health Organization expresses concern that people in developing countries do not get enough fat; they recommend that they increase their fat intake to 15–20% of kcalories. We Americans have more cause to be concerned about too much fat in our diet. In the United States in 1985 and 1986, the typical consumption of fat accounted for approximately 36% of total kcalories; this is the lowest estimate among several large surveys (National Research Council, 1989). However, the 1989 RDA subcommittee and the National Research Council (1989) recommend a limit of 30% of kcalories from fat. Guidelines for reducing risk of heart disease and cancer make the same recommendation, as was discussed earlier.

In addition to the potential benefits of reducing the risk of disease, lowering fat intake has been shown to have a positive effect on overall nutrient content of the diet. In a 100-day study in which people changed their diets from the typical U.S. high-fat diet to a diet containing approximately 25% of energy as fat, subjects increased their consumption of carbohydrates and many vitamins and minerals (Dougherty et al., 1988). This suggests that Americans could benefit in more than one way by lowering their fat consumption.

Assessment 7.1 shows a practical way of getting 30% of kcalories from fat without having to do lengthy daily calculations. The Nutrition for Living section suggests what kinds of changes in food intake can help reduce your intake of fat.

Determining Your Daily Fat Budget and Discretionary Fat Allowance

Most recommendations for total fat in the diet suggest that you limit your intake to 30% of kcalories.

Assessment 5.2 showed how to analyze your day's diet for the percentages of energy that came from each nutrient. Useful as that technique is retrospectively, it is not very practical when you need to make on-the-spot decisions about whether eating particular foods will result in excessive fat intake.

You may find it more convenient to have in mind a *daily fat budget in grams*. That gives you a numerical reference point against which you can compare the fat content (shown in grams on the nutrition label) of particular items you are considering.

Steps 1 through 3 below show you how to determine your daily fat budget; use a form similar to the one shown in Sample Assessment 7.1.

Assessment 7.1

1. Retrieve an earlier estimate of your approximate daily kcaloric intake. (Use the value from Assessment 2.1; or, if your weight is stable, you can use the estimate of your daily energy needs from Assessment 5.1.)
2. Calculate 30% of that figure.
3. Divide by 9, the number of kcalories in a gram of fat. The answer is your daily fat budget.
4. Next, you will find it useful to know how much fat you take in routinely (your habitual fat intake). You can estimate this based on the fat content of foods you eat every day: for example, how much (and what kind of) milk are you likely to drink? How much meat do you eat?

This type of information is called *food frequency data*. Notice that it does not necessarily include everything you eat every day, as the food records in other assessments do. Food frequency questionnaires emphasize foods that contain the nutrient(s) in question; for example, our focus here is on fat. Fried vegetables (a source of fat) are considered, whereas other vegetables (containing little fat) are not. The items that vary in your diet from day to day will be considered in step 5.

The chart in Sample Assessment 7.1 lists commonly consumed sources of fat. Fill it in to reflect your habitual intake. If you consume other fat sources regularly, add those foods to the chart, using fat contents from Appendices E and F.

5. Now subtract your habitual fat intake from your fat budget for the day. This figure gives you the number of grams of fat available for other things—your discretionary fat allowance.

You can "spend" your discretionary fat allowance as you wish. You may decide to keep your per-item intake of fat to low or moderate levels for most other foods you eat. On the other hand, there may be certain high-fat items that you want to have occasionally, for which you can compensate by selecting other low-fat items for the rest of the day. The person in the sample assessment, for example, might want to have a fast-food quarter-pound hamburger on some days to use her discretionary fat allowance; on other days, she may want to spend it on more butter or salad dressing.

1. Enter approximate daily kcaloric intake ___2700 kcals___

2. Calculate 30% of kcaloric intake ___× 0.3___

   Equals kcalories allowed from fat ___810 kcals___

3. Divide by 9 (kcalories per gram) ___÷ 9___

   Equals daily fat budget in grams ___90 grams___

4. Calculate your usual daily fat intake

Sample Assessment 7.1 Determining your daily fat budget and discretionary fat allowance

Basic Food	Serving Size	Approximate Fat (grams) Per Serving	Servings You Consume Per Day	Daily Fat (grams) from This Food
Fruits and vegetables				
Potatoes, French fried	10 pieces	8	1	8
Potato chips	1 ounce	10		
Grain products				
Bread, yeast	1 slice	1	3	3
Corn chips	1 ounce	9		
Muffin, bran	1	5		
Popcorn, unbuttered	3 cups	1	1	1
Snack crackers, many kinds	1 ounce	8–10		
Milk and milk products				
Milk, whole	1 cup	8		
Milk, 2%	1 cup	5		
Yogurt, made with 2% milk	1 cup	4		
Cheese	1⅓ ounces	12		
Cottage cheese, creamed	2 cups	20	¼	5
Ice cream, reg.	1½ cups	21		
Meats and meat alternates				
Lean meats	2 ounces	6	1	9
Medium-fat meats	2 ounces	10		
Legumes	1 cup	1		
Nuts	½ cup	35		
Combination foods				
Hamburger sandwich	"quarter-pound"	24		
Pizza, cheese	⅛ of 15"	9		
Limited extras				
Oil, butter, margarine, mayonnaise	1 teaspoon	5	3	15
Regular salad dressing	1 ounce	18	1	18

HABITUAL FAT INTAKE (GRAMS)   63

5. Calculate your discretionary fat allowance

   Daily fat budget ___90 grams___

   Minus habitual fat intake ___63 grams___

   Equals discretionary fat allowance ___27 grams___

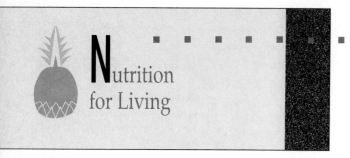

Nutrition for Living

Reducing Fat in Your Diet

Excess dietary fat (or its kcalories) appears to be involved in the development of several of life's major miseries: overweight, heart disease, and cancer. If you want to reduce your fat intake (and, consequently, kcalories), here are some steps you can take:

■ Gradually cut down on fried foods such as fried chicken, fried fish, french fries, and fried chips because frying food usually adds at least 2 teaspoons of fat per serving. Substitute roasted, broiled, baked, steamed, and simmered foods.

■ Try using milk that is lower in fat than your current choice. One cup of whole milk contains the equivalent of 2 teaspoons of butter, 2% milk has 1 teaspoon per cup, 1% milk has half of that, and skim milk is almost fat-free.

■ Reduce the amount of fatty extras you add at the table. These extras include butter and margarine (which are almost pure fat), oily salad dressings, mayonnaise, and other rich sauces. You might try substituting less-fatty alternatives: teaspoon for teaspoon, sour cream only has about 25% as much fat as butter, cream cheese has about 33% as much as butter, and low-fat mayonnaise has about 50% as much fat as regular mayonnaise. Some salad dressings are reduced in fat, and others are almost fat-free.

■ If you snack often, think about your choices. Many snack foods—such as rich snack crackers, nuts, fried chips, cheese, ice cream, and most cookies—are high in fat. Consider substituting fresh fruit; crackers that are less greasy; re-duced-fat cheese food products; ice milk or low-fat frozen yogurt; cereal with low-fat milk; or a bagel with a thin spread of cream cheese or jelly.

■ Eat more fish and poultry and less red meat and high-fat processed meats. When you buy any kind of meat, look for lean cuts. Trim off obvious fat in any case. Cook it without added fat or with as little fat as possible. To reduce fat even further, prepare chicken without skin.

■ Gradually cut back on fat and make substitutions for some high-fat ingredients in recipes. For example, try using low-fat yogurt, buttermilk, or blender-whipped cottage cheese instead of sour cream or mayonnaise. (Caution: You can go only so far in modifying favorite recipes. In some cases, you may be better off to look for new low-fat recipes that have been pretested; such cookbooks are available.)

■ If you have a family history of heart disease and want to cut down your cholesterol intake, restrict your consumption of egg yolks and liver, since these have the highest amount of cholesterol. Egg whites can be used without restriction.

Not all these ideas will suit everybody, but each person may find some that could be worked into his or her lifestyle. As with all intended dietary changes, make your changes gradually so they are more likely to last. For example, you may realize from the above suggestions that many fast-food items are high in fat. If you now eat at fast-food restaurants daily, you cannot expect yourself to suddenly and totally abandon the habit. Instead, begin by changing your habits one or two days each week by eating elsewhere or carrying a lower-fat meal. Gradually make your fast-food meals occasional events.

Finally, to address the other end of the spectrum, note that we are *not* suggesting that people try to totally eliminate fat; it performs many vital functions for us. Moderation is the key.

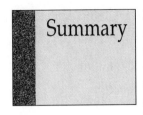

Summary Because of their chemical structure, **lipids** generally do not dissolve in water but do dissolve in such substances as ether. **Fats** and **oils** are common lipids. People think negatively about lipids but enjoy eating them, and evidence of these conflicting attitudes is everywhere.

Lipids have six important functions: (1) they provide energy, stored in compact form as **adipose tissue;** (2) they provide the essential nutrient **linoleic acid;** (3) they carry fat-soluble vitamins into the body; (4) they form body components such as cell membranes and some hormones; (5) they insulate the body in the form of **subcutaneous fat;** and (6) they are deposited in places where they can protect internal organs.

Glycerides are the most common forms of lipids, and consist of one, two, or three **fatty acids** attached to the 3-carbon compound **glycerol.** Triglycerides (having three fatty acids) account for about 90% of the weight of lipids in foods. Fatty acids vary in chain length and in their degree of **saturation** with hydrogen atoms: at room temperature, triglycerides containing long, saturated fatty acids are usually solid (fats), whereas those containing short or unsaturated fatty acids are usually liquid (oils).

Other lipids common in nature are **phospholipids,** such as the **lecithins** present in cell membranes, and **sterols,** such as **cholesterol** and vitamin D.

Food science has developed many ways of modifying food fats, such as separating fats and oils from their natural sources, and **hydrogenating** unsaturated fatty acids to make them firmer. Many **fat substitutes,** such as **sucrose polyester** and *Simplesse,* have been developed for commercial and retail uses. They are at various stages of the approval process, with *Simplesse* having been approved for limited use early in 1990.

The amounts of lipids in different foods vary considerably and are not always obvious on inspection. Foods naturally higher in triglycerides are many dairy products, many meats, and nuts. Cholesterol occurs in variable amounts in food of animal origin and is present in amounts much smaller than triglycerides. Cholesterol is also synthesized in your body.

Lipids take many forms during digestion, absorption, and transport. Triglycerides are broken down into their components by **lipases** and then, along with **bile** salts, are incorporated into micelles and transported to the intestinal wall cells. Cholesterol also reaches intestinal cells by this route. Once in the cells, these non–water-soluble substances are packaged along with proteins into water-soluble **lipoproteins,** which can be carried readily in the bloodstream. Lipoproteins are also synthesized in the liver. There are four major categories of lipoproteins: **chylomicrons, very low density lipoprotein (VLDL), low density lipoprotein (LDL),** and **high density lipoprotein (HDL).**

Lipids concentrate in specific kinds of body substances. Triglycerides are either used immediately for energy or stored as body fat. Phospholipids are found mainly in cell membranes. The fate of cholesterol in the body is currently being studied intensively. Some cholesterol is secreted in the bile; other cholesterol remains in the blood; and some remains in body cells, including the linings of blood vessels. Generally, high levels of LDL cholesterol increase a person's risk of atherosclerosis.

Lipids are involved or suspected of involvement in the development of several major health problems. **Atherosclerosis** is the major disease affecting the blood vessels and is one of the most common causes of death in North America. Although no clear proof of cause and effect is currently available, a variety of evidence suggests that dietary lipids play a role in its long-term development. **Strokes** and **heart attacks,** caused by interruptions of blood flow to the brain and heart, respectively, are serious consequences of atherosclerosis. Many risk factors have been studied intensively in an attempt to learn more about the cause and prevention of this disease. **Cancer,** a general term for many diseases characterized by uncontrolled cell growth, also may be influenced by dietary lipid consumption. Excess fat intake is also implicated in overweight.

Many experts recommend limiting overall fat intake to 30% of kcalories. Assessment 7.1 and this chapter's Nutrition for Living give practical advice for modifying fat intake.

References

Abbott, R.D., P.W. Wilson, W.B. Kannel, and W.P. Castelli. 1988. High density lipoprotein cholesterol, total cholesterol screening, and myocardial infarction: The Framingham Study. *Arteriosclerosis* 8:207–211.

Addis, P. 1986. Occurrence of lipid oxidation products in foods. *Food Chemistry and Toxicology* 24:1021–1230.

Addis, P. and S.W. Park. 1989. Role of lipid oxidation products in atherosclerosis. In *Food toxicology: Perspective on the relative risks,* eds. S.L. Taylor and R.A. Scanlon. New York: Dekker.

American Heart Association. 1988. Dietary guidelines for healthy American adults: a statement for physicians and health professionals from the Nutrition Committee. *Circulation* 77:721A–724A.

Anderson, K.M., W.P. Castelli, and D. Levy. 1987. Cholesterol and mortality: 30 years of follow-up from the Framingham Study. *Journal of the American Medical Association* 257:2176–2180.

Berry, E.M. and J. Hirsch. 1986. Does dietary linolenic acid influence blood pressure? *The American Journal of Clinical Nutrition* 44:336–340.

Bjerregaard, P. and J. Dyerberg. 1988. Mortality from ischaemic heart disease and cerebrovascular disease in Greenland. *International Journal of Epidemiology* 17:514–519.

Boissonneault, G.A., C.E. Elson, and M.W. Pariza. 1986. Net energy effects of dietary fat on chemically induced mammary carcinogenesis in F344 rats. *Journal of the National Cancer Institute* 76:335–338.

Bonanome, A. and S.M. Grundy. 1988. Effect of dietary stearic acid on plasma cholesterol and lipoprotein levels. *The New England Journal of Medicine* 318:1244–1248.

Bray, G.A. 1987. Obesity—A disease of nutrient or energy balance? *Nutrition Reviews* 45(no.2):33–42.

Brown, M.S. and J.L. Goldstein. 1986. A receptor-mediated pathway for cholesterol homeostasis. *Science* 232:33–47.

Burr, M.L., J.F. Gilbert, R.M. Holliday, P.C. Ellwood, A.M. Fehily, S. Rogers, P.M. Sweetnam, and N.M. Deadman. 1989. Effects of changes in fat, fish, and fibre intakes on death and myocardial reinfarction: Diet and reinfarction trial (DART). *The Lancet* 1989:757–761.

Committee on Diet, Nutrition, and Cancer. 1982. *Diet, nutrition, and cancer.* Washington, DC: National Academy Press.

Committee on Nutrition, American Academy of Pediatrics. 1986. Prudent life-style for children: Dietary fat and cholesterol. *Pediatrics* 78:521–525.

———. 1989. Indications for cholesterol testing in children. *Pediatrics* 83:141–142.

Committee on Technological Options. 1988. *Designing foods.* Washington, DC: National Academy Press.

Council on Scientific Affairs, American Medical Association. 1983. Dietary and pharmacologic therapy for the lipid risk factors. *Journal of the American Medical Association* 250:1873–1879.

Donato, K. and D.M. Hegsted. 1985. Efficiency of utilization of various sources of energy for growth. *Proceedings of the National Academy of Sciences USA* 82:4866–4870.

Dougherty, R.M., A.K. Fong, and J.M. Iacono. 1988. Nutrient content of the diet when the fat is reduced. *American Journal of Clinical Nutrition* 48:970–979.

Dreon, D.M. B. Frey-Hewitt, N. Ellsworth, P.T. Williams, R.B. Terry, and P.D. Wood. 1988. Dietary fat: Carbohydrate ratio and obesity in middle-aged men. *American Journal of Clinical Nutrition* 47:995–1000.

Expert Panel. 1988. Report of the National Cholesterol Education Program expert panel on detection, evaluation, and treatment of high blood cholesterol in adults. *Archives of Internal Medicine* 148:36–69.

Expert Panel. 1990. Report of the expert panel on population strategies for blood cholesterol reduction. Press conference. February 27, 1990.

Graham, S., J. Marshall, B. Haughey, A. Mittleman, M. Swanson, M. Zielezny, T. Byers, G. Wilkinson, and D. West. 1988. Dietary epidemiology of cancer of the colon in western New York. *American Journal of Epidemiology* 128:490–503.

Grundy, S.M. 1989. Monounsaturated fatty acids and cholesterol metabolism: Implications for dietary recommendations. *Journal of Nutrition* 119:529–533.

Hammond, E.G. 1988. Trends in fats and oils consumption and the potential effect of new technology. *Food Technology* 42:117–120.

Harper, A.E. 1988. Nutrition: From myth and magic to science. *Nutrition Today* 23(no.1):8–17.

Harris, C.M., M.W. Dysken, P. Fovall, and J.M. Davis. 1983. Effect of lecithin on memory in normal adults. *American Journal of Psychiatry* 140(no.8):1010–1013.

Harris, W.S. 1989. Fish oils and plasma lipid and lipoprotein metabolism in humans: A critical review. *Journal of Lipid Research* 30:785–807.

Havel, R.J. 1988. Lowering cholesterol. *Journal of Clinical Investigation* 81:1653–1660.

Hunter, D.J., I. Kazda, A. Chockalingam, and J.G. Fodor. 1988. Fish consumption and cardiovascular mortality in Canada: An inter-regional comparison. *American Journal of Preventive Medicine* 4:5–10.

Isles, C.G., D.J. Hole, C.R. Gillis, V.M. Hawthorne, and A.F. Lever. 1989. Plasma cholesterol, coronary heart disease, and cancer in the Renfrew and Paisley survey. *British Medical Journal* 298:920–924.

Jones, D.Y., A. Schatzkin, S.B. Green, G. Block, L.A. Brinton, R.G. Ziegler, R. Hoover, and P.R. Taylor. 1987. Dietary fat and breast cancer in the National Health and Nutrition Examination Survey I epidemiologic follow-up study. *Journal of the National Cancer Institute* 79:465–471.

Kantor, M.A. 1989a. Nutrition, cholesterol and heart disease Part II: Structure and functions of lipoproteins. *Nutrition Forum* 6(no.2).

———. 1989b. Nutrition, cholesterol and heart disease Part III: How diet affects blood cholesterol levels. *Nutrition Forum* 6(no.3).

Kinsella, J.E. 1988. Food lipids and fatty acids: Importance in food quality, nutrition, and health. *Food Technology* 42:124–145.

Koch, D.D., D.J. Hassemer, D.A. Wiebe, and R.H. Laessig. 1988. Testing cholesterol accuracy: Performance of several common laboratory instruments. *Journal of the American Medical Association* 260:2552–2557.

Kris-Etherton, P.M., D. Krummel, M.E. Russell, D. Dreon, S. Mackey, J. Borchers, and P.D. Wood. 1988. The effect of diet on plasma lipids, lipoproteins, and coronary heart disease. *Journal of the American Dietetic Association* 88:1373–1400.

Kritchevsky, D., M.M. Weber, C.L. Buck, D.M. Klurfeld. 1986. Calories, fat, and cancer. *Lipids* 21:272–276.

Kromhout, D., E.B. Bosschieter, and C.L. Coulander. 1985. The inverse relation between fish consumption and 20-year mortality from coronary heart disease. *New England Journal of Medicine* 312:1205–1209.

Kwiterovich, P. 1989. *Beyond cholesterol.* Baltimore: The Johns Hopkins University Press.

Laboratory Standardization Panel. 1988. Current status of blood cholesterol measurement in clinical laboratories in the United States. *Clinical Chemistry* 34:193–201.

Lands, W.E. 1986. Renewed questions about polyunsaturated fatty acids. *Nutrition Reviews* 44:189–195.

Linscheer, W.G. and A.J. Vergroesen. 1988. Lipids. In *Modern nutrition in health and disease,* eds. M.E. Shils and V.R. Young. Philadelphia: Lea and Febiger.

Lipid Research Clinics Program. 1984. The lipid research clinics coronary primary prevention trial results: Reduction in incidence of coronary heart disease. *Journal of the American Medical Association* 251:351–364.

Love, R.R. 1988. Dietary fat and human breast cancer: Epidemiological evidence. *Food and Nutrition News* 60(no.3):13–15.

Mannes, G.A., A. Maier, C. Thieme, B. Wiebecke, and G. Paumgartner. 1986. Relation between the frequency of colorectal adenoma and the serum cholesterol level. *The New England Journal of Medicine* 315(no.26):1634–1638.

Mattson, F.H. 1989. A changing role for dietary monounsaturated fatty acids. *Journal of the American Dietetic Association* 89:387–391.

McNamara, D.J. 1987. Effects of fat-modified diets on cholesterol and lipoprotein metabolism. *Annual Review of Nutrition* 7:273–290.

McNamara, D.J., R. Kolb, T.S. Parker, H. Batwin, P. Samuel, C.D. Brown, and E.H. Ahrens, Jr. 1987. Heterogeneity of cholesterol homeostasis in man. *Journal of Clinical Investigation* 79:1729–1739.

Mensink, R.P. and M.B. Katan. 1989. Effect of a diet enriched with monounsaturated or polyunsaturated fatty acids on levels of low-density and high-density lipoprotein cholesterol in healthy women and men. *The New England Journal of Medicine* 321:436–441.

Mills, P.K., W.L. Beeson, R.L. Phillips, and G.E. Fraser. 1989. Dietary habits and breast cancer incidence among Seventh-day Adventists. *Cancer* 64:582–590.

Moore, T.J. 1989. *Heart failure.* New York: Random House.

National Dairy Council. 1986. Diet, nutrition, and cancer: New findings. *Dairy Council Digest* 57(no.2):7–12.

National Research Council. 1989. *Diet and health.* Washington, DC: National Academy Press.

Ney, D.M. 1990. The cardiovascular system. In *Clinical nutrition and dietetics,* ed. F.J. Zeman. New York: The MacMillan Publishing Company.

Nutrition Reviews. 1987. New findings on palm oil. *Nutrition Reviews* 45:205–207.

O'Connor, T.P. 1985. Dietary fat, calories, and cancer. *Contemporary Nutrition,* July, 1985.

Pariza, M.W. 1986. Calories and energy expenditure in carcinogenesis. *Contemporary Nutrition* 11(no.4).

RDA Subcommittee. 1989. *Recommended dietary allowances.* Washington, DC: National Academy Press.

Roberts, L. 1987. Measuring cholesterol is as tricky as lowering it. *Science* 238:482–483.

Rohan, T.E., A.J. McMichael, and P.A. Baghurst. 1988. A population-based case-control study of diet and breast cancer in Australia. *American Journal of Epidemiology* 128:478–489.

Romieu, I., W.C. Willett, M.J. Stampfer, G.A. Colditz, L. Sampson, B. Rosner, C.H. Hennekens, and F.E. Speizer. 1988. Energy intake and other determinants of relative weight. *American Journal of Clinical Nutrition* 47:406–412.

Sempos, C., R. Fulwood, C. Haines, M. Carroll, R. Anda, D.F. Williamson, P. Remington, and J. Cleeman. 1989. The prevalence of high blood cholesterol levels among adults in the United States. *Journal of the American Medical Association* 262:45–52.

Simopoulos, A.P. 1988. Omega-3 fatty acids in growth and development and in health and disease. Part II: The role of omega-3 fatty acids in health and disease: Dietary implications. *Nutrition Today* 23:12–18.

Surgeon General. 1988. *The Surgeon General's report on nutrition and health.* Washington, DC: U.S. Department of Health and Human Services.

Taylor, W.C., T.M. Pass, D.S. Shepard, and A.L. Komaroff. 1987. Cholesterol reduction and life expectancy. *Annals of Internal Medicine* 106:605–614.

Toma, R.B., D.J. Curtis, and C. Sobotor. 1988. Sucrose polyester: Its metabolic role and possible future applications. *Food Technology* 42:93–95.

Törnberg, S.A., L.E. Holm, J.M. Carstensen, and G.A. Eklund. 1986. Risks of cancer of the colon and rectum in relation to serum cholesterol and beta-lipoprotein. *The New England Journal of Medicine* 315:1629–1633.

Willett, W.C., M.J. Stampfer, G.A. Colditz, B.A. Rosner, C.H. Hennekens, and F.E. Speizer. 1987. Dietary fat and the risk of breast cancer. *The New England Journal of Medicine* 316:22–28.

8

Proteins

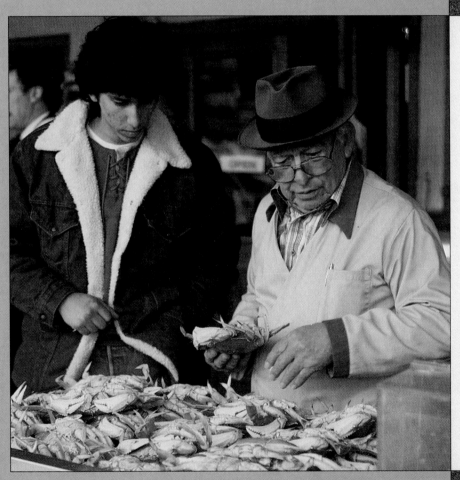

P lay the word association game for a few seconds. *Protein.* What words do you think of? Meat? Lean? Lively? Strong . . . fit . . . energetic? . . . Many people associate protein with muscle, vitality, and fitness. It's true that protein is related to life and vitality, because protein is a critical component of every cell. The cells of your body, a bacterium, an apple, a pine tree, a rhinoceros—every living thing contains protein.

A very inadequate intake of protein for a long period of time will result in loss of muscle tissue, poor physical and mental performance, and a gradual breakdown of vital organ tissues, impairing their functioning. If the diet is grossly deficient in kcalories at the same time—which is the usual situation when protein intake is low—death may result. People in the developing countries face this double deficit much of the time. Such lessons cannot fail to impress us with the importance of getting enough protein and kcalories.

Perhaps our knowledge of this vital need has influenced Americans to value protein above other classes of nutrients. Just page through a household magazine to see how protein and its most popular sources are treated: most meals are planned around the primary protein source; people spend hundreds of dollars and devote backyard and kitchen space to grills that are designed primarily to cook meats; and most people spend the largest portion of their food dollars on meats, fish, and poultry, the most popular sources of protein. There is no question about the status protein enjoys in our society. The name itself reinforces the priority we give it; the Greek word *protos,* from which the word protein is derived, means "first."

This supervaluing of protein has led to another predictable phenomenon: *we tend to give it credit for more than it can deliver.* Look at the ads in various sports magazines for protein supplements that are claimed to improve performance, or at articles about diets that imply that protein will melt fat off your body. In light of scientific evidence, it is clear that these claims have *over*rated protein.

To get a more thorough understanding of what protein is and what it does, we should look first at its structure.

Figure 8.1 Amino acid structures. (a) Generalized structure of amino acids. All amino acids have both an amino ($-NH_2$) group and an acid ($-COOH$) group; they differ only in the makeup of their R groups (green). (b)–(d) Specific structures of three amino acids. The simplest (glycine) has an R group consisting of a single hydrogen atom. An acid group in the R group makes the amino acid more acidic. An amine group in the R group makes it more basic.

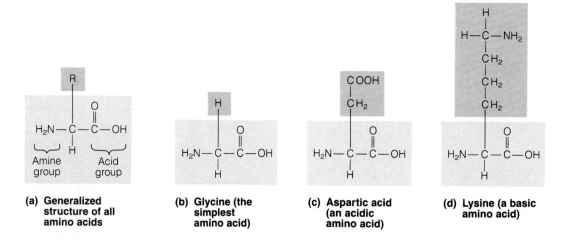

(a) **Generalized structure of all amino acids**

(b) **Glycine (the simplest amino acid)**

(c) **Aspartic acid (an acidic amino acid)**

(d) **Lysine (a basic amino acid)**

Proteins Have a More Complex Structure Than the Other Macronutrients

Protein is an umbrella term that includes thousands of related substances. In the body, some of them are solids, and others are found dissolved within fluids. The major unifying feature shared by the thousands of different proteins is that they are all composed of building blocks called **amino acids.**

The Structure of an Amino Acid

An amino acid, being an organic substance, contains carbon, hydrogen, and oxygen. Unlike other organic nutrients, amino acids also contain nitrogen as a necessary part of their structure, and sometimes sulfur as well.

Approximately 100 amino acids exist in nature, but only 20 of them are used to build proteins. Human cells can produce certain amino acids needed for protein synthesis, as long as the right ingredients are present—compounds containing carbon, hydrogen, oxygen, and nitrogen. Since carbon, hydrogen, and oxygen are liberally available from various dietary sources, the cell has no trouble coming up with those elements, but it has a critical need for nitrogen sources in order to synthesize amino acids.

Figure 8.1 shows the general structure of an amino acid and several examples.

To form proteins, amino acids are linked together by **peptide bonds.** If two amino acids have been joined, the resulting substance is a *dipeptide;* three amino acids create a *tripeptide.* A larger number of connected amino acids constitutes a *polypeptide.* A protein may be made up of one or more polypeptides.

The Structure of a Protein

The structure of a protein is infinitely more complicated—there are sometimes hundreds of amino acids in a single protein molecule. These molecules are bent, folded, or coiled into very specific three-dimensional configurations; Figure 8.2 gives an example. The shape of the molecule is provided by the various cross-linkages formed between amino acids at different places in the chain. The same amino acids may appear many times in a single molecule of a protein, and their order is critical: if one is in the wrong place, or if one amino acid substitutes for another, a different protein may result.

An analogy using letters and words demonstrates the point. Let's say that the letters *A, E, M, S,* and *T* each represent a different amino acid. If you combine these "amino acids" in different ways, you can make different "proteins," such as *steam, mates, teams,* and *meats.* If you add other letters—like an *R* and another *S*—you can then make *masters* and *streams.* Omitting

proteins—thousands of related nitrogen-containing organic substances that have structural, regulatory, and energy-providing functions

amino acids—the approximately 20 "building block" molecules the body uses to construct proteins

peptide bonds—the linkages that hold amino acids together

some of the letters, you can make *stem, same, mesas, rate,* and so on. All are distinctly different "proteins," although they were all derived from the same six "amino acids." This analogy breaks down when we consider molecule size: our "proteins" should have hundreds of letters.

The cells of every living organism have the capability of synthesizing their own proteins, provided they have the right amino acids available. All species of plants and animals construct the unique proteins they need for supporting their own life and growth.

How does the body know how to assemble its different proteins? The answer is found in the nucleus of every body cell, where materials called *deoxyribonucleic acid (DNA)* and *ribonucleic acid (RNA)* contain the information that governs the synthesis of each protein. To extend the letter analogy, DNA and RNA direct the "spelling" of proteins.

When a cell needs to make a particular protein, it draws from the assortment of amino acids available to it at that time. If a cell needs to continue making a certain protein but it runs short of one of the constituent amino acids, it cannot synthesize any more of that protein. The amino acid or acids that are in particularly short supply are called the *limiting amino acid(s).*

The foods we take in contain proteins, but not exactly the same ones that make up our own bodies. The fact that food proteins are not identical to human proteins is not a problem: digestion dismantles food proteins so we can use the components for reassembling our own body proteins (more on this topic later).

Now let's take a more specific look at exactly what it is that humans need from dietary protein.

Figure 8.2 An example of protein structure. This artist's rendering shows two structural patterns—the helix and the pleated sheet—that shape protein molecules. Both patterns depend on hydrogen bonding along the polypeptide chain. The R groups of the amino acids are not shown.

Dietary Protein Needs Are Actually Needs for Nitrogen and Essential Amino Acids

It is something of a misnomer for us to speak of "protein needs": more accurately, we first and foremost need sufficient *nitrogen* from food proteins. Second, we need enough of *certain amino acids* that are necessary for human

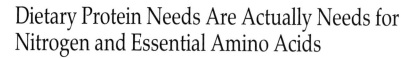

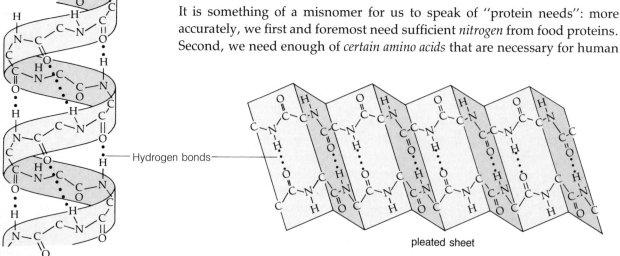

pleated sheet

protein synthesis and that cannot be produced within the body; these are called **essential amino acids.**

These two concerns are often referred to as issues of protein *quantity* and *quality*.

essential amino acids—those the body needs for protein synthesis but cannot produce for itself and so must obtain from foods

Quantity of Protein—Adequate Nitrogen

Recall our earlier statement that living cells can synthesize some amino acids if they have a nitrogen source; and then, once they have the amino acids, they can synthesize their own unique proteins. In a practical sense, then, the most important protein intake issue is quantity: getting enough protein in the diet to provide the necessary nitrogen for amino acid production.

Table 8.1 shows the protein contents of various foods, grouped according to the Basic Food Guide. You can see that, in general, dairy products, meats and meat alternates, and foods made from these offer the greatest amount of protein per serving. But notice that most foods (except some of the limited extras) offer at least *some* protein.

When you see that protein is in almost all of the foods in the four basic groups of the Basic Food Guide, you can see why protein intake and kcalorie intake are so closely related. If your diet is very low in kcalories, it is also likely to be low in protein and therefore nitrogen. On the other hand, if you eat enough of the basic foods to satisfy your energy needs, you will usually get enough protein at the same time. If, however, a large proportion of your kcalories comes from the foods in the very low-protein limited extras group, your protein intake may be inadequate.

Quality of Protein—Adequate Amounts of Essential Amino Acids

The second protein intake issue is one of quality. To be judged of good quality, a food protein must contain adequate amounts of essential amino acids the body needs for protein synthesis but cannot produce by itself.

Nine amino acids are essential in the diet (RDA Subcommittee, 1989). Table 8.2 lists them, as well as the 11 nonessential amino acids (the ones the body can produce).

Not only have scientists learned that these 9 amino acids are indispensable, but they have also estimated what amounts of most of them are needed by the human body. Figure 8.3 illustrates our relative needs for specific essential amino acids. To be judged of good quality, a good protein should contain the essential amino acids in those approximate proportions. In fact, one way of indicating protein quality is for scientists to calculate a *chemical score,* which reflects the amount of the most limiting amino acids compared with a *reference protein* of excellent quality such as egg or milk protein. In such a system, the proteins with the most desirable proportions of amino acids earn the highest scores.

Table 8.1 Amounts of Protein in Standard Servings of Various Foods

RDA for 19–24 year-old male: 58 grams/day
RDA for 19–24 year-old female: 46 grams/day

Protein (grams) — scale: 0, 5, 10, 15, 20, 25

Food	Household Measure	Protein (grams) — bar graph
Fruits and vegetables		
Fruit, all kinds	$\frac{1}{2}$ cup	~0
Peas	$\frac{1}{2}$ cup	~4
Corn, potatoes	$\frac{1}{2}$ cup	~2
Lettuce, green beans	$\frac{1}{2}$ cup	~1
Grain products		
Bread, roll	1 slice, 1	~2
Cookies, small	4	~2
Pasta, cooked cereal	$\frac{1}{2}$ cup	~3
Popcorn	3 cups	~3
Tortilla, waffle	1	~2
Milk and milk products		
Milk, all kinds	1 cup	~8
Cheese, hard	$1\frac{1}{3}$ ounces	~8
Cheese, processed	2 ounces	~11
Ice cream	$1\frac{1}{2}$ cups	~8
Pudding	1 cup	~8
Meats and meat alternates		
Beef, lean	2 ounces	~15
Chicken breast, roasted	2 ounces	~15
Fish	2 ounces	~12
Eggs	2 medium	~11
Peanuts	$\frac{1}{2}$ cup	~19
Peanut butter	$\frac{1}{4}$ cup	~19
Tofu	6 ounces	~12
Combination foods		
Cheese pizza	$\frac{1}{8}$ of 15" pie	~14
Chicken and noodles	1 cup	~18
Bean burrito	6 ounces	~12
Spaghetti with meat	1 cup	~14
Macaroni and cheese	1 cup	~13
Cream of mushroom soup	1 cup	~4
Beef soup with noodles	1 cup	~4
Limited extras		
Butter, salad dressing, carbonated beverages		
Cream cheese	$1\frac{1}{3}$ ounces	~3
Gelatin dessert	$\frac{1}{2}$ cup	~2

Table 8.2 Essential and Nonessential Amino Acids

Amino Acids Essential in the Diet	Amino Acids Not Essential in the Diet
Histidine	Alanine
Isoleucine	Arginine
Leucine	Asparagine
Lysine	Aspartic acid
Methionine	Cysteine[a]
Phenylalanine	Glutamic acid
Threonine	Glutamine
Tryptophan	Glycine
Valine	Proline
	Serine
	Tyrosine[a]

[a]The amino acids cysteine and tyrosine are not essential, but can substitute in part for methionine and phenylalanine, respectively.

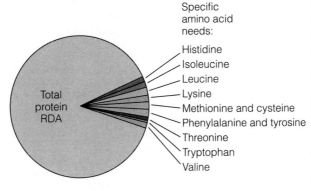

Specific amino acid needs:
Histidine
Isoleucine
Leucine
Lysine
Methionine and cysteine
Phenylalanine and tyrosine
Threonine
Tryptophan
Valine

Total protein RDA

Figure 8.3 Relative amounts of essential amino acids and total protein needed by adults. This figure makes two points: the first is that, all together, the essential amino acids represent only a small portion of the recommended total amino acid (protein) intake. The other is that the essential amino acids are not all needed in the same amounts. (RDA Subcommittee, 1989; Young and Bier, 1987.)

In reality, protein quality reflects not only amino acid content but also how well the body can make use of what is present. To determine this, scientists have found it useful to feed a particular protein to an animal and assess the biological effects (Munro and Crim, 1988).

The simplest and crudest test of this type involves measuring the weight gain of a laboratory rat fed a particular test protein compared to another rat fed a reference protein; this yields a value called the *protein efficiency ratio*. Another method consists of giving a known amount of a specific type of protein and then determining how much protein was deposited in the animal's body tissues; this is *net protein utilization*. In humans or animals, a test of *biological value (BV)* can be done by feeding known amounts of a specific food protein, measuring excreted nitrogen (the indicator for protein) in urine and feces, and then calculating the percentage of nitrogen—and ultimately protein—that was retained. Although these methods yield different numerical results, they all suggest that the protein quality in some types of foods is better than others.

The results of these tests all indicate that food proteins from animal sources are generally of higher quality than proteins from plant sources. The following are some representative foods and their biological values: egg protein, 100; cow's milk, 93; fish, 76; beef, 74; soybeans, 73; whole wheat, 65; peas, 64; peanuts, 55. The proteins that match human needs *best* are found in eggs and milk, but meats, fish, poultry, cheese, and soybeans (a notable plant source) also have protein of *good quality*. The proteins in other legumes, nuts and seeds, most grains, and vegetables get a *fair* rating. A protein of unquestionably *poor* quality is gelatin; note that the poor quality of this animal protein is an exception to the general rule.

These ratings correspond generally with information about the essential amino acid content of these foods; the greater the number of *limiting amino acids* a food has, and the more severe the limitations, the lower the quality of its protein. Table 8.3 lists the amino acids most likely to be in short supply and identifies some foods in which their levels differ substantially from human needs.

Knowing that animal products provide both a higher quantity and a higher quality of protein, one might think that we would advise against **vegetarian eating styles,** since they avoid animal products to one degree or another. Not so, although we need to make a couple of qualifications.

There are many different types of vegetarians. Other than their common trait of avoidance of some or all animal products, their food intakes (and other lifestyle practices) may be widely different from one another (Ameri-

vegetarian eating style—eating habits that avoid some or all animal products

Table 8.3 Status of Limiting Amino Acids in Some Foods

	Cystine	Methionine	Lysine	Threonine	Tryptophan
Cheese, eggs, milk, meat			X	X	
Corn			—	—	—
Legumes	—	—	X	X	—
Whole grains (with germ)		X	X	—	
Nuts, seed oils, soy beans		—	X	X	
Sesame seeds, sunflower seeds	X	X	—		X
Peanut protein		—	—	—	
Green leafy vegetables, leaf protein		—			
Gelatin		—	—		—

Symbols: X = High amount of amino acid present in that food.
— = Low amount of amino acid present in that food.
Blank spaces indicate a general good balance of amino acids in the food.

Adapted from Erhard, D. 1971. Nutrition education for the "now" generation. *Journal of Nutrition Education,* 3:135.

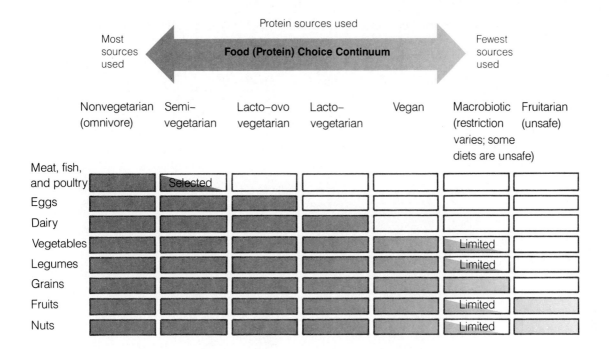

can Dietetic Association, 1988). Vegetarians are usually further defined according to *which* protein-containing foods they use or avoid. The better-known variations are as follows:

- **semivegetarian**—avoids only certain kinds of meat, fish, or poultry
- **lacto-ovo vegetarian**—avoids eating any animal flesh, but uses dairy products and eggs
- **lacto-vegetarian**—avoids eating animal flesh and eggs, but uses dairy products
- **vegan**—avoids *all* foods of animal origin, even dairy products and eggs
- **macrobiotic vegetarian**—progresses through ten dietary stages, starting with widely inclusive, then becoming increasingly restricted
- **fruitarian**—includes only fruit, nuts, honey, and/or olive oil

The differences between these eating styles are shown graphically in Figure 8.4. Note that the first three groups do not totally avoid animal products; they all include milk, a protein source of very high quality. When the diets of these vegetarian groups are evaluated, they are generally found to contain as generous amounts of protein as do the diets of people who eat all types of food, who are called **omnivores**. Like many North Americans, they are likely to take in almost double the protein they need, which gives them a glut of both essential and nonessential amino acids.

The fourth group on the list, vegans, rely exclusively on foods of plant origin. Even most vegans can easily meet their protein needs. Various food group plans have been developed for vegan use that supply adequate intakes for adult vegans (Mutch, 1988). Early in this book, Table 2.5 adapted

Figure 8.4 Some types of vegetarianism. The term *vegetarian* means different things to different people. This figure identifies some types of vegetarians according to how great a variety of protein sources they allow themselves. Note that the fruitarian and many macrobiotic diets are so restricted that they are unsafe.

omnivores—people who eat all kinds of food

the Basic Food Guide for the needs of the vegan. In this chapter, Table 8.4 reiterates the guide and shows a sample menu.

Table 8.4 Basic Food Guide for the Adult Vegan

The recommended intakes of foods from the Basic Food Guide are shown below with a sample day's menu. The guidelines are *minimum* recommendations; some vegans will need to eat more to meet their needs for energy.

Summary of Recommendations	Est. Protein per Serving (grams)	Approx. Total (grams)
Fruits: 1–4, including 1 raw vitamin-C	0	0
Vegetables: 4, including 2 or more dark leafy greens	2	8
Grain products		
Whole-grain yeast bread: 4 slices	2	8
Other grains: 3–5	2	6–10
Meat alternates		
Legumes: 2 servings	15	30
Nuts or Seeds: 1 serving	15	15
	TOTAL	67–71

SAMPLE DAY'S MENU

Breakfast

½ cup orange juice
1 cup cooked oatmeal with raisins, dried apples, and cinnamon
2 slices whole-grain toast
2 tablespoons peanut butter

Lunch

1 cup split pea soup
1 whole-wheat English muffin with butter or margarine
1 cup spinach salad with French dressing
2 medium oatmeal cookies

Dinner

Mixed entree of:
  1 cup lima beans
  ½ cup onions, celery, and water chestnuts
  ½ cup tomato sauce
½ cup buttered broccoli
1 cornmeal muffin with butter or margarine
1 cup apple juice

Snacks

3 cups popcorn
grapes
¼ cup mixed nuts

Two principles that apply to the use of any food group plan but that have special significance for the vegan are *to select variety within the food groups* and *to eat sufficient amounts of food.* The reason we emphasize variety for the vegan is that humans need essential amino acids in particular proportions, as we have mentioned. It isn't important that the amino acids present in any one individual food match the pattern that represents human needs, as long as the assortment available from everything eaten during the day does fulfill those needs (American Dietetic Association, 1988). The amino acids from the foods we eat become part of a general pool of circulating amino acids from which amino acids are drawn as needed; as long as enough of the essential amino acids enter the pool to restore those used during the day, the body is able to continue normal protein synthesis.

This means that even though a given plant protein has one or more limiting amino acids, a more generous amount of that amino acid from another food or foods can make up for the shortfall in the first; this principle is called **complementing** (from the root word *complete*) or **mutual supplementation.** Figure 8.5 gives examples of foods whose amino acids substantially complement each other within the same dish. Many of these combinations have been commonly used in various world cultures—from the familiar American peanut butter sandwich (the peanut is actually a legume) to the more exotic *hummus* of the Middle East. Note that although it is not necessary to get all the right proportions of essential amino acids within the same meal, these dishes promote healthy variety in protein sources that will satisfy the overall daily need for amino acids.

Another perspective on the issue becomes clear when looking at Figure 8.3; notice what a small proportion of the total recommended intake for amino acids needs to come from essential amino acids. If you consume your RDA for protein, even from all-plant sources, you are likely to get as much as you need of the essential amino acids. The important principle here is *to eat enough food from the basic food groups* to fulfill your overall needs for energy and protein.

complementing (mutual supplementation)—eating together foods whose amino acids are *collectively* in proportion with human needs, although individually they are not

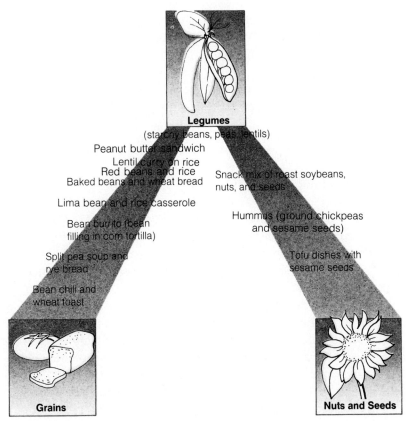

Figure 8.5 Complementary protein relationships important to some vegans. Low-quality protein in a plant food can be made more biologically valuable by combining it with another food that makes up for its amino acid shortfalls. Generally, legumes have complementary relationships with grains and with nuts and seeds.

Some groups of vegans find that meeting their needs for optimal amounts and proportions of essential amino acids is a challenge: these are people whose bodies need to make more protein but whose overall food intake may be too low to supply the necessary basic ingredients. The classic examples are pregnant and lactating vegan women, whose bodies need protein for added maternal tissues, for the fetus, and for milk production. For the pregnant or lactating vegan, it is a wise safeguard to intentionally complement protein intakes over the course of the day while generally increasing overall food consumption. This can be accomplished by using a special eating guide (given in Chapter 16) that will help her meet her increased needs for not only protein but also other nutrients.

Children who are vegans are another consideration. Vegan children, like all children, need extra energy, protein, and other nutrients to achieve normal growth. They also need more protein of higher quality: almost half of their recommended protein intake should be composed of essential amino acids (Young and Bier, 1987). Since foods of plant origin tend to have lower-quality proteins and lower concentrations of them (and of some other nutrients) compared with an equal volume of foods of animal origin, the vegan child may need to eat a larger quantity of food than he or she wants to consume. Unfortunately, some children who consume vegan diets fail to thrive (Williams and Worthington-Roberts, 1988). Therefore, although it is *possible* for vegan children to meet nutritional needs if they eat sufficient quantities of a well-planned plant-based diet, the practicalities suggest that children are likely to be better nourished if they include some animal sources of protein in their diets. Fortunately, vegan parents often see the wisdom of this approach and provide their children with lacto-ovo or lacto-vegetarian diets.

Before we leave the topics of protein quantity and quality, we should discuss how protein is shown on a nutrition label, since it relates to both matters.

Nutritional Labeling of Proteins

Labels will change during the 1990s, but as this book is going to press, the top of nutrition labels lists the number of grams of protein and other macronutrients in a serving of food. The bottom part of the label indicates what percentages of the U.S. RDA for protein and some other nutrients are present in a serving of the food.

To account for the differences in protein quality between foods, two standards exist in the U.S. RDA for protein: one that is used for foods that have higher-quality protein, and one for those of lower quality. Since theoretically the body can make better use of the higher-quality protein, its U.S. RDA is set at 45 grams. For the lower-quality protein, the U.S. RDA is 65 grams.

Changes in how protein quality is evaluated for labels have been proposed. Both now and in the future, when the protein content of a food is expressed as a percentage of the standard, the consumer does not need to have any knowledge of what quality of protein is present, since it is already taken into account.

Protein and Its Derivatives Have All Three Major Functions

One way of underscoring protein's crucial role in the body is to note its involvement in all three general types of functions nutrients can have. Proteins constitute body structure, regulate various body processes, and are an energy source. In this section we look at examples of how protein performs each of these functions.

Constituting Structure

Protein is a part of every living cell: it is part of the cell membrane (along with phospholipids and cholesterol), the cytosol, and the small organelles floating in the cytosol, including the nucleus. Therefore, it is a key component in the structure of the body.

Proteins that give structure and definition to the body are prominent in such tissues as skin, muscles of internal organs, skeletal muscle, connective tissue, and the matrix (framework) of bones and teeth. Many different kinds of proteins make up these tissues.

To a certain extent, the composition of body proteins is also variable from one person to another, depending on the DNA code inherited. For example, a slight difference in normal proteins results in individuals having A, B, AB, or O blood types. Occasionally, an organism is genetically programmed to make a consistent error in protein synthesis. For example, small variations in the amino acid content and arrangement of the blood protein hemoglobin can result in serious blood diseases, such as sickle-cell anemia (Figure 8.6). In this condition, red blood cells are misshapen and unable to function normally. The course of this disease, which is found predominantly in blacks, is a painful one that often results in early death.

Regulating Processes

Proteins influence a variety of *metabolic functions.* You have already learned that enzymes, which are proteins, are critical to the process of digestion. But that is not the only function they perform: there are thousands of different types of enzymes in the human body that accomplish many different tasks. Without them, biochemical reactions would occur so slowly that life as we know it could not be supported.

Figure 8.6 Serious consequences of an error in protein synthesis: sickle cell anemia. This photograph shows both healthy red blood cells (disk-shaped) and sickle cells (crescent-shaped), which are unable to perform the normal oxygen delivery function of hemoglobin. This drastic difference occurs as a result of one incorrect amino acid in the hemoglobin structure.

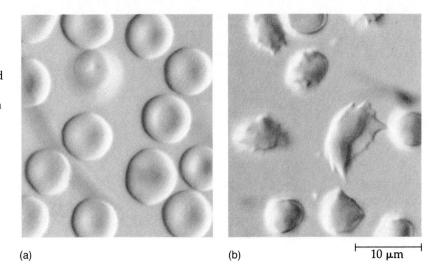

(a)

(b)

⊢———10 μm———⊣

Other proteins influence metabolic reactions. For example, *hemoglobin* is a blood protein that carries oxygen to be used for energy production in body cells. *Myoglobin* is a related protein present in muscle. If the levels of these proteins in the body are low, the amount of oxygen that can be delivered to cells will also be low, and energy production will be compromised. There are many soluble proteins in the body that serve as carriers for nutrients.

Hormones, some of which are proteins or peptides, are chemical messengers produced in one part of the body to affect a process in another region. Among the many processes that hormones affect are metabolism and reproduction. Insulin is an example of a protein hormone.

Proteins are also critical to the body's *defense network.* Because proteins are present in skin, they are part of the body's first line of defense against infection. However, the skin is just one of several protein-dependent defenses.

If disease-causing bacteria attempt to enter the body via any of its various openings, they are likely to be destroyed by bactericidal substances found in mucosal secretions. But if disease-causing bacteria or viruses gain entry anyway, other aspects of the body's immune system take over. The body recognizes that the invading organisms consist of unfamiliar proteins (called **antigens**), and it produces its own proteins (called **antibodies**) to search and destroy the organisms. If a person's protein intake has been inadequate for an extended period of time, the immune system is not able to function as well, and the person is more likely to develop an active case of the disease (Myrvik, 1988).

Proteins affect *mineral balance* and *fluid balance.* The proteins in cell membranes function as gatekeepers that control the access of certain electrolytes to the cell. For example, sodium ions are actively pumped out of the cell by these proteins, whereas potassium ions are pumped in. The appropriate location of these electrolytes is critical to the function of nerves and muscles. Without the right balance of these minerals in intracellular and extracellular fluids, such vital functions as the beating of the heart cannot take place. The

antigens—foreign substances, such as proteins, that can provoke an immune response

antibodies—proteins that protect the body against antigens by binding to and inactivating them

location of these minerals affects distribution of body water, as you learned in Chapter 4.

Protein is involved in fluid balance in a more direct way as well. In Chapter 4 you learned that water tends to move across membranes to equalize the concentration of particles on the two sides. Soluble proteins, along with electrolytes, are among the dissolved particles that influence fluid shifts. For example, albumin, the most abundant soluble protein in blood, helps maintain the fluid volume within blood vessels. If blood protein levels fall from severely inadequate protein intake for several weeks, some fluid will move from the blood into interstitial spaces. This condition is called *edema*.

Another function of proteins is to help maintain *acid–base balance*. Body systems require their fluid environments to have a specific pH in order to function normally; Figure 8.7 shows the different pH of various fluids needed in the body. The strong hydrochloric acid produced by the stomach provides the low pH the stomach enzyme *pepsin* needs to begin protein digestion; at any higher pH, the function of pepsin would be compromised. The pH of the bloodstream, on the other hand, must be maintained between the narrow range of 7.35 and 7.45, or basic metabolic processes will cease (Marieb, 1989). In the most severe cases of acid–base imbalance, death results.

How can the pH of various body environments be maintained so precisely? Essentially, there are three mechanisms by which the healthy body accomplishes this: the respiratory system, the kidneys, and chemical buffer systems. Of the chemical buffer systems, the *protein buffer system* is the most powerful.

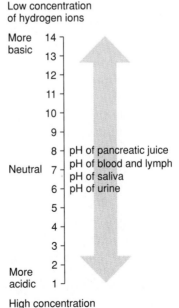

Figure 8.7 Normal pH of various body fluids.

A buffer, as you learned in Chapter 4, is a substance that minimizes changes in pH by releasing or binding hydrogen ions. Soluble proteins, notably those within body cells, are very effective buffers because of the activity of parts of their side groups (R groups). As the pH drops into the realm of 3 to 5, the acid group on glutamic acid or aspartic acid, for example, can accept hydrogen, thereby raising the pH. If the pH rises above 8, amino groups on amino acids such as lysine and arginine are important releasers of hydrogen ions, thereby lowering the pH. These changes can occur within a fraction of a second and are therefore the first line of defense when conditions occur that could affect pH (Smith, 1983).

Proteins are also important in *nerve impulse transmission*. At least three amino acids, *tryptophan, tyrosine,* and *glutamic acid,* are known to be neurotransmitters or precursors of neurotransmitters. (We discussed another neurotransmitter precursor, choline, in Chapter 7 [on lipids].) As with choline, researchers are working to learn how diet may affect the production of these neurotransmitters, and how they in turn may affect behavior and nervous system function within the space of a few hours.

The fact that diet can influence these important biochemicals leads people to fantasize about the possible effects of controlling behavior or mental function by eating certain types of foods. (Wouldn't you like to be assured that your memory and thought processes would be in top form if you ate certain foods before an exam?) However, this area is still highly experimental; it is too early to suggest applications of most of these theories to real-life situations.

serotonin—a neurotransmitter having several functions, including the ability to promote sleepiness

Researchers Judith and Richard Wurtman suggest that diet might affect behavior via the neurotransmitter **serotonin,** which is made within the brain from the essential amino acid tryptophan. Among the many physiological functions of serotonin is its ability to promote sleepiness. If the level of tryptophan in the brain is increased, the production of serotonin is increased, and sleepiness ensues.

Since tryptophan is an amino acid, and proteins are rich in amino acids, one might think that high-protein foods would therefore cause sleepiness. The Wurtmans suggest that this is not the case. They hypothesize that after a high-protein meal, many amino acids compete with tryptophan to get into the brain, so the amount of tryptophan that gains entry is not particularly high. However, after a high-carbohydrate meal, insulin lowers the blood levels of these competing amino acids, just as it lowers blood glucose. This may enable tryptophan to get into the brain more easily, where it produces serotonin and promotes sleepiness.

The nonessential amino acid tyrosine is a precursor for the neurotransmitters *dopamine* and *norepinephrine*. These substances are known to have an effect on blood pressure and depression. Studies are in progress to determine what the practical applications of such relationships might be.

The nonessential amino acid *glutamic acid* functions as a neurotransmitter that excites brain cells to higher levels of activity (Barinaga, 1990); in excess, it can actually stimulate nerve cells to death. The amounts of this amino acid that occur in the proteins of common North American foods are usually not dangerous, but some naturally occurring chemical relatives of glutamic acid have caused serious problems: in 1987, about 150 Canadians became seriously ill from eating mussels high in this type of chemical. Four people died, and twelve survivors suffer permanent memory loss. Fortunately, these are very rare occurrences.

Providing Energy

Like carbohydrates and lipids, proteins can be metabolized for energy; they yield 4 kcalories per gram. However, as you learned in Chapter 5 (on energy), the body primarily uses available carbohydrates and fats, saving proteins for their unique uses as much as possible. Estimates regarding what proportion of a day's energy use might come from protein range from 1% to 15% (Goodman, 1988).

There are several circumstances in which the body increases its use of protein for energy. If carbohydrate and fat are insufficient to meet the body's energy needs, protein will be broken apart and *deaminated* (have amino groups removed) and be metabolized in place of carbohydrate (Figure 5.7). Or if the central nervous system needs glucose but no carbohydrate is available from any source, the same process occurs. (This reemphasizes the protein-sparing function of carbohydrates.)

Somebody who is on a weight-reduction diet that severely restricts both kcalories and carbohydrate is likely to metabolize some body protein to make up the excessive energy deficit. Some evidence also exists that during the early weeks of a demanding conditioning program, especially in untrained individuals, protein usage for energy increases.

The Body Handles Protein Very Efficiently

Although the structure of protein is complex, the body has no trouble dismantling it. In fact, the body treats proteins pretty harshly, beginning in the stomach; obviously the treatment is effective since 95% or more of the proteins that arrive in the small intestine are absorbed (Ganong, 1989).

Before we discuss the digestion of protein, it is important to point out that food is not our only source of this nutrient; our own bodies provide a substantial amount of protein for internal recycling every day. Both digestive juices and the cells that line the digestive tract (which are sloughed off and replaced every couple of days) contain proteins that are digested and absorbed along with the proteins from food. Some experts estimate that as much as 70 grams of protein per day are made available from these sources, compared with 100 grams of protein per day from the average American diet (Munro and Crim, 1988).

Digestion, Absorption, and Transport of Dietary Proteins

After being chewed and swallowed, the proteins in food meet their first chemical challenge in the stomach. Here, hydrochloric acid begins the process of taking apart the large protein molecules. The first step in unfolding protein structure is called **denaturation.** (Proteins can be denatured outside the body, too, by heat, alcohol, and certain other chemicals.)

denaturation—unfolding of the three-dimensional structure of a protein

In addition, the stomach enzyme pepsin breaks some of the long protein strands into polypeptide units containing many amino acids. We mentioned earlier that pepsin is specially designed to work in the harsh acid climate of the stomach. Most of the body's other enzymes would themselves be digested by stomach acids, but this one finds the acid environment ideal. In fact, if the stomach juices are not acid enough, pepsin cannot function.

Pepsin has its limits, though; it just begins breaking down proteins so they are more vulnerable to the battery of enzymes they will face in the small intestine. In the small intestine, many other **proteases** from the pancreas and intestinal wall cells take up the task of dividing the long, unraveled protein and polypeptide strands into units suitable for absorption. The enzymes succeed in reducing most proteins to tripeptides, dipeptides, and single amino acids. There is evidence that some large polypeptides, and even intact proteins, escape digestion in the healthy GI tract and are able to be absorbed; however, these are thought to represent a minor proportion of proteinaceous substances absorbed (Gardner, 1988).

proteases—protein-digesting enzymes

After absorption, these substances travel via the portal vein to the liver and then are carried into the general circulation. Table 8.5 summarizes the steps of digestion and absorption.

Table 8.5 Summary of Phases of Protein Digestion and Absorption

	Proteins
Mouth	—
Stomach	Unraveling of protein strands by acid; hydrolysis by enzyme pepsin to polypeptides
Small intestine	Hydrolysis of most proteins by pancreatic enzymes and enzymes from intestinal wall cells to amino acids, dipeptides, tripeptides; absorption
Large intestine	—

Food Allergies—An Irregularity in the Body's Handling of Proteins?

For many years, food allergies have been presumed to be the consequence of a "leaky" gut that allowed large polypeptides or intact proteins to be absorbed and enter the circulation, where they were recognized as antigens; as a consequence, the immune system produced antibodies, and some sort of allergic reaction ensued.

Now that scientists know that at least a small amount of intact protein *normally* enters the bloodstream of a healthy person, it is apparent that had the original explanation been adequate, we would all have allergies (Gardner, 1988). From what we currently know, it is likely that genetic predisposition has something to do with food allergies (allergies tend to cluster in families), and environmental factors—such as foods fed during infancy—may also have an effect. Even though there is much we don't know about how allergies develop, the methods by which allergists (physicians specialized in the treatment of allergies) have traditionally identified and treated their patients are still appropriate.

Allergies can manifest themselves in surprising ways. An allergy may cause symptoms far removed from the gastrointestinal tract. A person with a food allergy might experience respiratory symptoms (such as asthma or sneezing); skin symptoms (rash, hives); nervous system symptoms (headache, dizziness); cardiovascular symptoms (rapid heartbeat); urinary symptoms (blood in the urine); or gastrointestinal symptoms (vomiting, diarrhea).

Food allergies may be difficult to diagnose, not only because they can take so many forms, but also because the symptoms may take several hours to occur. On the other hand, some people react to offending foods almost immediately.

Opinions vary somewhat as to which foods most commonly lead to allergic reactions. The American Academy of Allergy and Immunology lists cows' milk, egg white, peanuts, wheat, and soybeans as the most common protein allergies in the United States. Shrimp, tomato, codfish, and crab also have been implicated (Thompson, 1986).

Because food allergies are more likely to occur in infants, the best practice is for the mother to breastfeed her baby and to delay introducing the common allergens into an infant's diet. This is an especially wise tactic for an infant with a family history of allergies (International Life Sciences Institute, 1986).

If an infant does develop food allergies, is he or she saddled with them forever? Usually food allergies subside by about the age of 5. In an allergic child, however, the possibility always exists that other types of substances, such as inhaled pollens or dust, may result in sensitivities when the child is older.

We have a few final cautions about food allergies. Because they manifest themselves with such a wide variety of symptoms, some people are tempted to ascribe any puzzling adverse physiological or behavioral symptoms—such as arthritis or mental or emotional illness—to food allergy, without having an adequate scientific basis for such a connection. If such people severely restrict their diets for a long period of time in an attempt to avoid presumed allergens, they may develop nutritional problems if their "allergy diet" ignores basic nutritional needs. Self-diagnosis and dietary self-treatment can also become a serious problem if it prevents such people from getting an accurate diagnosis of their condition, which should be the basis for treatment.

People who suspect they have food allergies are advised to seek out a physician with specialized training in allergy diagnosis and treatment, such as a member of the American Academy of Allergy and Immunology (AAAI). Skin-prick tests and challenge tests (ingesting the suspect food or substance in measured amounts under controlled conditions) are the most accepted means of diagnosis. Cytotoxic testing (mixing food extracts with a person's white blood cells in a laboratory dish) and sublingual challenges (placing a bit of the suspect food or substance under the tongue) are regarded as questionable in their accuracy (Anderson and Sogn, 1984).

Once a food allergy has been diagnosed, an allergist can help a patient learn how to avoid the offending substance (the preferred approach to treatment) and/or prescribe a medication for relief of symptoms.

The AAAI estimates that less than 2% of the American population have true food allergies. An additional small proportion has food sensitivities, which produce symptoms similar to allergies but are not caused by invasion of foreign proteins.

Food Technology Can Make or Modify Proteins and Their Derivatives

Now that you are familiar with how the body handles protein, you have the background for understanding a discussion of the technological modifications of protein. The reason it is important to have the physiological information first is that some objections have been raised about what processed proteins and their derivatives might do in the body.

New and old processes provide us with a whole range of products that Nature never thought of—from processed proteins shaped into entirely new foods to isolated amino acids. And as with technological modifications of carbohydrates and fats, there are potential advantages and disadvantages to their use.

Processed Proteins

Soybeans are a high-protein food that is processed in many different ways. For example, recent technology enables soy protein to be separated from most of the other soybean components into *soy protein isolates*. These can be spun into strands of texturized vegetable protein and then shaped and flavored into *meat analogues* that resemble foods such as hot dogs, veal cutlets, or meatballs. Sometimes the manufacturer improves on the protein quality of these products by adding limiting amino acids.

Soy protein concentrates, another derivative, are also produced by removing some of the nonprotein components of soybeans, but not as many as are removed to make isolates. Soy protein concentrates are used to provide texture and to aid in emulsification, fat absorption, and water absorption.

The practice of modifying soybeans to produce new forms of food is far from new; Oriental cultures have done so since antiquity. *Tofu* is a curd product made from water in which soybeans have been soaked; the soy proteins in the water are separated and pressed into a cake, resulting in a product with a texture resembling soft cheese. People who use it should realize that a large serving—6 ounces—is needed to provide as much protein as a 2-ounce serving of meat. *Miso,* an Asian soybean paste that is used as a flavoring ingredient or condiment, also is a soy-protein-containing food. However, it does not usually contribute much protein to the day's diet, since only small amounts of it are likely to be used at once.

Fish is another high-protein food that can be remodeled into new forms. Although it is an ancient Japanese practice, there has been recent commercial interest in the production of *surimi,* a slurry made from minced, fresh fish. First it is washed to remove the fishy taste, then seasoned, flavored, and shaped into look-alikes of lobster, shrimp, and other seafood (Martin, 1988).

Another protein that is commercially isolated is *casein,* a cow's milk protein. Casein or its derivative, *sodium caseinate,* is used as an ingredient in foods such as frozen dessert toppings and coffee whiteners. *Hydrolyzed vegetable protein* is used as a flavoring component. Figure 8.8 shows some examples of proteins or their derivatives as found in processed foods.

Figure 8.8 Examples of protein or protein derivatives in two processed foods.

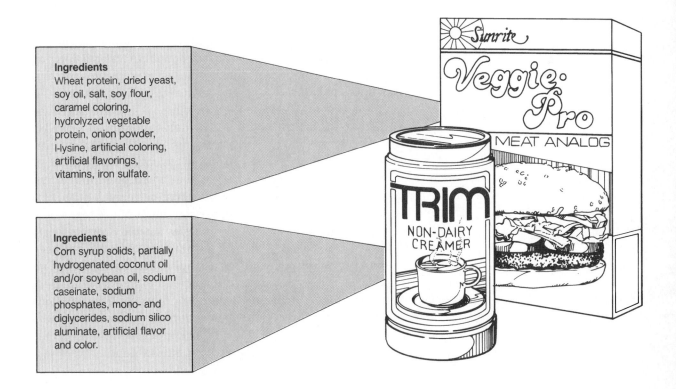

Ingredients
Wheat protein, dried yeast, soy oil, salt, soy flour, caramel coloring, hydrolyzed vegetable protein, onion powder, l-lysine, artificial coloring, artificial flavorings, vitamins, iron sulfate.

Ingredients
Corn syrup solids, partially hydrogenated coconut oil and/or soybean oil, sodium caseinate, sodium phosphates, mono- and diglycerides, sodium silico aluminate, artificial flavor and color.

Processed Amino Acids

Food technologists are also able to isolate individual amino acids and produce dipeptides. The use of these products, however, has met with varying degrees of success. Some amino acids have been added selectively to grain products to enhance their protein quality; the intention was to improve the protein quality in diets of people in developing countries, especially those whose diets were based on one staple grain product. Although this application may seem to have merit, in practice it didn't help much. That is because the major problem in these countries was an *overall shortage of food*; if sufficient food to supply the amount of energy needed for growth and activity had been available, enough protein would have been present also. Since their kcalorie intake was inadequate, most of the protein in their diets was metabolized for energy.

Monosodium Glutamate (MSG)   An amino acid derivative that has been in widespread use for decades is *monosodium glutamate (MSG)*. MSG is made from *glutamic acid*, mentioned earlier as a neurotransmitter. It has been available for decades as the flavor enhancer "Accent"; it is present in many commercially prepared foods and can be purchased for home use. There has been some question about whether the amounts added to foods might be sufficiently high to approach toxicity in some people, especially young children.

This question was first raised more than 20 years ago, when a researcher demonstrated that a single dose of MSG given orally by itself to rats or monkeys caused damage in one region of the brain, especially in infant animals. Concerned that the same effects might occur in human babies, he crusaded to have the Food and Drug Administration (FDA) take action preventing the use of MSG. The FDA, armed with test results showing that MSG given to animals *with food* (which dilutes the MSG) does not have the same effect, refused to ban MSG from the food supply—but the baby food industry voluntarily removed the additive. The debate continues today because MSG is present in relatively large amounts in a few products that might be fed to young children, such as instant soups. Other neuroscientists share some concern on this issue, recognizing that when present *in excess*, this neurotransmitter "can actually stimulate nerve cells until they die." However, the exact amount of glutamate or the conditions of use that would cause this to happen in humans have not been determined (Barinaga, 1990).

That has not been the full extent of MSG's troubles: MSG also has been implicated (but not proved to be at fault) in a condition called *Chinese restaurant syndrome (CRS)*. CRS is the name given a group of symptoms experienced by a few people when they ingest Chinese or other food that contains large amounts of MSG. For several hours after eating the offending food(s), these people complain of some or all of the following: severe tightness in the chest, asthma, sensations of warmth and tingling, stiffness and/or weakness of the limbs, headache, lightheadedness, heartburn, and gastric discomfort. Although the symptoms of CRS are not life threatening, they can be unpleasant—and frightening—if mistaken for more serious problems.

Although a considerable amount of circumstantial evidence has been accumulated against MSG in regard to this condition, other studies refute it. For example, in one study six people who claimed to have CRS were given different beverages on two occasions, one containing MSG, the other containing salt. Four people had *no reaction to either drink,* whereas the other two reacted to *both.* Apparently, then, it takes more than MSG to trigger this syndrome, but it is possible that MSG acts in concert with something else (Kenney, 1986).

Aspartame   Another use of amino acids involves the dipeptide **aspartame,** which is marketed under the names *Nutrasweet* and *Equal.* It was accidentally discovered to be a sweet compound when scientists were synthesizing a product for ulcer therapy late in 1965.

Aspartame, which is 180–200 times as sweet as sucrose, is composed of phenylalanine and aspartic acid. Being a protein derivative, it provides 4 kcalories per gram; but since it is such a potent sweetener, only small amounts are needed to achieve a sweetening effect equivalent to much larger amounts of sugar, making it a very low-kcalorie substitute for sugar. Aspartame is used in the United States as a tabletop sweetener and in soft drinks, dry beverage mixes, cocoa, instant coffees and teas, milk and shake mixers, cereals, chewing gum, puddings, fillings, gelatin mixes, yogurt, fruit juice beverages, and more.

The amino acids in aspartame occur normally in proteins we consume every day: a 4-ounce hamburger has about 12 times more phenylalanine than a can of aspartame-sweetened soda. Despite this, it was necessary to test carefully whether aspartame might have negative effects, based on the concern mentioned earlier that purified amino acids (or in this case, the products of the breakdown of a dipeptide) might cause unwanted effects.

After testing by its manufacturer, aspartame was approved in 1981 by the Food and Drug Administration for use up to a level established as the *acceptable daily intake* (ADI). Later, the American Medical Association and the Centers for Disease Control stated they also thought it was safe. According to the FDA, if aspartame were to replace all the sugar and saccharin (an unrelated artificial sweetener) in the diet, the highest consumption would be far below any level even suspected of causing negative effects (Institute of Food Technology, 1986). A subsequent test with six normal adults who drank the equivalent of 3 (12-ounce) cans of aspartame-sweetened beverage every hour for 8 hours had no significant effect on blood plasma levels of aspartate or its metabolites (Steginks et al., 1989). The number of aspartame-sweetened beverages and other products that could be consumed by children before they would reach the ADI for their body size have been calculated: for a 6-year-old, it would be 4 beverages and 7 other products, and for an 11-year-

aspartame—a sweet dipeptide composed of phenylalanine and aspartic acid; used as a low-kcalorie sweetener

old, it would be 8 beverages and 10 other products (Thomas-Doberson, 1989). Unfortunately, experts fear that some children in the United States consume close to or in excess of the ADI for aspartame.

Nonetheless, some adults claim to have experienced problems such as dizziness, panic attacks, skin hives, swelling of throat tissue, gastrointestinal symptoms, migraines, seizures, and eye damage from aspartame. Some researchers believe there may be a scientific basis for certain complaints. The dispute is far from over. To provide further data, the FDA has contracted for a three-year study on the behavioral effects of this and other amino acids.

In the meantime, what should people do? Should they avoid aspartame, or can they safely consume it?

One small group of people has always been advised to avoid it; those are people with *phenylketonuria*, an inborn error of metabolism that results in brain damage if too much phenylalanine is consumed. It is for the benefit of these people (who are usually diagnosed at birth) that all products containing aspartame must be so labeled.

But what about other people? What guidelines apply?

For individuals who suspect that aspartame has a harmful effect on them (perhaps due to an unusual sensitivity to this compound), it makes sense to stop consuming it or at least to limit intake. Similarly, a very cautious approach for a pregnant woman or a small child would be to avoid it. Most adults, however, would be unlikely to experience any negative effects if consuming a moderate amount of aspartame as part of a mixed diet.

Other Amino Acid Products Although MSG and aspartame have been the major amino acid products used in the food supply, many others have appeared on the market. Some formulas designed for weight loss and consisting of amino acids, vitamins, and minerals have been available; Chapter 10 (on body fatness) will deal with the inadvisability of using such products. A product consisting of a mixture of amino acids has also been marketed as a protein supplement for athletes; it is discussed in Critical Thinking 8.1 on p. 263.

Amino acids are also sold individually and are readily available over the counter. The Food and Drug Administration (FDA) classifies amino acids as dietary supplements, because they are naturally occurring components of food. However, most people who take them do not need them to meet their recommended intake for protein; rather, they are using them—sometimes in very high doses—to try to achieve drug-like effects. When individual amino acids are taken by themselves (not with foods), their activity in the body can be considerably different than when they are consumed as part of food. The problem is that the use of amino acids in this way is largely untested, in regard to both possible benefits and levels of toxicity. There are two sources of information—animal studies and case reports.

Animal studies have shown that taking disproportionate amounts of amino acids interferes with growth either from direct toxic effects or from interference with the function of other amino acids (Munro and Crim, 1988).

Animal studies are limited in their application to humans, in part because of species differences and also because many of the claims made for amino acids have to do with how people *feel* rather than with measurable physical effects.

The other source of information about the use of individual amino acids is case reports of human toxicity. Unfortunately, these are only occasionally published; it would be helpful if more were reported so that people could be alerted to the effects of overdoses and the levels of intake at which they occurred. It is only people who go to the doctor's office with their problem whose experience may become part of the medical literature—provided the doctor writes it up, submits it, and it is published. A cluster of occurrences late in 1989 had important public health implications, and therefore the reports about them received widespread dissemination in the media. It involved supplements of the essential amino acid tryptophan, which have consequently been recalled; it is discussed in the Slice of Life.

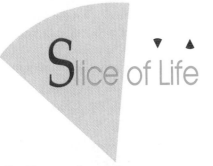

Slice of Life

The Tryptophan Mystery

During the bright New Mexico summer, Carol (not her real name) had been sailboarding and winning tennis tournaments. Then she began to experience pain—first in her temples and jaws, then spreading throughout her body until she was completely incapacitated (Steinbrook, 1989).

For several months, her case had doctors completely baffled. Despite extensive testing, there were few clues leading to the cause of her problem. The only abnormal finding was that she had a very high count of *eosinophils*, a type of white blood cell that is usually elevated when a parasitic disease or tumor is present, but she had neither.

While Carol lay in the hospital that fall, three similar cases developed in the area; within two more weeks 30 cases had been identified, some outside New Mexico. Physicians, consultants, and public health officials kept in close contact by phone. One of the doctors who had worked with

Carol noticed an odd similarity between the histories of the patients: all had been taking the amino acid *tryptophan* before they became ill. Although correlational data do not prove causation, it was compelling to note that within this small sample of patients, all had taken tryptophan. They notified federal authorities; in mid-November, 1989, the FDA warned the public to stop using tryptophan and asked manufacturers to recall tryptophan supplements and other products in which it was a major ingredient.

Far from being the end of either the problem or the mystery, this was just the beginning. By the end of 1989, almost 1000 cases were discovered in 48 states, and 1 death had resulted (Harvard Medical School Health Letter, 1990). Also by this time, the condition had acquired a name: *eosinophilia-myalgia syndrome*, referring to the elevated levels of eosinophils in the blood, and the muscle pain that was the principal symptom of the illness. Other symptoms were weakness, fever, joint pain, shortness of breath, rash, and inflammation of the lungs.

But why tryptophan? Why should this amino

acid, which had been taken by some people for several years without apparent consequence, be associated with a relatively sudden outbreak of serious—even life-threatening—problems?

One possibility that had to be considered was that tryptophan, in the amounts that were being consumed, might be toxic. However, most people in the United States ordinarily consume between 1 and 5 grams of tryptophan per day as a component of their usual diet, and the patients with eosinophilia-myalgia syndrome had consumed an average of 1.2 grams of purified tryptophan from supplements (with a few as high as 17 grams per day). Comparing the average supplemental intakes with the average dietary intakes, toxicity seemed an unlikely explanation; but it was still under consideration, since consuming an individual amino acid with water gives a different response than consuming the same substance in food. The presence of other amino acids and other compounds in food affects the absorption and utilization of an amino acid.

Another point of consideration was the possibility that some people's bodies are more sensitive to the amino acid in its pure form than others are. Because this product had been available for many years over the counter, however, it would seem that some people would have developed the problem before this latest series of cases.

Others noted that there is a variant of the tryptophan molecule that is known to cause eosinophilia. It is possible that some of this "off-form" developed in the product during processing, shipping, or storage, or it is possible that a highly toxic contaminant found its way into the tryptophan.

The front-running hypothesis is that a contaminant in certain brands of purified tryptophan was responsible. As we went to press with this book, the mystery had yet to be solved—if it ever will be. But as an additional safeguard, in late March of 1990, the FDA expanded its recall of *all* tryptophan-containing products, even those including very small dosages. ▼

Considering the serious lack of information about the effects of taking purified amino acids, the National Research Council advises against their use (1989). People who take them are experimenting on themselves. Those taking amino acids—or any other nutritional supplement, for that matter—who experience a health problem should be sure to report their use of the product to their health care professional.

Too Little or Too Much Dietary Protein Carries Some Risk

One of the themes of this book is that it is important to get enough of the essential nutrients—but not too much. For every class of nutrients, problems can occur with either underconsumption or overconsumption. Proteins are no exception.

Shortage of Protein

Although we have made the point that in our society it is usually quite easy to get enough protein, there are places in the world where the common foods are very low in protein or where there is simply an inadequate quantity of food of any kind. In either of these circumstances, concern about inadequate protein is legitimate.

"Pure" Protein Deficiency Protein deficiency by itself—that is, without accompanying *energy* deficiency—is a rare phenomenon. Protein deficiency is seen in its pure form in just a few places in the world, where the food choice is extremely limited and the staple food is extremely low in protein.

Cassava (a starch root) and yams are foods that have only about a third of the protein provided by grains on a weight basis. A study done in Nigeria, where these foods are staples, found that only 5–8% of the kcalories in people's diets came from protein (Worthington-Roberts, 1981). Protein deficiency manifested itself in low weight gains during pregnancy; low maternal milk production; high infant mortality (40% in the first five years); extremely low weights and heights in children; poor intelligence scores for children; and increased susceptibility to infections. When protein was supplemented, all of these abnormalities were reversed.

Protein–Energy Malnutrition (PEM) It is much more common to find long-term protein deficiency associated with severe underconsumption of other energy-producing foods: this condition is called **protein–energy malnutrition (PEM),** a fairly widespread situation in the developing countries. Usually the problem is that people simply do not have enough food. PEM would be relieved if these people had access to more of what their diet already contained.

PEM affects young children more than others, because their need for protein and other nutrients is greater per unit of body weight. PEM manifests itself in a variety of ways; two severe conditions are marasmus and kwashiorkor. Although kwashiorkor originally was thought to result from protein deficiency alone, more recent thinking is that it also involves inadequate energy intake. Experts in PEM, Benjamin Torun and Fernando Viteri, state, "The concept that marasmus or kwashiorkor is the end result of either severe energy or protein deficiency is too simplistic" (1988).

Marasmus is a condition in which a person becomes thinner and thinner from a progressive loss of fat and muscle tissue. People with marasmus are extremely weak and listless and have decreased resistance to infection. **Kwashiorkor** produces quite different physical symptoms; the body becomes swollen with fluid because there is less protein than is normal in the blood, and fluid from the bloodstream is thus allowed to migrate into the tissues. Sometimes the swelling makes the person look healthfully chubby, but other signs quickly disprove this image: dark hair has become red, a dermatitis (skin condition) has developed, and the person obviously feels miserable. Once again, resistance to infection is reduced. Liver damage is characteristic. A child with kwashiorkor is pictured in Figure 8.9.

It is not known exactly what determines which form of PEM will develop in an individual living under these circumstances; often, marasmus and

protein–energy malnutrition (PEM)—long-term protein deficiency associated with severe energy deficiency; fairly widespread in the less developed countries

marasmus—a serious form of PEM characterized by progressive fat and muscle loss

kwashiorkor—a serious form of PEM in which liver damage results in fluid shifts that create a swollen appearance

Figure 8.9 A child with kwashiorkor. Although this child may not appear malnourished to the casual observer, she is: the swelling caused by the fluid in her tissues camouflages her protein-energy malnutrition. The other signs are more obvious—her dark hair has turned reddish, she has a skin condition, and she is feeling great misery.

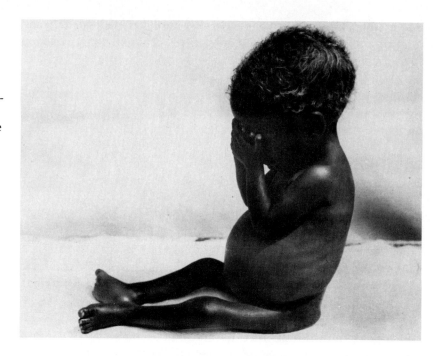

kwashiorkor occur together in the same group of children. However, children who develop kwashiorkor have often experienced additional stress from certain infections and parasites that have not plagued children with marasmus.

Susceptibility to Infection As stated previously, in its most severe forms, inadequate dietary protein results in poorer resistance to infection. However, even in milder dietary inadequacies of energy and/or protein, the body's defenses for dealing with invading microorganisms are weaker and/or slower to respond (Myrvik, 1988).

Because infection raises the body's need for both kcalories and protein, it creates an even wider gap between what the body needs and what the diet supplies. For this reason, PEM and infection create a downward spiral in the health of many people in developing countries. Diseases such as measles, which would run a short course in well-nourished populations, become killers among the poorly nourished.

Of course, people in the developing countries are not the only ones who ever experience this decrease in disease resistance: it can also happen to people in developed countries who seriously shortchange themselves on kcalories and protein because of disease, medication, or deliberate attempts to maintain an unrealistically low body weight. The effect can be the same—a disease that would have been easily resisted under normal circumstances may establish itself and be difficult for the victim to shake.

Fatty Liver If the liver had inadequate access to protein due to long-term dietary deficiency, fats can accumulate in the liver. (Recall from Chapter 7 [on lipids] that the body uses protein to create lipoproteins, the form in which lipids are transported in the body.)

Protein deficiency can also occur among alcoholics in the developed countries if their intake of alcohol replaces a large part of their food intake. However, in alcoholics, the development of fatty liver is also influenced by the fact that alcohol is toxic to the liver, and in alcoholics this damage allows fat to be deposited (Shaw and Lieber, 1988).

Excess of Protein

It is not uncommon for Americans to consume more than twice what the recommendations suggest, so it is appropriate to consider what the consequences of such overindulgence might be. As with any of the macronutrients, an excess of protein can result in the creation of *additional body fat*, if total kcalories consumed exceed the kcalories needed.

Another problem with excessive protein intake is that many commonly consumed high-protein foods are also high in fat. If you have a high intake of high-protein/high-fat foods, the total fat content of your diet will be high, making you a candidate for the problems associated with high fat intake. On the other hand, you can obviously be deliberate about choosing the lower-fat/high-protein foods. Table 8.6 gives you examples of options within dairy, flesh (meat, poultry, fish) protein, and plant protein foods. For a more comprehensive picture of which high-protein foods are high or low in fat, refer back to the Basic Food Guide sections on milk products and meats and meat alternates.

Table 8.6 Fat Levels That Accompany 7–8 Grams of Protein in Various Kinds of Foods

Food	Protein (grams)	Fat (grams)
Milk and milk products		
Skim milk	8	0
Cheddar cheese	7	9
Animal protein sources		
Haddock, broiled	7	2
Beef ribeye	7	13
Plant protein sources		
Lentils	8	0
Peanuts	8	15

Another possible problem is dehydration. When very high levels of protein are consumed, the body dismantles the amino acid surplus. The separated amino groups are metabolized into urea, which is excreted in the urine. These processes demand more work of the liver and kidneys.

A sizeable volume of water is needed to excrete urea in the urine. To metabolize 100 kcalories of protein, the body uses 350 grams of water, whereas 100 kcalories of carbohydrate or fat use only 50 grams (Worthington-Roberts, 1981). This means that if a person who consumes a great deal of protein does not also consume a lot of water, dehydration is a possibility. This is the reason why high-protein weight-reduction diets often recommend consuming large volumes of water. It also explains why athletes consuming high-protein diets are in double jeopardy of dehydration—because of both urinary losses and perspiration.

Calcium Loss   Some studies show that people who consume protein at levels at least twice as high as the amount recommended by the RDA excrete more calcium. For reasons not entirely understood, the intake of high amounts of protein prompt the kidney to release more calcium into the urine than it normally would. This may lead to negative calcium balance (net loss of calcium from the body) if a person consumes less than the RDA for calcium.

In theory, this means that the person who eats a lot of meat but avoids the recommended number of servings of dairy products per day *may* be slowly but steadily losing bone calcium. (Many other factors, such as level of dietary phosphorus, gender, age, and activity level can also affect this situation; Chapter 13 [on minerals] will discuss this more thoroughly.) However, epidemiological data do not exist to support this theory. Therefore, many experts question whether high protein intakes contribute to **osteoporosis,** a condition in which gradual loss of bone mass causes weakening of bone (National Research Council, 1989; RDA Subcommittee, 1989).

osteoporosis—condition in which bone mass decreases, thereby weakening the bone

Assess Your Own Protein Intake Compared with Recommendations

Since protein has so many important functions, you would surely not want to shortchange yourself. However, you will probably be surprised at how easy it is for a healthy adult to get the amount of protein he or she needs. That is, it is generally easy to get what you need if you eat enough food to match your energy expenditure. Those who restrict their energy intake may not automatically get enough protein.

How Scientists Determine Protein Needs

How do scientists know how much protein is enough for a healthy adult? In essence, they have measured the amount of protein that is lost from the body in a day's time to find out how much should be replaced. The major losses occur via the urine. Urinary *nitrogen* is measured; from this value, it is possible to calculate how much *protein* has been discarded, since protein is 16% nitrogen. Much smaller amounts of protein are lost in the feces, sweat, skin, hair, and nails; collection and analysis of these amounts present their own challenges.

But it is not enough to measure the body's losses: intake of dietary protein is another important part of the equation. Some of the urinary nitrogen may come from excess protein that was in the diet. If a person has eaten more protein than his or her body needs for replacement of worn tissues, the unneeded amino acids are either metabolized for energy or are converted to fat and stored. In either case, the nitrogen from the surplus is excreted in the urine along with the *un*recycled nitrogen from worn internal tissues.

Protein needs, then, are determined using **nitrogen balance studies** that measure both intake and output of nitrogen. If output and intake are equal, the person is said to be "in balance." If output is greater than intake, the person is losing protein, or is in "negative balance"; this occurs with injury, surgery, illness, and starvation. If intake is greater than output, the body is creating new protein and is in "positive balance"; this occurs during growth, pregnancy, lactation, healing, and muscle-building.

nitrogen-balance study— biochemical test that determines whether protein is being lost, gained, or simply maintained; involves comparing nitrogen intake with loss of nitrogen from all body routes combined

There have been thousands of studies about protein metabolism. They have shown that people's protein needs vary slightly from one individual to another; this is consistent with the generalization we made in Chapter 1 about people's unique needs for levels of nutrients. The studies also show that there is a strong relationship between the need for protein and the need for kcalories: a person who is losing weight needs more protein to stay in balance than a person who is maintaining body weight (Munro and Crim, 1988). This is because some of the protein is used for energy.

When the RDA committee members considered recommendations for protein intake, they took into account as many of these factors as they could. To allow for individual variation, they included a generous margin in the recommendation. They also added a margin to cover for the fact that people's diets are made up of proteins of varying quality; the recommendations do assume, though, that the proteins will come from both animal and plant sources. However, be aware that the protein RDAs are not adequate for a person who is losing weight rapidly or who is ill. During illness and after surgery or serious accidental injury, the appropriate recommendation for protein could be double or more the amount recommended for the healthy person, depending on the nature of the illness and/or the extent of the surgery or injury (Munro and Crim, 1988).

Recommended Protein Intakes for the Healthy Adult

The RDA committee advocates that you calculate your recommended daily protein intake based on body weight. (If you are substantially overweight or underweight at the moment, use your ideal body weight in the calculation; your protein needs are based primarily on lean body tissue and do not change much when your body contains different amounts of fat.) First convert your weight to kilograms; then multiply it by 0.8 gram per kilogram to get the recommended daily intake. Note that this corresponds with the figures in the RDA table; 58 grams of protein per day for the 72-kilogram man and 46 grams for the 58-kilogram woman.

People who are developing new tissue need more dietary protein. According to the 1989 RDA, the pregnant woman should consume 60 grams each day during pregnancy. During the first six months of lactation she should consume 65 grams per day and thereafter 62 grams per day.

Children's needs vary according to their ages; in the first six months after birth, they should take in 2.2 grams of protein per kilogram of body weight. As they get older, the recommendation per unit of body weight gradually drops until it gets to the adult level of 0.8 gram per kilogram.

Assessment 8.1 outlines a method for determining adequate protein intake; this chapter's Nutrition for Living offers guidelines to follow to get the protein you need.

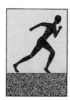

Recommended Protein Intakes for Athletes

Do athletes need more protein? For many centuries, it was believed that a high-protein diet would help a person excel at physical activity, because protein was thought to be the major fuel required by muscle. For this reason, some of the original Olympic contenders ate meals primarily of high-protein foods, such as meat, milk, and eggs (Hickson and Wolinsky, 1989).

In 1866, however, two German scientists published the results of experiments proving that protein was *not* the preferred energy substrate for the working muscle. Many studies have reinforced those early findings: fat and carbohydrate are undeniably the major energy sources for both athletes and nonathletes.

Nutrition scientists and exercise physiologists in recent years have learned that during strenuous athletic activity, protein may contribute up to 15% of energy (Goodman, 1988), especially when carbohydrate intake is low and/or exercise is prolonged (that is, over two hours). Furthermore, after such a bout of exercise, the body synthesizes more protein. These factors suggest that the serious adult athlete might benefit from more than the 0.8 gram per kilogram recommended for the average adult.

How much is the right amount? There is considerable disagreement on this point. Opinions range all the way from scientists who insist that 0.8 gram per kilogram is adequate for the athlete (they remind us that the RDA has a built-in safety factor) to a few who promote as much as 3 grams per kilogram.

There are many reasons for such disparities. To begin with, some of the studies that people hold up as proof of protein needs are of poor quality. For example, a study was conducted on two groups of high school boys who were involved in a standard physical training program. Every day, boys in the experimental group were given a beverage containing 25 grams of pro-

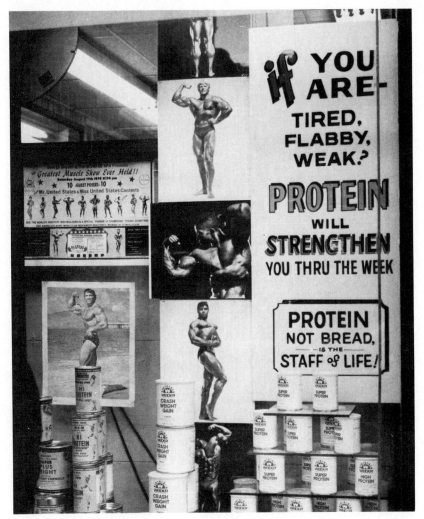

IF YOU ARE— TIRED, FLABBY, WEAK?

PROTEIN WILL STRENGTHEN YOU THRU THE WEEK

PROTEIN NOT BREAD, —IS THE— STAFF of LIFE!

Promises that can't be kept. Protein or amino acid powders are often marketed for muscle building. They are neither necessary nor effective; only a regular, graduated body building program can add muscle mass within genetic limits.

tein and 375 kcalories; boys in the other group received a placebo almost devoid of protein and kcalories. At the end of the 8-week study, all boys had made gains in body weight, total weight lifted, and muscle girth, but the boys receiving the protein and kcalorie-rich drink progressed more.

This study has been cited by some to prove that extra protein is needed for physical activity and muscle building. But in a review of this study, a notable shortcoming was pointed out: no records were kept of the boys' dietary intakes, so it is impossible to know whether their diets met standards for adequacy to begin with (Hickson and Wolinsky, 1989). It is possible—given the inclination of some teenagers to skip breakfast and eat other meals irregularly—that the experimental beverage was simply making up for deficits in the boys' dietary intakes, because the gains experienced by the experimental group were about as much as would be expected from normally healthy, adequately fed, growing boys in a training program of this type. Keep in mind that in all studies regarding protein needs, overall energy intake must be considered, because when energy intakes (or carbo-

Determining Protein Intake Adequacy

To find out how your protein intake compares with your needs, follow the steps below.

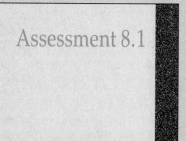

Assessment 8.1

Calculation of Recommended Daily Intake

1. Convert ideal body weight from pounds to kilograms, using as an example a person whose ideal weight is 165 pounds:

$$\text{Body weight in kilograms} = \frac{\text{ideal body weight (lb)}}{2.2 \text{ lb/kg}} = \frac{165 \text{ lb}}{2.2 \text{ lb/kg}} = 75 \text{ kg}$$

2. Circle the basic standard and extra need that applies to you:

Basic standards

Older teen (nonathlete)	0.9 g/kg body weight
Adult (nonathlete)	0.8 g/kg body weight
Older teen (athlete)	0.9–1.8 g/kg body weight
Adult (athlete)	0.8–1.6 g/kg body weight

Extra needs

Pregnant	Add 10 grams to prepregnant recommendation.
Lactating	Add 15 grams to prepregnant recommendation for first six months and 12 grams thereafter.

3. Calculate the amount of protein recommended for you:

$$\text{Recommended daily protein intake} = \left(\text{body weight in kg} \times \text{basic standard} \right) + \text{extra need}$$

$$= (75 \text{ kg} \times 0.8 \text{ g/kg}) + 0 \text{ g}$$

$$= 60 \text{ g of protein}$$

Determination of Actual Intake for One Day

1. Keep a record of your intake for 24 hours, as shown in Sample Assessment 8.1.
2. Using Appendices E and F and information from food labels, determine the amount of protein in each item consumed and enter values on the record.
3. Total the protein column.

Comparison of Recommendation with Intake

1. Calculate what percent of your recommended intake you actually consumed, using the following formula:

Percentage of recommendation = (intake ÷ recommendation) × 100

$$= (84 \div 60) \times 100$$
$$= 140\%$$

2. Compare the percent you calculated with guidelines that suggest too little or too much: if your intake is less than 70% or more than 200% of your recommendation (and this is typical for you), you run the health risks described in this chapter.

Food or Beverage	Amount	Protein (grams)
Chili con carne	1 c	15
Crackers, sesame	4 squares	1
Sandwich:		
White enriched bread	2 slices	4
Turkey	2 oz.	16
Mayonnaise	2 T.	tr
Hamburger:		
Beef patty	2 oz.	14
Bun	1	4
Green beans	½ c	2
Sloppy Joe sandwich:		
Meat (ground beef)	2 oz.	14
Bun	1	4
Tomato sauce	2 T.	tr
Ice milk	2 c	10
		84

Sample Assessment 8.1 Determining protein intake adequacy

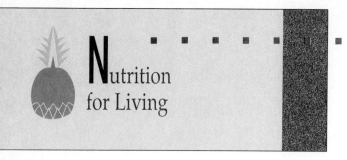

Nutrition for Living

Meeting Your Protein Needs

An adequate supply of protein is critical, but you don't need to eat huge servings of meat to get it. Most Americans who eat a mixed diet easily get more than they need, although people who have very low energy intakes or avoid all foods within a certain category may not get enough protein.

Here are some examples of what it takes to meet various people's protein needs. Note that there is a wide variety of protein sources—and a wide variety of forms, tastes, textures, and costs—associated with these sources.

■ Use the groups of the Basic Food Guide to get the protein you need. The minimum suggestions of the Basic Food Guide for adults probably provide enough protein to meet recommendations for you:

Servings of Basic Foods	Approximate Grams of Protein
5 fruits and vegetables	0–10
6 grains	12
3 milks through age 24; 2 thereafter	16–24
2 meats or meat alternates	30
Total for the day	58–76

Most people eat more than this in a day.

■ Develop an accurate mental picture of serving sizes of meats and meat alternates to know what you're getting; each serving of the following defined sizes provides approximately 15 grams of protein. For meats, 2 to 3 ounces is a serving; that would be a piece without fat or bone about the size of a deck of cards. (A fast-food quarter-pound hamburger with cheese has 30 grams of protein.) Most processed presliced sandwich meats weigh less than an ounce per slice, so three thin slices constitute a serving. Two eggs provide about as much protein as 2 ounces of meat. Because plant foods are less concentrated in protein, serving sizes need to be larger: it takes 1 cup of cooked legumes, $\frac{1}{2}$ cup of nuts, $\frac{1}{4}$ cup of nut butter, or 6 ounces of tofu ($\frac{3}{4}$ cup) to provide approximately that amount of protein.

■ Realize that with protein, you don't necessarily get what you pay for: cost and benefit may not be proportional. An expensive steak at $5 per pound does *not* contain better protein than a cheaper cut of meat or poultry or fish. Plant sources provide protein at just a fraction of the cost of flesh proteins, which makes them an excellent nutrition buy. (They also have the benefit of often being low in fat while generous in some other nutrients.) Highly processed protein sources such as tofu (from soybeans) or surimi (from fish) are more expensive than the foods from which they were made. The most costly of all sources of protein are protein supplements, which can cost far more per gram of protein than tenderloin and sometimes even more than lobster.

hydrate intakes) are seriously inadequate, protein will be diverted from its unique roles and will be used in greater amount for energy.

There are other reasons that studies yield different results. Exercise physiologists have learned that protein and amino acid metabolism is affected by the nature and duration of the activity being done (Goodman, 1988); for example, the protein needs of a runner and a weight lifter may be different. Since the vast majority of studies on protein needs during exercise have been done for endurance activity such as bicycling or running, these results may not be on target for other kinds of activities.

Another issue concerns the selection of subjects for experiments. Exercise physiologists know that when people who are not accustomed to much physical activity start an aerobic training program, they metabolize an increased amount of protein for energy; this causes some body protein to be lost initially. But after a couple of weeks on a program, their metabolism adapts and this prevents further losses over time (Hickson and Wolinsky, 1989). Thus, if studies are done with people who are unaccustomed to exercise, their apparent "needs" will be considerably higher than they were before or will be again; the short-term needs indicated by these studies are not representative of the ongoing needs of the person who is regularly very active.

The timing of data collection can be important as well. As we mentioned above, exercise physiologists have learned that *during* endurance exercise, some protein is broken down and used for energy production; but in the hours *after* a bout of exercise, the body gradually begins to *synthesize* protein. Therefore, it makes a great deal of difference as to *when* body substances such as blood or muscle tissue samples are taken: if you take them in the midst of an exercise session, you might conclude that activity has a destructive effect, whereas if you take samples later, it may seem that exercise promotes formation of protein. It is important not to draw conclusions about overall protein nutrition based on one brief glimpse of protein metabolism at an isolated moment.

Another problem in doing these studies has to do with how the breakdown of body protein is measured. If researchers want to know whether body protein is being lost, they might look for a biochemical "marker" as evidence of muscle tissue destruction. One marker that has been used in many studies, a substance called *3-methylhistidine,* is not a perfect marker for skeletal muscle breakdown (Goodman, 1988); therefore there is room for some disagreement about the recommendations that come from studies in which 3-methylhistidine measures were the basis for the advice.

Other studies of protein utilization during exercise have been done using *nitrogen balance studies.* As you read earlier, nitrogen balance is determined by comparing nitrogen intake with nitrogen losses. This type of study is difficult to apply to the athlete because during physical activity, a significant amount of nitrogen is lost in sweat, and those losses are very difficult to collect and measure. In order to recover nitrogen lost by this route, scientists have to rinse the subject with deionized water (containing no dissolved materials) after exercise and rinse the perspiration from clothes; then they analyze all the rinse water for nitrogen. If such care is not taken to accurately determine all losses, studies of nitrogen balance in athletes misrepresent their protein status and needs.

When all of these factors are considered, you can see why different recommendations for protein intake for physical activity cover such a wide range. Fortunately, one scientist has recently evaluated the existing studies and reported the findings from the best of them (Goodman, 1988). He points out that several well-designed studies show that the RDA recommendation of 0.8 grams of protein per kilogram of body weight is sufficient to maintain the existing lean body mass of a physically active adult and to provide the raw materials for building additional muscle tissue. However, some other well-conducted studies suggest that intakes between 1.0 and 1.5 g/kg body weight are necessary. There is general agreement that more studies should be done (Williams, 1985; Astrand and Rodahl, 1986; Hickson and Wolinsky, 1989), especially for athletes in their preteen and early teen years, who still need sufficient protein for growth (Goodman, 1988).

Caution is advised regarding the upper end of the intake range: since there are no known benefits of consuming very large amounts of protein and since there are possible negative consequences to health of doing so, it makes sense not to take in excessive amounts. The 1989 RDA recommends that people should not take in more than double their RDA for protein, which would be 1.6 g/kg body weight for the adult and 1.8 g/kg body weight for the older teen.

It is easy for an athlete to get this amount of protein in food. The eating guideline for the athlete, first shown in Table 2.5 and repeated in this chapter in Table 8.7 with a sample menu, provides 70–96 grams of protein. If these recommendations are followed by a young adult weighing 150 pounds (68 kg), he or she would get 1.3 g of protein/kg body weight. Many athletes, especially those of larger body size and those who train many hours per day, are likely to need more kcalories and therefore should eat more than this menu provides. As they increase their intake of food, their intake of protein generally will increase as well.

Table 8.7 Basic Food Guide for the Young Adult Athlete

The recommended intakes of foods from the Basic Food Guide are shown below with a sample day's menu. The guidelines are *minimum* recommendations; many athletes need to eat more to meet their needs for energy. A person who eats more will also get more protein.

Summary of Recommendations	Est. Protein per Serving (grams)	Approx. Total (grams)

Fruits and vegetables
   1 vitamin A
   1 vitamin C
   Others to make group total of 5
	2 for vegetables;
	0 for fruit
		0–10

Grain products: 6–12 or more as needed	2	12–24
Milk and milk products: Three servings through age 24; after that, 2 servings per day	8	16–24
Meats and meat alternates: 2 servings	15–21	30–42
	TOTAL	58–100

SAMPLE DAY'S MENU

Breakfast

$\frac{1}{2}$ cup orange juice
1 oz. breakfast cereal
1 cup 2% milk
1 slice of whole-wheat toast
   with butter and jelly

Lunch

Sandwich of:
   2 slices bread
   2 oz. sliced turkey
   lettuce
   low-fat mayonnaise
2 plums
$1\frac{1}{2}$ cups milk
2 oatmeal cookies

Afternoon Snack

12 crackers
Carbonated beverage

Dinner

Mixed entree of:
   $1\frac{1}{2}$ cup macaroni
   3 oz. lean ground beef
   $\frac{3}{4}$ oz. cheese
   $\frac{1}{2}$ cup tomato sauce
1 slice French bread
$\frac{1}{2}$ cup green beans
$\frac{1}{2}$ cup fruit salad

Evening Snack

3 cups popcorn
1 cup fruit-flavored drink

This menu contains approximately 90 grams of protein. If it was consumed by a person weighing 150 pounds, the menu would provide 1.3 g protein/kg body weight.

Despite the fact that it is easy for most physically active people to achieve protein intakes within the recommended range from their usual diets, some athletes take protein supplements. Critical Thinking 8.1 examines this practice.

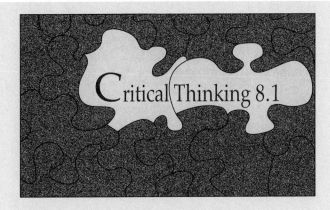

Are Protein Supplements Helpful to the Athlete?

The situation

You've always been an active person. You use your bicycle for transportation much of the time, and almost every day you participate in some sort of sports activity. Last month, you joined a soccer team that plays two games per week, and recently you've become interested in weight lifting. You've decided you'd really like to excel at these two activities.

Some of the soccer players and weight lifters you've met are really into nutrition. Several of them take different types of protein supplements; they are convinced the supplements help their performance, and they're encouraging you to try them. A couple of people have showed you the products they use. One of the packages suggests a daily protein intake of 2 g protein/kg of body weight; another supplement label recommends 3–3.5 g protein/kg body weight. You wonder whether you should give these products a try.

Is the information accurate and relevant?

■ Experts in protein research recommend protein intakes of from 0.8 g/kg body weight to 1.6 g/kg for the adult; for the older teenager, the recommended range is from 0.9–1.8 g/kg body weight. More is not better; in fact, the 1989 RDA advises against anybody going above these ranges (see text).

■ Research has shown no additional beneficial effects on strength, power, hypertrophy of muscle, or physiological work capacity from taking protein supplements (Williams, 1989), provided a person has eaten an adequate diet.

■ Unless an athlete is consuming a low-kcalorie diet, it is unlikely that protein intake will be low; in 1985, the average man and woman in the United States ate a diet containing 97 and 66 grams of protein, respectively, which more than meets their needs.

■ If a diet is low in protein nonetheless, a protein supplement may make up the deficit.

What else needs to be considered?

Essentially, there are three types of protein-based supplements marketed for the athlete: whole (intact) protein supplements, mixtures of amino acids, and individual amino acids.

Whole-protein supplements are generally made from proteins of milk or soybeans. When you use these products, you are getting protein without getting other nutrients the original foods contained. This can be an advantage if you need protein and you want to get it for the fewest possible additional kcalories. A disadvantage to using this type of product is that it is often more expensive than the whole food would be.

Mixtures of amino acids are essentially "predigested proteins." They are promoted as being easier to absorb than whole proteins because they are already in the simplest possible form. However, the normally healthy GI tract easily digests and absorbs over 90% of dietary proteins; in fact, protein experts generally believe that the healthy gut *prefers* dealing with whole proteins. It absorbs the variety of protein particles produced by digestion (amino acids, dipeptides, tripeptides, and even some larger polypeptides and whole proteins) bet-

ter than it absorbs material reduced entirely to amino acids. (The only circumstance in which such products have valid use are when a person's gut is *not functioning normally:* they are sometimes used in hospitals for patients with severe GI disorders.)

The third category of protein supplements is individual amino acids. Some athletes take certain amino acids hoping they will have anabolic (muscle-building) effects; some pseudoscientific publications have suggested that certain amino acids serve as "growth hormone releasers" (Hickson and Wolinsky, 1989). But early studies demonstrated that adding amino acids above the requirement level did not promote positive nitrogen balance. No studies have been done to assess the long-term effects of taking high levels of these individual purified amino acids. Therefore, taking them in high doses is like taking untested drugs (see text).

What do you think?

■ Option 1   You decide to evaluate your current diet for protein by doing Assessment 8.1. If your intake is within the range recommended for athletes your age, you will continue to eat as you have been.

■ Option 2   You decide that if your intake of protein is not high enough, you will eat more high-protein foods to bring it into the range scientists recommend.

■ Option 3   You decide that if your intake is not high enough, you will supplement your diet with a whole-protein type of supplement.

Do you see any other adequate and safe options? Which suits you best?

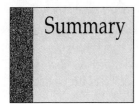

Summary

▶ We tend to value protein far above the other classes of nutrients, to the point of giving it credit for more than it can deliver.

▶ There are thousands of different **proteins** that differ widely in complexity and function. However, all consist of **amino acids** joined together by **peptide bonds.** Every amino acid consists of an amino group, an acid group, and a characteristic side group. Approximately 20 amino acids are used to synthesize proteins, and every living cell can produce some of them if it has the necessary raw materials.

▶ Dietary protein needs are actually needs for nitrogen (to make those amino acids the body can produce itself) and for **essential amino acids** (those the body cannot produce, but must obtain in foods). Protein is widespread in our food supply, but not all protein is of the same quality; in general, animal sources are better than plant sources in terms of matching human needs for essential amino acids. However, different foods eaten within the same day often contain—*in combination*—acceptable proportions of amino acids, a phenomenon known as **complementing.**

▶ Protein's crucial role in the body is evident from its many functions: (1) constituting cell and tissue structure; (2) regulating a wide variety of body processes including metabolic reactions, hormonal activity, body defenses, mineral and fluid balance, acid–base balance, and nerve impulse transmission; and (3) providing energy (in emergencies, or if present in surplus).

▶ Proteins can be modified by food technology just as the other macronutrients can. Soy protein isolates and concentrates commonly turn up as meat analogues and texturizers, respectively. Protein supplements of various kinds are marketed for several purposes, few of which are really legitimate. The amino acid derivative **monosodium glutamate (MSG)** is a commonly used flavor enhancer, and the dipeptide **aspartame** is an increasingly common sugar substitute.

▶ The body handles dietary protein very efficiently. **Denaturation** (unfolding) and digestion begin in the stomach with the action of pepsin, and other **proteases** take over the breakdown process in the small intestine. Secreted proteins and proteins from sloughed cells of the GI tract are also digested. Then amino acids, dipeptides, and tripeptides are efficiently absorbed. Occasionally large peptide fragments are absorbed. In some cases these absorbed proteins provoke an immune response, in which case the susceptible individual is said to have a food allergy (the symptoms of which can occur in body sites far removed from the digestive tract). The body is also very efficient at recycling many of its own proteins.

▶ As for the other nutrients, there is an optimal range of protein intake. Pure protein deficiency is rare, but in the less developed countries **protein–energy malnutrition,** a result of general food shortage, is fairly widespread. Two severe forms of this disorder are **marasmus** and **kwashiorkor.** In addition to its other consequences, inadequate protein intake can lead to increased susceptibility to infection and to fatty liver. Excess protein in the diet can lead to an increase in body fat and in some cases to dehydration.

▶ A healthy adult can easily meet his or her protein needs by eating a balanced diet. Protein intake guidelines are usually based either on body weight or on the total number of kcalories consumed. Needs vary among individuals; athletes have been shown not to benefit from consuming protein far in excess of the RDAs, though people who are recovering from illness or injury may need considerably more than the recommended amount.

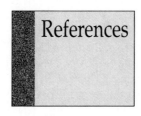

References

American Dietetic Association. 1988. Position of the American Dietetic Association: Vegetarian Diets. *Journal of the American Dietetic Association* 88:351–355.

Anderson, J.A. and D.D. Sogn, eds. 1984. *Adverse reactions to foods.* NIH Publication no. 84-2442. Washington, DC: U.S. Department of Health and Human Services.

Astrand, P.O. and K. Rodahl. 1986. *Textbook of work physiology*. New York: McGraw-Hill Book Company.

Barinaga, M. 1990. Amino acids: How much excitement is too much? *Science* 247:20–22.

Ganong, W.F. 1989. *Review of medical physiology*. Norwalk, CT: Lange.

Gardner, M.L. 1988. Gastrointestinal absorption of intact proteins. *Annual Reviews of Nutrition* 8:329–350.

Goodman, M.N. 1988. Amino acid and protein metabolism. In *Exercise, nutrition, and energy metabolism*, eds. E.S. Horton and R.L. Terjung. New York: The Macmillan Company.

Harvard Medical School Health Letter. 1990. Tryptophan: Natural disaster. *Harvard Medical School Health Letter* 15(no. 4):1–2.

Hickson, J.F. and I. Wolinsky. 1989. Human protein intake and metabolism in exercise and sport. In *Nutrition in exercise and sport*, eds. J.F. Hickson and I. Wolinsky. Boca Raton, FL: CRC Press.

Institiue of Food Technology. 1986. Sweeteners—alternatives to cane and beet sugar. *Food Technology* 21:116–128.

International Life Sciences Institute (ILSI)-Nutrition Foundation (NF). 1986. Food allergies. Washington, DC: ILSI-NF.

Kenny, R.A. 1986. The Chinese restaurant syndrome: An anecdote revisited. *Food and Chemical Toxicology* 24:351–354.

Marieb, E.N. 1989. *Human anatomy and physiology*. Redwood City, CA: The Benjamin/Cummings Publishing Company.

Martin, R.E. 1988. Seafood products, technology, and research in the U.S. *Food Technology* 42(no. 3):58–62.

Munro, H.N. and M.C. Crim. 1988. The proteins and amino acids. In *Modern nutrition in health and disease*, eds. M.E. Shils and V.R. Young. Philadelphia: Lea & Febiger.

Mutch, P.B. 1988. Food guides for the vegetarian. *American Journal of Clinical Nutrition* 48:913–919.

Myrvik, Q.N. 1988. Nutrition and immunology. In *Modern nutrition in health and disease*, eds. M.E. Shils and V.R. Young. Philadelphia: Lea & Febiger.

National Research Council. 1989. *Diet and health*. Washington, DC: The National Academy Press.

RDA Subcommittee. 1989. *Recommended dietary allowances*. Washington, DC: The National Academy Press.

Shaw, S. and C.S. Lieber. 1988. Nutrition and diet in alcoholism. In *Modern nutrition in health and disease*, eds. M.E. Shils and V.R. Young. Philadelphia: Lea & Febiger.

Smith, E.L., R.L. Hill, I.R. Lehman, R.J. Lefkowitz, P. Handler, and A. White. 1983. *Principles of biochemistry: General aspects*, 7th edition. New York: McGraw-Hill Book Company.

Steginck, L.D., L.J. Filer, Jr., E.F. Bell, E.E. Ziegler, and T.R. Tephly. 1989. Effect of repeated ingestion of aspartame-sweetened beverage on plasma amino acid, blood methanol, and blood formate concentrations in normal adults. *Metabolism* 38:357–363.

Steinbrook, R. 1989. Tracking disease the old way. *The Los Angeles Times*, November 27, 1989.

Thomas-Dobersen, D. 1989. Calculation of aspartame intake in children. *Journal of the American Dietetic Association* 89:831–833.

Thompson, R.C. 1986. Food allergies: Separating fact from hype. *FDA Consumer* 20:25–27.

Torun, B. and F.E. Viteri. 1988. Protein-energy malnutrition. In *Modern nutrition in health and disease*, eds. M.E. Shils and V.R. Young. Philadelphia: Lea & Febiger.

Williams, M.H. 1985. *Nutritional aspects of human physical and athletic performance*. Springfield, IL: Charles C. Thomas.

Williams, M.H. 1989. Nutritional ergogenic aids and athletic performance. *Nutrition Today* 24: 7–14.

Williams, S.R. and B.S. Worthington-Roberts. 1988. *Nutrition throughout the life cycle*. St. Louis: Times/Mirror Mosby.

Worthington-Roberts, B.S. 1981. Proteins and amino acids. In *Contemporary developments in nutrition*, ed. B.S. Worthington-Roberts. St. Louis: The C.V. Mosby Company.

Young, V.R. and D.M. Bier. 1987. A kinetic approach to the determination of human amino acid requirements. *Nutrition Reviews* 45:289–298.

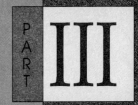

P A R T **III**

EATING TODAY:
CHOICES AND PITFALLS

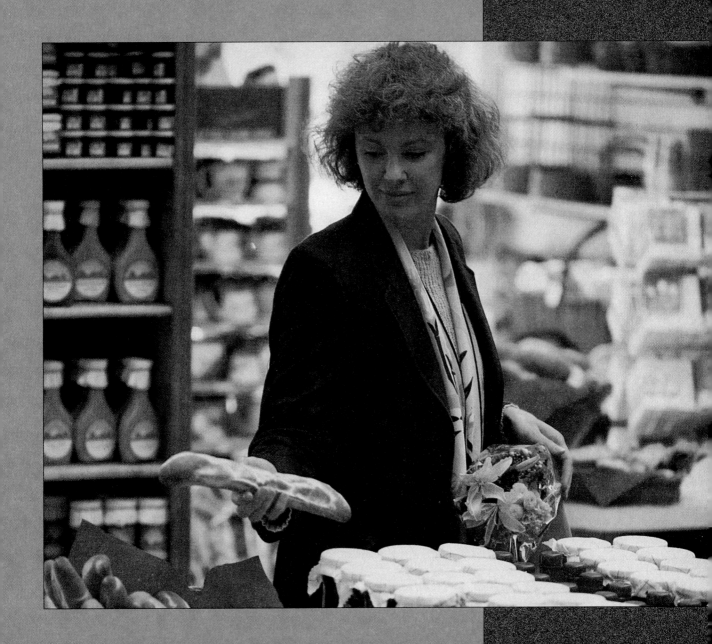

9

Why You Eat What You Do

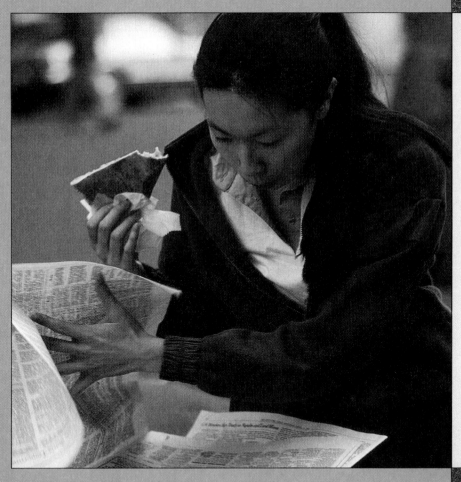

hy do you eat what you do? "That's simple," you may be thinking, "I eat what I eat because I *like* it." True, sensory appeal—especially taste—is very important to food choice, but there are many other factors that influence what you put on your plate.

We begin this chapter by acknowledging a fundamental truth that affects your opportunity to make food choices in the first place: *you can't eat what you don't have*. Therefore in the first half of our discussion, we will consider the *factors that affect food availability*. This means answering questions that relate to the big picture: What resources are needed to make food production possible? What is the demand for food? And do current circumstances allow for equitable distribution of food?

In the second half of the chapter, we'll concentrate on factors that influence *what you choose* from what is available to you. We are all affected by a few predispositions that are inborn. We are also substantially influenced by various cultural experiences—through our families, ethnic heritage, and religious affiliations, through the mass media that surround us, and so on. Ultimately, we choose what we eat based on very personal factors, such as what we like, what we can afford, what helps us feel good physically and emotionally, and what fits into the way we live.

While this chapter's organization may suggest that factors affecting availability operate independently from factors affecting our choices, that is not the case. As we will see, they are substantially interdependent. For example, just as availability affects our choices, choices (or our collective preference) influence decisions about food production to a certain degree. Figure 9.1 reflects this reciprocal relationship.

We conclude the chapter with a section on *making changes in eating behavior*, because we have found that while studying nutrition, many people want to make improvements in their diets. We are not suggesting that every reader *needs* to modify his or her food habits; many of you are discovering as you evaluate your current practices that they are already very healthful and are well worth continuing. But others of you will find some way(s) in which your eating could be improved, and you will want to do something about it. To that end, we offer some suggestions that may help you succeed at the challenging business of changing long-term eating habits.

Food Availability Is the Result of Food Production, Demand, and Distribution

Having access to food involves more than just its production. We also have to compete with others for that food, and we need to have a way of transporting it from farms, dairies, and ranches to where we are. Since our food supply comes literally from all over the world, this discussion will encompass global issues as well as more regional concerns; even matters that are limited to a seemingly distant geographical area ultimately affect us all.

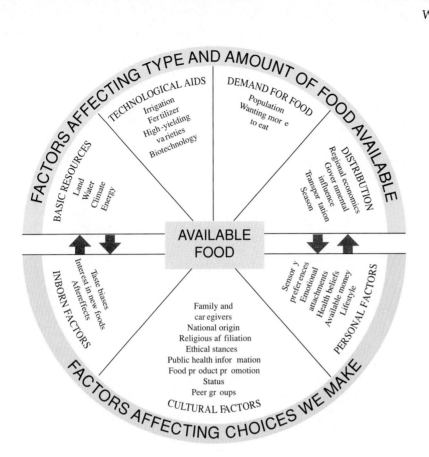

Figure 9.1 Factors affecting food availability and choice. Many factors influence what is available to us and what we select. Ultimately, the effects come full circle: food preferences (choices) also substantially affect what is produced, and exposure to a given food (its availability) helps to condition our preferences. (The size of the segment does not reflect its importance.)

Capacity for Production

Food production depends on basic agricultural resources, such as **arable** land and a favorable climate. Beyond what these resources can support naturally, the food supply can be substantially increased through the use of various technologies. Let's look first at what basic factors must come together to make food production possible.

Basic Agricultural Production Resources Four environmental resources must be suitable for producing food: land, water, climate, and energy. If any one of these is inadequate in a region, less food can be grown.

Land is basic to food production, but not all land is arable: it needs to have adequate topsoil to support growth. Topsoil supplies the chemical substances that plants need to grow and is therefore essential to the survival of all living things.

The amount of area planted in grain is a commonly used indicator of total food production capacity for a given season. As recently as the period between 1950 and 1981, the amount of worldwide acreage devoted to grain production expanded by almost 21% (Brown, 1988). However, between 1981 and 1988, it declined by 7%. This was due in part to the temporary idling of cropland under U.S. food supply management programs, but it was also

arable—fit for cultivation

Figure 9.2 Desertification in the Sahel. In the sub-Saharan region of Africa, overgrazing and cutting down of trees have resulted in losses of topsoil that could have supported crops.

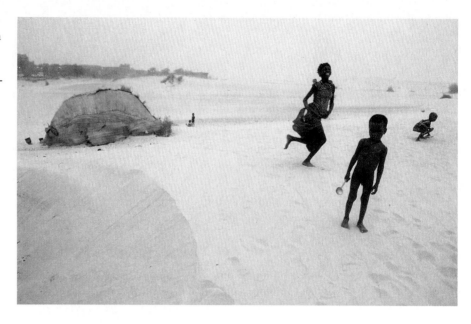

due to less recoverable losses from degradation of land in various parts of the world. There have been substantial losses of cultivable land in India and the sub-Saharan region of Africa, as denuding of the area has allowed the deserts to advance into once productive range and croplands (Figure 9.2).

Degradation of land has been even more extensive in the tropics, where an increasing population has driven many people into the rain forests to clear space, establish homes, and grow food for their families. Although this is believed to be the major cause of tropical deforestation, there are also cases in which people have slashed and burned large areas to raise beef or other cash crops for export to developed regions such as North America, Japan, and Western Europe. An estimated 15 million acres of moist tropical forests are cleared annually (World Resources Institute, 1988). Figure 9.3 shows the extent of deforestation in the tropics.

Many problems result from such practices. For one, after just a few years of intense cultivation or after seven to ten years of grazing, the topsoil becomes so depleted and eroded that it is no longer very productive. Since the soil can no longer yield enough to meet their needs, farmers in these regions stake out yet another area of forest, clear it, and use it until it, too, loses productive capacity. Methods of **sustainable agriculture** can be used in the rainforest, but pressing population growth, shortsightedness, and the temptation of quick gains have often encouraged the more destructive methods (Nations and Komer, 1986).

A serious environmental problem that results from deforestation is that the burning and loss of trees results in an increase in carbon dioxide (CO_2) in the atmosphere over the normal level (Detwiler and Hall, 1988). Why this is a problem will be discussed shortly.

Adequate water is another basic production resource. Water helps hold topsoil in place and provides the moisture plants need. The drought of the

sustainable agriculture— method of growing crops that assures the maintenance and continued productivity of the soil

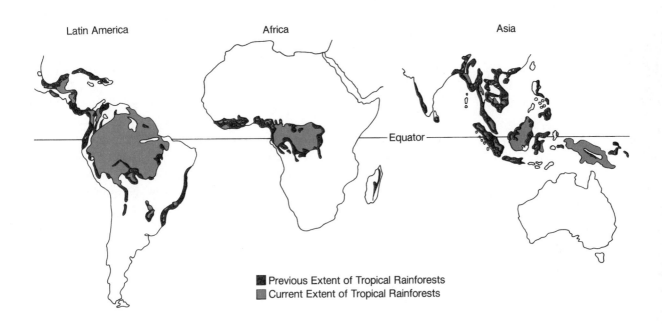

Latin America   Africa   Asia

—— Equator ——

■ Previous Extent of Tropical Rainforests
▨ Current Extent of Tropical Rainforests

summer of 1988 in North America was a searing testimony to the critical nature of water: grain production in the U.S. and Canada was reduced by almost one-fourth. This contributed to the most dramatic decline in annual grain harvest (an index of global food production capacity) that the world has ever known (Brown, 1988).

In areas where rainfall is consistently inadequate, the use of surface or groundwater for irrigation has enabled land to become productive. Between 1950 and 1982, irrigated area in the world nearly tripled (Brown, 1988); in 1985, about 30% of the world harvest came from irrigated cropland (World Resources, 1988). There are limits to the extent to which these water supplies can be tapped, though. In the U.S., irrigation is lowering the water table in some areas by 6 inches to 4 feet per year. Continuation of this trend would ultimately make irrigation impossible. Furthermore, poorly managed irrigation can cause land to become infertile through waterlogging or accumulation of mineral salts to toxic levels. More careful management can extend the land's productivity.

Water is also important as the natural habitat of certain animal foods: fish and shellfish from oceans, lakes, and rivers make important contributions to the diets of many people. We have come to learn, though, that food from these sources also has a limit. Therefore the technology of **aquaculture** or "fish farming" is being aggressively developed. It provides ideal conditions for fish and shrimp reproduction and growth and protects maturing fish

Figure 9.3 Tropical deforestation: so what if the trees disappear? Although clearing the rainforest temporarily provides land for farming and ranching, it adds to the serious long-term problems of land depletion and erosion, global warming, and decrease in biological diversity. (Smithsonian Institution, Tropical Rainforests: Disappearing Treasure, Traveling Ext. Service, 1988)

aquaculture—producing seafood in a protected environment from natural predators (Martin, 1988; Redmayne, 1989). As a result, the number of young that grow to an appropriate size for food is hundreds of times what nature would have allowed.

Suitable climate is also necessary for plants to grow; plants need particular temperatures and amounts of sunlight for their growth. Although it might seem that the tropics should be ideal for agriculture because of the region's year-round warmth and light, these conditions also foster weeds, pests, and diseases. The most productive areas to date have been lands in the temperate zone, where winter serves as an effective herbicide and pesticide (Myers, 1984).

By studying meteorological conditions of the past, however, scientists know that the climate of an area is not fixed for all time. Though they are not able to see clearly what lies ahead, they do agree that the makeup of the earth's atmosphere is changing and that pollution of the atmosphere with minute solid particles is also having an effect on climate.

Many scientists hypothesize that pollutants and changes in atmospheric gases (especially an increase in carbon dioxide) are forming an invisible "greenhouse" over the earth that will lead to higher temperatures, increased summer dryness, and a reduced grain crop (Brown and Young, 1988). Corn, which accounts for two-thirds of the U.S. grain harvest, is especially vulnerable to environmental changes and may experience wide swings in year-to-year production.

The most cautious experts point out that there is still a lot to learn about the intricate interactions of pollutants and their effects on the various strata of the atmosphere (World Resources Institute, 1988). Other scientists have suggested that the earth is gradually entering a cooling-off period; but the weight of scientific opinion is shifting to the belief that global warming is the trend.

Energy is the fourth basic production resource. Cultivation of a crop from planting to harvest requires the investment of human, animal, and/or mechanical energy (Figure 9.4). Farmers' decisions about what crops to plant are partly influenced by the availability of energy sources, whether humans, water buffaloes, or tractors and gasoline.

In the United States, the agricultural system is a highly mechanized one that relies heavily on fossil fuel use. This system allows a relatively small proportion of the population to produce food for the entire population. To grow 1 kcalorie of food, process it, and bring it to the table, however, we use about 9 kcalories of fossil fuel (Steinhart and Steinhart, 1978). In China, where human labor provides most of the energy, only 1 kcalorie of fossil fuel is used to produce about 20 kcalories of food. For every kcalorie produced, this is an almost 200-fold difference in need for a finite energy source.

In the United States it would be difficult to recruit the proportion of the population necessary for a manual system like that used in China. But it has been estimated that if the whole world used the energy-intensive agricultural methods that the United States does, the world's supply of petroleum

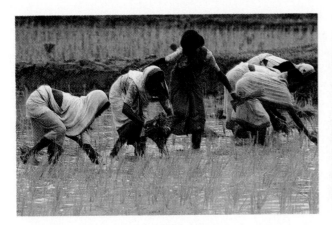 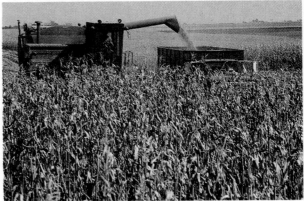

would be exhausted in a few decades (Pimental et al., 1978). Even if the U.S. alone continues its high use of fossil fuels, the supply will decrease, petroleum prices will rise, and food prices will increase as a result. When this happens, people all over the globe suffer the consequences: consumers in the developed countries pay higher prices for goods, and third-world farmers find it harder to feed their own families, to say nothing of competing in world markets.

For example, the production of chemical fertilizers requires energy. Appropriate application of fertilizers to an intensively farmed soil can increase crop production to many times what the yield from unfertilized soil would have been. But many farmers in developing countries simply don't have the money to buy chemical fertilizers. They therefore cannot realize the yields that might provide adequate food for their families and—possibly—surplus crops to sell.

Figure 9.4 Energy in agriculture. Energy from a variety of sources can be used to increase food production. Human labor was the original form used, and it is still the major source in many areas of the world today. Although machine-assisted production makes it possible for a small number of farmers to produce food for large numbers of people, agriculture that relies heavily on petroleum contributes to the depletion of a finite energy source.

Technological Aids to Production   Once the basic production resources have been employed to their natural limits, the way to produce more food is to increase yields with various technologies. Several already mentioned have been in widespread use for some time, such as supplementing natural rainfall by irrigation and enhancing the quality of the soil with fertilizers. Development of high-yielding grain hybrids has also greatly increased food production. The effectiveness of these three technologies was amply demonstrated in the 1960s, when they were employed as the major elements of the Green Revolution (Brown, 1989). This agricultural movement enabled many Third World nations, especially in Asia, to increase their food production many times over. The downside of the Green Revolution was that these intensive farming methods in some areas led to environmental degradation from overuse of pesticides and fertilizers (World Resources Institute, 1988). When new technologies are implemented, it is important to consider long-range environmental impacts as well as short-term production gains. Overall, the benefits of the Green Revolution are still being realized, but they have probably reached their limit: they are already in use in those areas where they are feasible.

biotechnology—the use of living systems for the production of useful products

A group of more recent technologies in which there is a great deal of interest are the biotechnologies. **Biotechnology** involves the use of living systems—including plants, animals, microbes, or any part of these organisms—for the production of useful products (Harlander, 1989). Although the term *biotechnology* has been coined quite recently, the practice itself has been going on for more than 8000 years. For example, cheese, yogurt, alcoholic beverages, vinegar, and sourdough all depend on bacteria for their production, thereby fitting the definition of biotechnological processes.

More recent applications involve the extensive use of enzymes by the food processing industry to produce high-fructose corn syrups, beverage clarifiers, meat tenderizers, and texture modifiers.

genetic engineering—making changes in the genetic makeup of plants or animals by incorporating genes from other species

The newest aspect of biotechnology involves making genetic changes in living systems. In a process known as **genetic engineering,** a gene that carries a desirable characteristic of a particular plant or animal is implanted into the genetic structure of a different plant or animal that lacks that trait. As far as plants are concerned, genetic engineering has the potential to confer resistance to insects, diseases, and herbicides (Gasser and Fraley, 1989), improving nutritional quality, reducing naturally occurring toxicants (Doyle, 1988), and reducing risk of damage from early frost. In animals produced for meat, genetic engineering has the potential to stimulate growth, promote feed efficiency, and reduce fat content while increasing lean muscle mass (Pursel et al., 1989).

One application that has received wide publicity is the use of bovine growth hormone (BGH; also called bovine somatotropin, or BST) produced by genetically engineered bacteria. Dairy researchers have found that the regular injection of cows with a small amount of this growth hormone, which is similar to that produced naturally in the cow's body, enhances milk production. The future use of this technology is debatable (Sun, 1989). Some opponents believe that it favors large agricultural operations rather than smaller family farms. Others believe that it is unreasonable because costly federal programs are already necessary to *limit* milk production and stabilize prices. Still others seem to fear the technology mainly because it is new. The net result is that legislatures in several states have limited or delayed the sale of milk produced with BGH.

Some of the changes mentioned above, such as promoting disease resistance, have been accomplished in the past with selective breeding programs. The advantage of genetic engineering over earlier methods is that the benefits can be accomplished far more rapidly and in a more controlled fashion. The potential of biotechnology and genetic engineering for the food production and processing industries is almost unlimited. Because it represents the unknown, however, it arouses many fears and anxieties—some justified, some not.

It is important to remember that genetic engineering and biotechnology are not inherently "good" or "bad"; it all depends on how they are used. Food scientists urge the development of clear and rational government policies for regulating bioengineered products (Institute of Food Technologists,

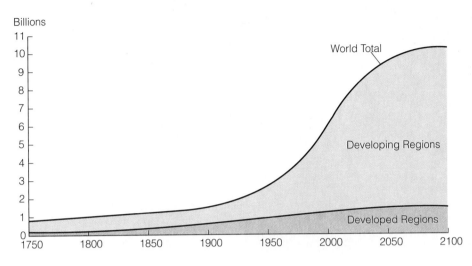

Figure 9.5 The past, present, and future of population growth. We are in the midst of a period of very rapid growth in world population, with the increases coming largely from the developing countries. With current population around 5 billion, estimates of how high it will go suggest 10 billion or even 14 billion. Can the food supply keep up with population growth? (Source: Thomas W. Merrick, et al: World Population in Transition: *Population Bulletin* Vol. 42, No. 2 (1986) Fig. 1, p. 4)

1988). They also urge the public to back the development of policies that will ensure maximal benefits and safety with the use of these technologies.

Demand for Food

The world's capacity for food production is of great concern, because the demand for food is increasing. One key aspect of demand is population: how many people need to be nourished? World population continues to increase at a rapid rate; after taking more than 100 years to double from 1.25 billion to 2.5 billion in 1950, population doubled again in only 37 years. The United Nations anticipates that the world population will reach 6 billion before the year 2000, more than 8 billion by 2025, and will finally stabilize at about 10 billion toward the end of the next century (World Resources Institute, 1988). Figure 9.5 shows this forecast; keep in mind that it is an estimate based on assumptions that fertility rates, especially in the developing regions (which currently account for three-fourths of the world's population), will decline as projected. More recently, in May of 1989, U.N. demographers predicted that world population will settle at 14 billion owing to failed family planning efforts (Brown, 1989). Attempts to decrease family size have

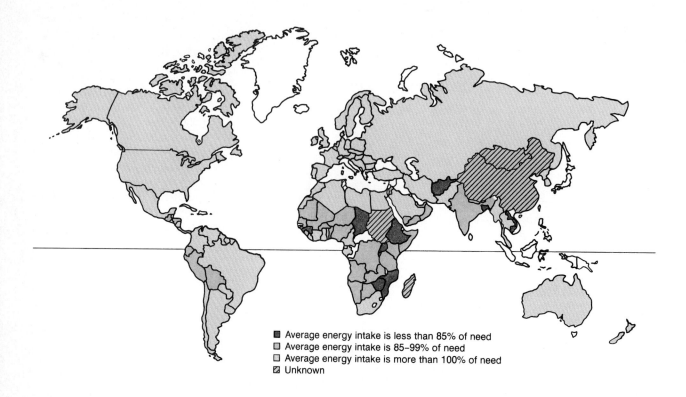

■ Average energy intake is less than 85% of need
□ Average energy intake is 85–99% of need
□ Average energy intake is more than 100% of need
▨ Unknown

Figure 9.6 Hunger and glut. The world's food supplies are very unevenly divided. With daily kcaloric needs of about 2400 for the moderately active person, average intakes range from less than 1500 kcalories in some developing regions to 3400 kcalories per person per day in the developed countries. (Source: Gaia, *An Atlas of Planet Management* (Anchor Press Book) London: Doubleday, pp. 48–49)

food security—having enough to eat now and the assurance of having enough in the future

been faced with a "Catch-22": while high population levels decrease the amount of available food, the lack of available food fosters higher birth rates. Why is this?

Historically, one factor that has been shown to help reduce the birth rate of a region is for its population to achieve a reasonable quality of life, including an adequate standard of living, a sense of well-being, and assurance of future economic security. That includes **food security;** that is, having reasonable confidence that food needs will be regularly met (Commoner, 1986). As long as people believe they must depend on their children to work and contribute to the family's welfare, they will continue to have more children. Population growth slows down only when people believe that factors other than family size can provide them with security and opportunity (Lappe and Collins, 1986).

You can see, then, that demand for food has two components: *the size of the population* and *the amount of food each person needs.* Figure 9.6 shows that in many countries, energy intakes are below the 2400 kcalories per day the average person needs for well-being and moderate physical activity.

Increases in population put stress not only on the food supply but also on the ecosystem. As population rises (especially in the developed countries), fossil fuel consumption increases. As we noted earlier, fossil fuel is the number one source of carbon dioxide production and contributes to the greenhouse effect. Furthermore, an increasing population in the developing tropical countries contributes to the destruction of the rainforest, the other major cause of increasing carbon dioxide (Balance Data, 1989). Therefore, an increasing population damages the ecosystem and ultimately has a negative effect on world food production capacity.

Distribution of Food

Once food production and demand have been considered, another major factor that determines what and how much food is available is distribution.

The importance of food distribution is underscored by the observation that at present no one in the world would starve if equal division of food occurred among all the inhabitants of the globe (World Resources Institute, 1988). In the last twenty years, during which time per capita food production has increased overall, the number of hungry people has actually been growing. This is because wealth is very unevenly distributed; the number of poor people is increasing, and the root causes of hunger are economic and/ or political powerlessness.

Economic and Social Structures   Lack of money results in hunger both because poor farmers cannot afford the agricultural supplies and technologies that could improve their food production, and because poor people do not have enough purchasing power to buy adequate food directly. Nations with a per capita income of $400 or less account for about 80% of the world's undernourished; the hungry are found primarily in the developing nations of South Asia and Africa (World Resources Institute, 1988).

When the economy of a poor country improves, there is a predictable effect on its demand for food: not only do people want more food, but they also want to eat the types of food more affluent people eat. That means that as people become more prosperous, they tend to eat less starch and more sugar, less plant protein and more animal protein, and more fat. Although it is certainly positive that hungry people get *more* to eat, the changes they make in *type of food* are not necessarily in their best health interest. If they actually were to achieve the diets of the developed countries, they likely would also adopt the health problems of affluence.

There are also people who starve in the midst of plenty in the developed countries (Figure 9.7). In a cross-sectional nutrition survey of the United States in the mid-1980s, approximately 15% of the people interviewed said "yes" to the question, "Do you ever go to bed hungry?" Of course, since there are other reasons why a person might be hungry—such as being on a severe weight-reduction diet—this percentage may not properly reflect the proportion of people who are involuntarily hungry.

Obtaining a good estimate of the extent of hunger is difficult. Hunger is hard to define, and hungry people can be difficult to locate; how can you get an accurate census of homeless, for example? Population sampling methods

Figure 9.7 Hunger in the midst of plenty. Even in the developed countries, where average intakes of food are more than adequate, some members of the population do not have enough to eat.

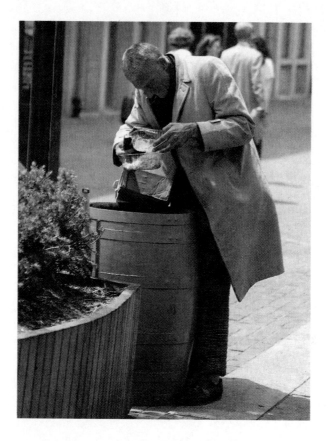

are being developed to deal with this issue (Sudman et al., 1988), and attempts were made to directly count people on the street during the 1990 census. Statistical difficulties notwithstanding, the increase in the number of emergency food relief sites and the number of people served by them testify to the fact that hunger is increasing in the U.S. (Thompson et al., 1988).

Experts are particularly interested in hunger among children because of its long-term effects on physical and mental development. The child poverty rate in the United States is estimated to have increased from 15% to 20% of all children between 1970 and 1987. In their study of poor children in rich countries, Smeeding and Torrey (1988) noted that childhood poverty is at least twice as high in single-parent families as in two-parent families. They also noted that poor children in the United States are worse off than children in any of the five other wealthy industrialized countries studied; a higher percentage of U.S. children (almost 10%) lives below 75% of the poverty line than are found in other countries (Smeeding and Torrey, 1988).

Governments and Institutions All political powers can influence both how much and what kinds of food are available to a population, but governments vary in the extent to which they influence the production and distribution of food. The most extreme position would be for a government to take total control of the production process and later also collect and distribute the crop; it is doubtful that any government exercises such complete control. Other governments have allowed just a few wealthy people to own most of the arable land, knowing they would use it for production of cash crops that would advance their own financial circumstances as well as the coffers of the government or its officials. Whatever the case, the effect of government on food availability can be substantial. Most governments, whatever their level of involvement, try to strike a balance between meeting indigenous needs and having sufficient currency to purchase needed foreign goods.

In countries that find themselves chronically at the brink of food inadequacy, periodic bad weather or political unrest can ultimately result in widespread famine. Experience has shown that sound government policies and adequate disaster plans can help stabilize such situations and avoid the worst-case scenarios (Glantz, 1987). For example, although Bihar, India experienced several years of successive crop failures, deaths due to starvation were minimized by the implementation of previously conceived management plans that included reinforcing local administration, improving communications, increasing public works programs, expanding rationing, giving inoculations, and providing agricultural support (Mellor and Gavian, 1987). On the other hand, African countries have been less able to avert disasters because of a combination of inadequate planning, civil unrest, and scarce human and/or material resources. Ethiopia serves as a stark example.

Sometimes the governments or humanitarian agencies of developed countries provide economic and technological assistance to developing countries. This can be extremely helpful, provided the technology is appropriate and sustainable by the recipients. Unfortunately, there are still instances of good intentions gone awry: sometimes donated equipment falls into disuse for lack of parts or skilled labor to repair it, or programs miss the mark because the donors do not understand the region's cultural constraints. For example, in some African countries, aid designed to help increase food production has been given mainly to men because the aid was distributed to landowners, and women are not able to own land there (Jacobson, 1988). Further, since women were responsible for securing the resources and producing the food, their failure to receive aid resulted in failure to increase agricultural production.

Most developed countries also have government programs designed to help domestic food producers. In the United States, programs provide various measures of government control in the production and marketing of certain crops such as peanuts, corn, rice, wheat, sorghum, barley, oats, and dairy products. Decisions about the production and marketing of other crops such as vegetables, some fruits, and nuts are determined by growers (or growers and handlers) through administrative committees that function with the help of federal guidelines (National Food Review, 1988). The effect of such programs and organizations is that producers have more income stability than if prices were determined entirely by free-market forces.

Figure 9.8 Per capita food production in developing and developed regions. This illustration shows that although the developed countries and some developing countries have improved their per capita food production over the last 25 years, Africa has steadily been losing ground in its fight to feed itself. (Source: United Nations Food and Agriculture Organization 1987 Country Tables, pp. 312–336)

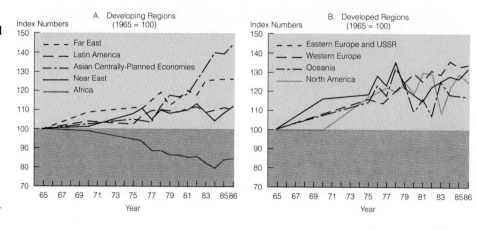

infrastructure—the basic framework of a system or organization

Transportation   The mechanics of distribution depend on an adequate transportation **infrastructure** including passable routes, functional vehicles and fuel, and sufficient labor; it also takes somebody to pay the freight. Transportation, whether by oxcart or airplane, makes it possible for people to gain access to a greater quantity of food and a more diverse diet. The more varied the food supply and the more that is available per capita, the more likely it is that the population overall will be well-nourished.

Transportation can be expensive, but expense can sometimes be moderated if food is put into the lightest and most compact form before shipping. Consider the following data assembled by agricultural economists who compared the cost of fluid milk shipped from Wisconsin to Florida, to the cost of milk that had been dried, transported as dry powder, and then commercially reconstituted: fluid milk cost $13.14 per hundredweight, whereas the dried milk after reconstitution cost only $8.83 (Jesse and Cropp, 1987).

Current Status and Projections

So, where do we stand in the relationship between the production, demand, and distribution of food?

In recent decades, in most areas of the world except Africa, production has increased at a faster rate than population (Figure 9.8), thanks largely to the Green Revolution (Brown, 1988). But trends in per capita food availability do not indicate whether the population is hungry or satisfied. Many do not have adequate food: it is estimated that one-fifth of the people of the world are hungry (World Resources Institute, 1988), and that 38,000 children under the age of 5 die each day from frequent infection and undernutrition (UNICEF, 1988).

What is the situation likely to be in the future? Trends in world agricultural production, consumption, and trade suggest abundant supplies during the coming decade. Some developing countries are becoming more self-sufficient, but a number of African and Latin American nations are likely to experience a widening gap between production and needs (Trostle, 1989). This situation puts such regions at greater risk of not only chronic hunger but also acute **famine.** That is because they lack what one expert believes to be the basic elements of famine prevention: surplus production, a highly developed transportation network, and a democratic form of government (Mellor, 1986).

famine—food scarcity so severe that many people die as a direct result of malnutrition

Beyond the year 2000, if the U.N.'s population estimates are correct, food production will need to increase dramatically again. How can this be accomplished? With most arable land already in use, irrigation nearly pushed to the limit, and a worldwide climate that is likely worsening, can technology feed the world's future population? The benefits of the Green Revolution have already been widely realized. Can newer technologies do even more?

The experts are divided in their opinions. Some say that in the near future we are unlikely to see advances on a par with those of the Green Revolution (Brown, 1989; Trostle, 1989). Others take a much more optimistic stance, believing that "biotechnology is destined to become a central force in the world's food system" (Doyle, 1988) and that "[genetic engineering] has provided an unparalleled opportunity to modify and improve crop plants" (Gasser and Fraley, 1989).

But we cannot rest our hopes for adequately feeding the world's population in the future on just one strategy such as the use of biotechnology. We must do our best to encourage the many interrelated factors that ultimately foster food security for all people—stable and cooperative governments, a healthy ecosystem, sustainable agricultural methods, and reliable and equitable distribution systems.

Now that we have considered many of the elements that influence our *access* to food, it is time to focus on the matter of what causes us to *choose* what we do from among the foods available to us.

Innate, Cultural, and Individual Factors Influence Food Preferences

The vastness of the food marketplace appears to be a mixed blessing. A student who grew up in Mexico and now lives in the United States expressed it one way when she said, "It's a lot harder to eat a good diet here than it was in Mexico; here, there is so much more to choose from."

We cope with the enormous number of food options with which we're confronted largely by settling down to a core group of foods on which to rely. The experts estimate that in the United States, only 100 generic items account for 75% of the total amount of food consumed (Molitor, 1980). Let's look now at the variety of factors that influence food preferences.

Inborn Factors

Psychologists who have studied why people select certain foods have identified some genetic influences, although they are relatively weak (Rosin, 1988). Of the four tastes (sweet, sour, bitter, and salty), infants react in consistent ways to two of them. A second tendency is to be both interested in, and cautious about, an unfamiliar food. Then, too, we seem to have the inborn ability to make a mental connection between the foods we have eaten and how we feel afterward. The upcoming section expands on these ideas.

Taste Biases   All babies and young children like sweet foods; babies who are tested in their first few days of life uniformly respond happily when they are given sweetened water. On the other hand, water with a bitter taste will bring scowls or crying. Although appreciation for sweetness may decline as people age, the predilection for some degree of sweetness persists throughout life. Psychologists suggest that this has been important to our survival, since the naturally sweet (sugar-containing) foods that early humans encountered were a source of life-sustaining energy.

In recent years, sweet foods have been cast in a dim light because of social pressure to be slim. Sugar-containing foods are now thought by some people to be "bad" (Executive Summary, 1986). How do people cope with this, given the liking they have for sweet things? The answer is that a relatively new industry—the sugar substitute industry—has been developed to resolve the conflict between our inborn liking for sweetness and the socially inspired rejection some people now have for sugar.

The bitter taste, as stated above, is rejected by infants (Rozin, 1988). Psychologists suggest that this may stem from the fact that many bitter substances in nature are toxic; those people who avoided toxic foods survived long enough to be our ancestors.

Some inborn biases can be modified, and they often are, by experience and conditioning. For example, some people acquire a taste for foods that are decidedly bitter. Others come to like foods so spicy that their mouths burn and eyes water when they eat them. One psychologist dubbed this behavior of eating foods that produce somewhat unpleasant sensations as "benign masochism," because it provides the thrill of apparent danger although it is really harmless (Rozin and Vollmecke, 1986).

Cautious Interest in New Foods   By nature, we are interested in new foods; at the same time, we tend to be cautious about trying them. This inborn trait allowed early humans to gradually expand their dietary variety in relative safety. Don't think of this interest in new foods as relegated to early humans

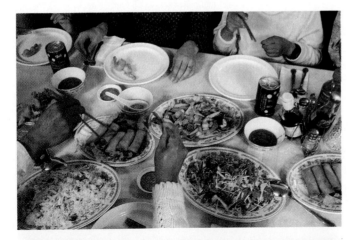

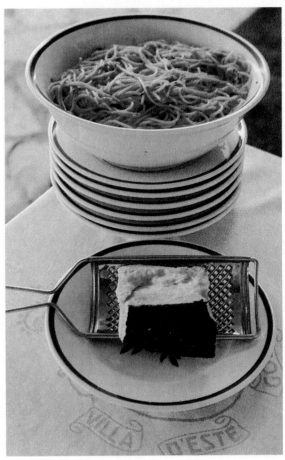

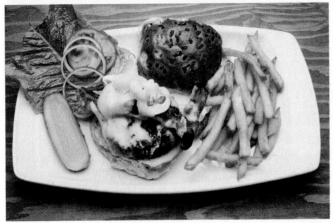

in the distant past, though; we are still experimenting. The fact that ethnic restaurants are flourishing is a prime example of our interest in trying cuisines other than our own (Figure 9.9).

Such interest is also evidenced by the introduction into the food supply of exotic items such as flower blossoms sometimes used in salads or as condiments. If this sounds appealing, trust your instinct to be cautious, and learn first which varieties are safe to eat (Environmental Nutrition, 1987).

Of course, people vary considerably in the extent to which they like to try new foods. Individual personal traits determine which way the balance tips. At the extremes, we describe people as **neophilic** (liking newness) or **neophobic** (rejecting it).

Ability to Associate Foods with Effects   People have a general ability to associate foods with their short-term effects on how they feel (Rozin, 1988). For example, under certain conditions we develop a liking for foods that relieve our hunger quickly, such as sweet foods. We may also make a connection between eating a certain food and relief of stomach pain. On the other hand, if we think that something we ate made us feel sick, we are very

Figure 9.9 No wonder ethnic restaurants are popular! Ethnic foods can appeal to us for a variety of reasons. One type of food might be from your culture of origin; another might meet your specifications for good health. You might especially like the flavors of a particular cuisine and find it surprisingly affordable. Exotic foods may appeal to your sense of adventure; and they are trendy.

neophilic—liking new things

neophobic—disliking new things

likely to avoid that food in the future, or to find it distasteful if we eat it unintentionally. This is such a powerful effect in some people that they have been able to condition themselves to avoid a particular food simply by *imagining* that the food would make them feel sick.

Cultural Factors

Wherever we are, the people and cultures around us influence our food choices. Anthropologists point out that in all societies, eating is the primary way of initiating and maintaining human relationships: eating and socializing experiences are inextricably intertwined with each other.

Family and Caregivers Starting with its first feeding, an infant is usually given food and affection at the same time by its caregivers. Therefore infants experience both physiological and emotional satisfaction and security when eating; this reinforces our interest in eating from the start.

The positive association between food, caregivers, and feelings of security lingers on in the form of our appreciation of things that appear homemade. The food industry has picked up on this, and offers us "Grandma's Pies" and "stew as good as Mom's." Ironically, this is one reason some imported foods are selling well in the U.S.: they look more homemade than domestic products. Certain British imports especially are perceived as "nurturing," "warm," and "cozy" (Food Technology, 1987).

Unfortunately, the connection between food and security can also be misapplied, as when people eat excessive amounts of food to make themselves feel better emotionally. This is maladaptive behavior, since the overeating fails to deal effectively with the cause of the emotional distress, and the weight gain that inevitably results may compound the original problems. Chapter 10 (on body weight) and Chapter 11 (on eating disorders) will deal extensively with this issue.

Families and caregivers seem to have more of an influence on a child's general attitudes about food and the world than they have on his or her specific food preferences. Studies show only a weak correlation between the foods liked by parents and those liked by their children (Rosin, 1988). (See Chapter 17 for a more thorough discussion of factors that influence children's eating patterns.)

cultural ecology—the study of how social and environmental factors produce unique cuisines and eating customs

National Origin Ethnicity is the best cultural predictor of food preference. Ethnic groups and nationalities have developed their unique cuisines through a combination of environmental and social factors. A discipline called **cultural ecology** involves the study of these influences (Grivetti, 1981). Each ethnic group encourages the use of some of the foods available to it while discouraging the use of others, even to the extent of designating them "taboo" (Bryant et al., 1985). Sometimes a food that is accepted or even prized by one culture may be deemed unacceptable or even disgusting by another. For an example, see how you react to the Slice of Life ''Foods of Zaire'' about a Peace Corps volunteer's experience in Africa.

Cultures often have a very basic **superfood** that has been the key to their survival over the ages and around which the rest of their cuisine has developed. The rice of the Orient and the wheat bread of Europe are examples of cultural superfoods. To testify to their importance, cultures often give mystical meanings to these foods. For example, the Mayan word for corn, ''ixim,'' literally means ''the grace of God.''

superfood—staple food of a culture

Food myths can arise from the belief that the characteristics of what is eaten can be acquired by the eater (a rather literal interpretation of ''You are what you eat''). For example, some primitive peoples have believed that eating part of an animal known for its ferocity will make a person brave; certain Eskimos believe that if a lactating mother eats duck's wings, her child will grow up to be a good paddler. Such mythical thinking is an attempt to explain and gain control over an environment that is often hostile (Harper, 1988).

Slice of Life

Foods of Zaire

When Nicholas was a Peace Corps volunteer in Zaire, he learned first-hand that various cultures make very different decisions about what is suitable to eat. Before going to Africa in 1988, his home had been in the Midwestern United States, and although he had eaten many international cuisines in ethnic restaurants, these meals had not prepared him for some of the foods of his adopted African culture.

Here's an excerpt from a letter to his family after several months in Zaire:

> A few days ago, I ate palm grubs which, I have to admit, are rivaled in taste only by a certain bright green grasshopper which is around just once a year. They remind me of that chewing gum with liquid in the middle that squirts out when you bite it . . . what's it called?
>
> This is *makelele* season, named after a big ugly bug resembling a grasshopper. It burrows into the sand and makes a lot of noise at night. (*Makelele* means ''noise'' in Kikongo.) Kids particularly like to dig them up, leaving holes in the ground all over the place. They wrap them up in leaves and put them on wood coals. It is good to see the kids eating these bugs, since they contain more protein than they usually get. They eat caterpillars here, too, and I have got so I can eat them. It's been a lot easier to get used to some of the local fish and vegetables, though, which really are quite good . . . even with my cooking, Mom.
>
> Although there isn't much food, people are generous and invite me to dinner sometimes. They serve everything in covered dishes. Once the father set a dish in front of me, smiled politely, lifted the cover, and there was a little cooked mouse. It was on its back, feet up, hair charred off by the fire. The family was very polite, and so was I. Yes, I did have a little bit of the mouse.

If the thought of eating bugs and mice makes you cringe, your cultural conditioning is showing. Insects and rodents are pests to most of us in the modern world, and we wouldn't think of eating any, even though they are nutritious. But given a different time, place, or set of circumstances— such as an African village with an extremely limited food supply—we might eventually accept them. Of course, the people of Zaire undoubtedly would initially find some of our foods detestible, too. ▼

Figure 9.10 Efficiency of converting grain to other forms of food. For animals to produce food for human consumption, they sometimes eat plants that could have been consumed directly by humans. This illustration shows how many pounds of grain (or grain and soy) are consumed by an animal in producing one pound of the stated product.

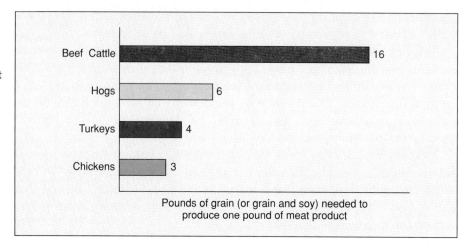

Pounds of grain (or grain and soy) needed to produce one pound of meat product

Much can be learned about a culture from its foods: the climate, economy, political situation, and religions of a country are reflected in its diet. In the United States, a mosaic of cultures, we have the opportunity to reaffirm our own roots and to learn about other cultures through folk fairs, international food clubs, and ethnic restaurants.

Religious Affiliation Some religions have developed dietary practices that are so elaborate and important to the group that they refer to them as "laws." For example, there are kosher (Jewish) dietary laws (Regenstein and Regenstein, 1988) and Moslem dietary laws (Twaigery and Spillman, 1989).

It is not always easy to discern what originally motivated particular dietary practices; very likely a combination of factors came into play. There are recurrent themes, though, such as ethical considerations, food safety, health maintenance, and symbolic values. The Seventh Day Adventists avoid eating animal flesh because they do not want to sustain themselves at the expense of another animal's life; the Latter Day Saints (Mormons) prefer not to consume caffeine, because they view the body as a temple of God, and the drug effects of caffeine may harm it.

Whatever their origins, these practices tend to be a prominent feature of the group's identity. Jewish scholars suggest that the primary reason for maintaining their practices is that they engender the sense of oneness with other Jews—both now and in the past—and the sense of uniqueness as a people.

Ethical Stances Decisions about what to eat can have an ethical basis independent of religion. Environmentalists, for instance, are concerned about eating behaviors that cause unnecessary stress on the ecosystem. They point out that the production of grain-fed beef cattle is wasteful, because in order to produce one pound of muscle (meat), 16 pounds of grain and soy are used (Figure 9.10) (Lappe, 1982). If people ate the plant products themselves instead of using them to feed animals, less acreage would need to be cultivated and there would be less depletion of soil nutrients. This has led some

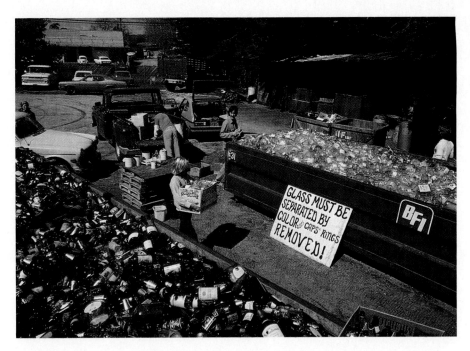

Figure 9.11 Recycling starts at home. In some communities, mandatory separation of trash into plastic, paper, metal, and glass enables once-used materials to be used again repeatedly.

people to avoid grain-fed beef. Range-fed cattle, on the other hand, are often grazed on domestic land that would be unsuitable for other forms of agriculture; therefore they *add* to the food supply.

Eating beef that has been imported from tropical regions is also viewed with disfavor by environmentalists. That is because sometimes rainforest has been cleared to create land for grazing cattle, thereby increasing destruction of the rainforest (Nations and Komer, 1986). In addition to the problems resulting from tropical deforestation already mentioned in this chapter is the concern that many species of plants and animals are destroyed as their habitat disappears; the decrease in biological diversity has both ethical and practical implications for our ecosystem (World Resources Institute, 1988).

The *energy* issue is also an ethical one. The food processing industry uses a large amount of fossil fuel for moving ingredients and products in and out of processing plants and distribution centers and for elaborate packaging of products. This suggests that if people used fewer convenience foods, considerable energy could be saved. While this may be the rule, there are exceptions. As we saw earlier, the shipping of dried milk powder for reconstitution—instead of fluid milk—can save on energy consumption.

The *solid waste* issue enters into the ethical picture as well. Space for disposal of solid waste is becoming scarce in most heavily populated areas of the world, especially in the developed countries. Some people concerned with this issue avoid using elaborately packaged foods; others urge food producers to use recyclable containers, lighter packaging, and biodegradable materials. Some trash collection departments now require citizens to separate their refuse according to its recycling potential (Figure 9.11). Critical Thinking 9.1 explores this issue more thoroughly.

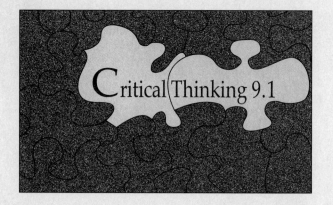

Fast Foods and Solid Waste

The situation

You have a couple of friends who decided to quit eating fast foods because they object to the type and quantity of packaging materials used. They say that fast-food packaging is contributing to the problems with solid waste disposal: the styrofoam containers used for some products are a problem because they are not biodegradable, and the amount of paper used is excessive.

You, on the other hand, eat fast foods quite often. You like the taste and consistent quality of the products, and their convenience and cost fit with the time and money you have available. However, you're beginning to feel pressured by your friends' convictions, and you wonder whether you should give up fast foods yourself.

Is the information accurate and relevant?

- It is true that styrofoam is not biodegradable. If used in landfill, it constitutes permanent refuse.
- You have been aware of double-packaging of some fast food products in past years, but you have observed lately in the places you eat that items are only single-wrapped.

What else needs to be considered?

While this issue is in the back of your mind, you find that information on solid waste pops up all over the place.

In the class you are taking on environmental issues, you learn that plastics, including styrofoam, represent about 7% of landfill. Styrofoam from fast food outlets would comprise some fraction of that; you asked, but the professor didn't have data as to what proportion it might be. In class you also learn that there is another environmental objection to styrofoam: that its manufacture involves the release into the atmosphere of chemicals that destroy ozone and contribute to the hole in the ozone layer. This, in turn, allows more of the harmful rays of the sun to reach the earth, causing effects potentially harmful to both animals and plants.

On the radio you heard that a researcher in "garbology" had found (when he took core samples at a garbage dump) that newspapers from ten years ago had not yet decomposed; so although paper biodegrades in time, if conditions are not

Human rights issues can also affect food choices. For example, the products of food producers with poor records for fair employment are being boycotted by some people. The abrogation of civil rights in South Africa has led some people to avoid the products of companies with subsidiaries and investments there, although others argue that this hurts the entire population, not just the oppressors.

Public Health Information and Nutrition Education Campaigns During the last decade, Americans have been on the receiving end of an increasing

conducive to its more rapid decomposition, it can take up landfill space for many years.

You saw in a news magazine that the industry has been experimenting with recycling plastics into items for which their stability is a virtue; some park benches and highway signs have been made from recycled plastics.

Your local paper carried a story about a neighboring community in which the town council decided to make separation of trash mandatory for citizens who have their garbage picked up by the town. Four different types of refuse—paper, glass, metal, and plastic—are to be recycled. A couple of days later in the "Letters to the Editor" column, several people had written in saying that your city should do the same.

On a kiosk on campus, you see a notice posted about a meeting on campus regarding the solid waste issue. You attend, and you learn that since the campus picks up its own trash, it would be possible for your institution to start its own recycling program.

Your values are another factor to consider. How much value do you put on the taste, convenience, and affordability of fast foods in your life right now? Do you believe that if you and your friends avoided fast foods, it would be a first step (albeit a small personal one) in helping to solve the solid waste problem?

What do you think?

You can see that there are a number of options in addition to the first two "all or nothing" positions currently practiced by you and your friends. Some options are:

- Option 1   You decide that at this time in your life, fast foods meet your needs very well, and the small amount of refuse you produce is insignificant compared with the total problem. Besides, by the time the problem gets really severe, there may have been a technological breakthrough to solve or at least substantially lessen the problem, so change now is not necessary.
- Option 2   You decide that your actions should reflect your belief that pollution is a big problem. You promise yourself that you won't use fast foods, realizing that you'll have to allow more time for food preparation.
- Option 3   You continue to eat *some* fast foods but avoid ordering items that come in styrofoam, or you boycott restaurants that use styrofoam.
- Option 4   You write letters of protest (even organize a letter-writing campaign) to the fast food restaurants that use styrofoam, stating your reasons for objecting to its use, and urging them to discontinue its use.
- Option 5   You get involved in the campus or city effort to make mandatory the separation of trash for recycling. This could help with the landfill problem without disruption of the fast food businesses.

Do you see other options? What is your stance?

---

amount of information about how the foods they eat (or don't eat) may affect their health (Lecos, 1988). These messages address four major health concerns: heart disease, cancer, high blood pressure, and osteoporosis.

Much of this educational outpouring has originated from various federal agencies and health organizations, such as the Food and Drug Administration, the National Institutes of Health, and the Surgeon General's Office. When surveys are done before and after an educational campaign, they usually demonstrate that people's knowledge about certain issues increases. For example, in the late 1970s, before there had been a concerted effort to acquaint people with the possible relationship between sodium and high blood pressure, only 12% of those surveyed were aware of it; by 1982, 34% knew of it. Substantial gains were also made in people's knowledge about heart disease through the use of educational campaigns.

To get their messages across, these agencies rely heavily on the mass media (Lecos, 1988); word is spread through press reports and public service announcements. Starting in the fall of 1984, the National Cancer Institute (one of the National Institutes of Health) allowed one of its health messages to be delivered in a new way—through product advertising. This was when the Kellogg Company first stated in its cereal ads that the National Cancer Institute recommended eating a high-fiber diet to reduce the risk of some types of cancer. The effectiveness of this campaign is evident: in a follow-up survey asking which foods are good sources of fiber, over two-thirds of those asked said breakfast cereals were (Lecos, 1988).

Although this ad delivered information very effectively to the American public, it opened a Pandora's box. Other food producers now make health claims for their products as well. Developing policies as to what can be said in order to inform and not mislead is providing to be a real quagmire. For one thing, the unique nature of each food makes it impossible for a generic policy to cover all cases easily. For another, experts question how much credit any one food should be given for being nutritious or for reducing risk of disease. After all, *health and nutritional status are affected by the total of what a person has eaten over a long period of time, not just by one food for a few weeks or months.*

Food Product Advertising and Promotion   Good advertising works to change public opinion, and that's the reason we see so much of it; but we need to be aware that some of the most aggressively promoted products are foods of relatively poor nutritional quality. About ten years ago, alcoholic beverages, frozen baked goods, cake and other dessert mixes, margarine, mayonnaise, and sweeteners were among the most heavily advertised products. On the other hand, many nutritious foods, such as meats, fish, poultry, canned vegetables, wheat flour, and cheese received much less promotion.

To some extent this situation seems to be changing. Increasingly, nutrition sells, and agencies such as the Cranberry Marketing Committee, the National Dairy Promotion and Research Board, and the National Livestock and Meat Board now advertise the nutritional merits of their products.

Some food companies have renamed existing products to cast an aura of good health around them. The interest in nutrition and health has influenced the development of new food products as well; now we see items on the market that would not have been imagined a generation ago: flour with added calcium, carbonated beverages with added nutrients, oat bran in almost any type of grain product you can name. Such products do not necessarily improve the nutritional quality of the total diet more than ordinary foods do. Unfortunately, sometimes the nutritional characteristics or benefits of a product are misrepresented in food advertising; in other instances, the dietary status of a promoted nutrient is already adequate for most Americans. However, in some cases products promoted for their nutritional quality provide nutrients to people whose intakes are low.

Status Foods that are scarce and expensive enjoy a higher status than other foods. In some circles, using them demonstrates to others that one is prosperous enough to afford them. You might order lobster tails rather than a steak—even if you liked them equally—to impress your companions or even the waiter. Somebody entertaining an important guest might choose a wine of rare vintage and high cost, not because his palate demanded it but because he could gain status in his guest's eyes because of his affluence and knowledge of fine wine.

Peer Groups Peer groups—subcultures distinguished by age, sex, occupation, or other common interests—can influence their members' food choices (Figure 9.12). Foods that become "in" with teenagers and restaurants that become popular with young professionals can credit their success to peer group influence.

A person may align her choices with those of an admired member of her group. When the most financially successful member of a group of business executives shows a preference for a particular brand of sparkling water or liquor, some associates are likely to recognize its "superiority" as well. Sexism also can have an influence: certain men may feel disinclined to eat salads or light cuisine in public because these have a feminine connotation to some people.

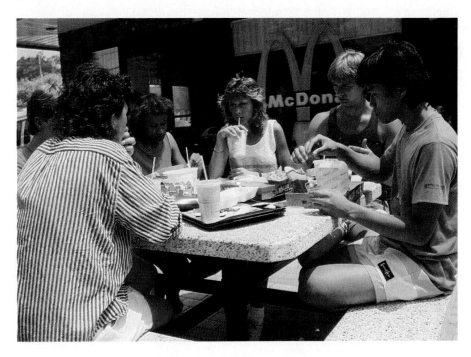

Figure 9.12 Peer groups can have a strong influence on food choice.

Unique Personal Factors

After the various inborn and cultural influences have had their effects, there are factors unique to you that also govern what foods you eat. These are the ultimate determinants of food choice.

Preferred Sensory Characteristics   Our food choices are heavily influenced by how food appeals to our senses. In almost every survey in which consumers are asked on what basis they chose a particular meal or why they selected what's in the shopping cart, *taste* is said to be the strongest determinant.

Technically, as mentioned earlier, there are just four basic *tastes*—sweet, sour, bitter, and salty—and our inclinations regarding them are affected by individual preference as well as by inborn and cultural influences. We also respond to certain food *smells*. The sensation of *flavor* is the combination of tastes and smells; this is what many people really mean when they use the term "taste." *Texture* also figures into the total picture of what we like: you may respond positively to foods that have crisp, soft, tender, chewy, granular, or smooth textures, for example. Other sensory characteristics that can affect preference are *temperature, moisture, color*, and the *shape and size of food pieces*.

Emotions   Emotions can play a large role in food intake. Most of us are influenced either to eat or not to eat by various emotional circumstances: a mood of celebration prompts most of us to want something to eat or drink. People are variously influenced to eat (or not to eat) when they are bored, lonely, tired, excited, or frustrated or when they want to delay or take a break from a less appealing activity. However, these factors often have more to do with the circumstances that initiate eating and the amounts of food people consume than they do with the particular types of food selected. Such emotional influences on eating will be discussed more thoroughly in Chapters 10 (on body weight) and 11 (on eating disorders).

Emotions *can* affect food choices to some degree. For example, psychologists suggest that when some people feel insecure or lonely, they may find particular appeal in foods associated with their relatively secure childhood. People may also reward themselves with certain types of foods if such foods were employed during early years to reinforce desired behaviors. This may explain why some people feel they "deserve" an ice cream cone or a candy bar after a demanding study session or a busy day at work.

Available Money   No matter what you would *like* to eat, the amount of money you have available for food controls what you *can afford to buy*. In the United States in 1988, people spent approximately 12% of their disposable incomes (after taxes) for food (Blaylock and Elitzak, 1989). Compare that proportion with the 61% that Americans spent for food in 1869. These figures indicate that personal income has risen much faster than food cost and consumption; food is truly a bargain *now*. It is also a bargain *here:* contrast our current situation with that in the developing countries, where food purchases often account for more than 50% of a household's income (Korb and Cochrane, 1989). Even compared to other developed countries, U.S. food is often less expensive. A Big Mac in Moscow costs 4 hours' wages; in the U.S., it only costs 32 minutes' wages.

No matter what the averages are, your own personal financial situation is the critical factor for you. If your household income is less than average, you will spend a larger proportion on food; in 1986, households with before-tax earnings below $5,000 spent almost 50% of it on food. On the other hand, households with incomes above $40,000 spent about 9% on food, as shown in Figure 9.13 (Dunham, 1987). That is, if your income is eight times someone else's, you will not buy eight times as much food or food that is eight times as expensive; food expenditure does not rise proportionately with income.

Lifestyle The way you live on a day-to-day basis can affect what you eat. For example, how much time do you have to spend on planning, buying, and preparing food? If you are consistently short of time, you will likely get into the habit of paying more for the convenience of processed foods. And how "food-centered" are you? For some people, meals are the most important events of the day, and these people deliberately give a lot of attention to food-related activities; others may forget about eating until hunger reminds them. If you're a real planner, you are probably more deliberate about getting what you would like to have. If you're very spontaneous, your intake may depend heavily on what happens to be around when you get hungry (Figure 9.14).

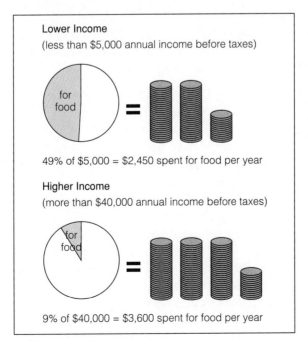

Lower Income
(less than $5,000 annual income before taxes)

for food

49% of $5,000 = $2,450 spent for food per year

Higher Income
(more than $40,000 annual income before taxes)

for food

9% of $40,000 = $3,600 spent for food per year

Figure 9.13 As you earn more, do you spend more for food? Yes and no. High-income households spend more *dollars* for food than do low-income households, but the *proportion* of income they spend is far smaller than that spent by low-income families. (Source: Dunham, D. *National Food Review*, 37:24, 1987)

Figure 9.14 Which pasta meal is "you"? Your lifestyle helps determine which form of food you will choose.

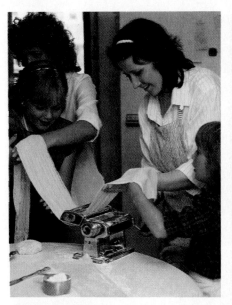
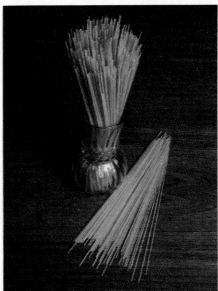
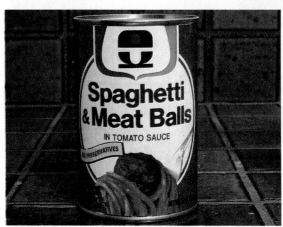

Beliefs About Long-Term Health Effects of Food In the discussion of cultural influences on food choices earlier in this chapter, we pointed out that knowledge about nutrition increases after a public education campaign. But such knowledge may not lead to behavior change: there is a considerable difference between *knowing what is wise to do* and actually *doing it*.

If you firmly believe that eating has long-term effects on health, what you know can influence your food choices. In surveys that ask consumers whether they have made any dietary changes for the sake of health, between one-half and three-fourths usually say, "yes."

People's concern about nutrition does not necessarily affect their choice of all food items in the same way. People are more attentive to nutrition when they are choosing main-course items than when selecting sweets or snack foods (Schutz et al., 1986).

What kinds of concerns do people have about nutrition? According to the Food Marketing Institute (1989), fat and cholesterol head the list, followed by salt, vitamins and minerals, sugar, and kcalories. As people age, they become increasingly concerned about these issues.

You Can Change Your Eating Habits

Now that you know about the biological, cultural, and personal influences on food choices, you may have the feeling that you have very little control over what you consume. Indeed, people who try suddenly to overturn their longstanding eating habits will find that failure is virtually guaranteed. But that doesn't mean that deliberate dietary change is impossible. What it takes is having good reasons for changing, strong motivation, attainable goals, and procedures to help you gradually form new habits. Therefore, you can see that you need to do quite a bit of *thinking* about your diet before you should start *doing* anything about it.

The first step is to *assess whether you really need to make any changes; we do not assume that you do.* What have the assessments in the preceding chapters told you about your eating habits? Does your diet generally meet the standards for good nutrition and health, or does it fall short (or is it excessive) in some way? Are there other reasons you want to make changes?

Secondly, are you *sufficiently motivated?* It takes energy to change habits, and a strong commitment can help you maintain your energy level. Experts recommend that people who are not highly motivated shouldn't even try to make changes, because they won't carry them through. Repeated failures can have negative mental and physical consequences (Kayman, 1989).

If you are convinced that you need to change your diet and are motivated to do it, then the next step is to use a process known to be helpful for achieving dietary change: it is **behavior modification.** This method was developed by psychologists to help people change many different kinds of behaviors including eating habits. Dietitians and nutritionists often teach clients to use such techniques (Holli, 1988), but you can implement them yourself. Behavior modification is described in Assessment 9.1.

behavior modification—process used to bring about gradual, sustainable changes in habitual behaviors

As you read about the process, note how important it is to set reasonable goals. Another important principle for success is to think positively throughout the program. Also consider whether you are a person who will benefit from social support; some do, some don't. Ways of enlisting support include telling your family and friends about what you are trying to do, asking them to praise you as they see you doing it, and urging them not to tempt you to deviate from your program. Some people make a written contract with a friend who will provide encouragement along the way. You have to know yourself in order to decide whether such measures would be helpful to you.

Even if you employ all the methods in Assessment 9.1, don't expect perfection; there will be times when you'll slip into your old behaviors. But don't despair or give up. When you experience an occasional lapse, renew your determination and "get back on the horse." Be proud of the successes you *have* achieved.

Using Behavior Modification Techniques to Change Food Habits

If you are highly motivated to change some aspect(s) of your diet, it helps to use a behavior modification program. Once you have designed yours using the techniques below, do not regard this list as iron-clad; while you are using your program, feel free to go back and make adjustments to its various features as needed.

What follows is an outline and explanation of each step in behavior modification. The "technique" steps should be followed regardless of the habit(s) you are attempting to change. For the purposes of the illustration, though, we have included an "example" for each step. In this example, you have chosen to increase your consumption of fruits and vegetables because you have been neglecting these foods for some time.

Assessment 9.1

Record Your Current Eating Habits

• Technique Find out what you are eating by keeping a record of your intake for several days. Make note of the time of day, the type and amounts of each food and beverages ingested, where you were at the time, who you were with, and what mood you were in (see Sample Assessment 9.1). This not only documents your current behavior to help you understand your eating pattern but also establishes a baseline against which you can compare your behavior as you change it.

Example You complete a diet record as shown in Sample Assessment 9.1. This day, you find you ate several servings of fruits and vegetables. On other days, you ate none or just one serving.

Set Realistic Goals

• Technique Decide what you want your eating habits to be. You have a general idea of this already—after all, you had something in mind when you decided dietary changes were in order—but now you need to get more specific. Are you trying to eat *more* of a certain kind of food? If so, how many servings do you eventually want to eat per day? Are you trying to eat *less* of something? What's your limit? Be sure that your goals are *attainable* and *maintainable*. The importance of reasonable goals cannot be overemphasized; evidence shows that they can be the most useful feature of a lifestyle change program (Berry et al., 1989).

Make sure your goals are written in terms of *behaviors* and not particular health *outcomes* such as a drop in blood pressure or lower body weight. *It is important to deal in behaviors here because they are under your control, whereas the rate at which the body responds is an individual variable not within your control.*

Surely, at some point you will want to find out whether you are achieving positive results from your changed behaviors, but there is no point in paying much attention to that at first.

Example   You decide you eventually want to consume five servings of fruits and vegetables per day, as recommended in the Basic Food Guide.

Evaluate Why You Practice Unwanted Behaviors

Technique   Psychologists point out that most eating behaviors, like many other types of behavior, consist of a chain of events: a *cue* brings you to think about the behavior, you *do it*, and then there is a *consequence*, either a reinforcement that encourages or a punishment that discourages that behavior in the future.

Generally, reinforcement has a stronger effect on future behavior than punishment. Reinforcers may either be positive (a good thing happens as a result of the behavior) or negative (a bad thing goes away as a result of the behavior).

If you understand what cue causes an unwanted behavior again and again, you can think of how to interrupt that chain of events and have more control over the consequence of your behavior.

Example   You realize that one reason why you don't eat many fruits and vegetables is that you think it's a nuisance to fix them for yourself. Furthermore, on several previous occasions when you bought fresh vegetables and put them in the drawer in your refrigerator, you forgot about them and they spoiled. Since you quit buying fresh produce, you have been glad not to have any more of those disgusting surprises and were thus reinforced not to purchase fresh vegetables.

Plan for Gradual Change and Then Do It

Design your strategy:

Technique   Decide which of your goals you would like to work toward first. If it represents a large departure from your current habits, plan to take it in stages. In other words, plan to get only part way there to begin with. After that has become a fairly comfortable habit, set your sights a little higher.

Example   To begin with, you decide to eat two servings of fruits and vegetables per day.

Technique   Now think of what cues commonly trigger the unwanted behavior. Are there features of your environment you can change to get away from the cues? Change them. Are there places or certain situations you should avoid? Stay away from them, at least until you form new habits. Are there situations you could set up for yourself that would serve as cues for your intended behaviors? Create those situations for yourself.

Example   You decide to buy types of produce that keep better, to store them properly, and to keep them more visible in the refrigerator so you will be reminded to use them. You realize that when you and your apartment-mate fix meals together, you don't mind fixing salads and cooked vegetables; he agrees to fix three dinners with you each week.

relapse prevention—planning how to cope successfully with situations that are likely to promote old behaviors you want to avoid

Technique   Practice **relapse prevention.** Some of the cues that trigger your unwanted behavior may be hard to avoid: stress and certain social situations can be troublesome. Think about those situations before they occur, and rehearse how you will handle them successfully. This doesn't absolutely guarantee a triumph, but it makes it more likely. Even if you have a *lapse* in your behavior, it doesn't need to result in *collapse* of your program. Focus on your successes, and go on.

Example   To practice relapse prevention, think about not wanting to fix vegetables at the end of an especially stressful day. Think about how you could carry through on meeting your goal. If you can afford it, you might go out for dinner and include a salad and/or cooked vegetable in the meal; or you could have some fruit that only needs washing; or you could open a can of vegetables that only need heating.

Technique   Next consider what reinforcements your new behaviors will provide, and design some rewards to give yourself even more reinforcement. One reward to use regularly is *positive self-talk;* that is, congratulate yourself every time you do as you intended. If you have asked people close to you for their support, this adds reinforcement. Plan other rewards, such as buying something you have wanted or taking time to do something you enjoy. Rewarding yourself as promptly as possible provides the best reinforcement.

Example   Immediately tell yourself that you did the job right, even though you didn't much feel like doing it at the time. Further reward yourself for meeting your dietary goals (and surviving the day!) by calling a friend and arranging to shoot baskets later.

Technique   Think positively, and practice "thought stopping" for negative ideas (Holli, 1988). Whenever you catch yourself with pessimistic or self-defeating thoughts, simply say "Stop" to yourself, and deliberately replace it with a more positive idea.

Example   At some points, you catch yourself thinking that in the whole scheme of things, eating enough fruits and vegetables isn't all that important. STOP. Change your thoughts to something like, "I know that there is nutritional benefit from doing this; and I know that soon it will be a habit, and I won't even have to think about it."

Monitor Your Progress and Fine-Tune Your Program

Technique   Check up on yourself as you go along. Periodically keep another series of diet records and compare them with your earlier records. Are you making progress? If so, keep up the program, or even step it up a bit. If it is not successful enough, analyze what is causing your lapses and modify your program.

Example   Next time you check your diet, you find that you're pretty consistently getting two fruits and vegetables per day, but sometimes only one or three. You decide to continue using the same techniques, but you advance to a goal of three servings per day.

Sample Assessment 9.1 Using behavior modification techniques to change food habits

Time	Food or Beverage	Amount Consumed	Location of Eating	Others Present	Mood
8:30 a.m.	Wheat cereal	2 c.	kitchen	——	?
	2% milk	1 c.			
	Coffee	1 c.			
11:00 a.m.	Sweet roll	1 medium	outside classroom	class members	tense (exam)
12:30 p.m.	Beef, macaroni tomato casserole	1 c	union cafeteria	friends	relaxed
	Bread	2 slices			
	Butter	3 pats			
	Cola	12 oz.			
	Chocolate pie	1 piece			
6:15 p.m.	Fried fish	5 oz.	kitchen	roommate	happy, relaxed
	Hash browned potatoes	1 c.			
	Lettuce salad	1 c.			
	2% milk	1½ c.			
	Frosted white cake	1 piece			
9:30 p.m.	Corn snacks	3 oz.	living room	——	pressured
	Root beer	12 oz. can			

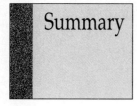
► The foods you eat reflect a whole spectrum of influences, ranging from what is *available* to you to what you *favor*. These influences continually interact with one another to affect how you make your food choices.

► One of the three major factors affecting food availability is the world's capacity for production. This, in turn, is affected by basic production resources including the amount of **arable land,** water, climate, and energy; technological aids such as **biotechnology** and **genetic engineering** can enhance production, and offer possibility for the future.

► Demand for food is the second major factor affecting food availability. Demand is increasing because population is increasing, and because people want to achieve **food security.**

► The third factor in food availability is distribution. A region's economic situation and social and governmental policies influence distribution; ultimately, an effective transportation **infrastructure** must be in place to get food to people.

► Residents of the United States and Canada are especially privileged regarding food availability, because we have a wide variety of nutritious foods reliably available all year round. However, an estimated one-fifth of the world's population is hungry, and the situation appears to be worsening in some African and Latin American countries, which periodically are at risk of **famine.**

► Food preferences are affected, first of all, by innate factors. We like sweet foods and dislike the bitter taste. The interplay between **neophilia** and **neophobia** gives us a cautious interest in new foods, and the ability to associate certain results with eating particular foods influences our future food choices.

► Culture is a second strong influence on food choices. Culture influences us through the people who take care of us as children, our ethnic/religious heritage (which may include a cultural **superfood**), ethical movements, health information, advertising, and our peers. The final screen through which our food choices sift is unique personal factors. Sensory preferences, emotional factors, finances, and lifestyle all have an impact on what we choose to eat.

► You can change your eating habits if you are determined to; **behavior modification** may help. Self-monitoring is the best way to see whether your habits are what you think they are; then, if you do decide to make changes, it is important to be realistic in your goals. Evaluate why you practice the unwanted behaviors; plan carefully for change, including strategies for **relapse prevention.** When you practice your new behaviors, give yourself rewards as soon as possible. Periodic monitoring will tell you how you are doing and give you insights about how to fine-tune your program.

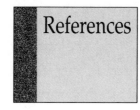
Balance Data. 1989. Global warming and population growth. *Balance Data* Number 26. Washington, DC: Population–Environment Balance.

Berry, M.W., S.J. Danish, W.J. Rinke, and H. Smiciklas-Wright. 1989. Work-site health promotion: The effects of a goal-setting program on nutrition-related behaviors. *Journal of the American Dietetic Association* 89:914–920, 923.

Blaylock, J. and H. Elitzak. 1989. Food expenditures. *National Food Review* 12:16–24.

Brown, L.R. 1988. The growing grain gap. *World Watch* 1:10–18.

Brown, L.R. 1989. Feeding six billion. *World Watch* 2:32–40.

Brown, L.R. and J.E. Young. 1988. Growing food in a warmer world. *World Watch* 1:31–35.

Bryant, C.A., A. Courtney, B.A. Markesbery, and K.M. DeWalt. 1985. The cultural feast. St. Paul: West Publishing Co.

Commoner, B. 1985. How poverty breeds overpopulation (and not the other way around). In *World Food, Population and Development*, ed.

G.M. Berardi. Totowa, N.J.: Rowman and Allanheld.

Detwiler, R.P. and C.A. Hall. 1988. Tropical forests and the global carbon cycle. *Science* 239: 42–47.

Doyle, J. 1988. Biotechnology and the food system. In *Consumer demands in the marketplace*, ed. K.L. Clancy. Washington, DC: Resources for the Future, Inc.

Dunham, D. 1987. Food spending and income. *National Food Review* 37:24.

Environmental Nutrition. 1987. Q: Are flowers edible? *Environmental Nutrition* 10(no.7):July, 1987

Executive Summary. 1986. International symposium on sweetness. *Nutrition Today* 21:16–17.

Food Marketing Institute. 1989. *Trends: Consumer Attitudes & the Supermarket.* Washington, DC: Food Marketing Institute.

Food Technology. 1987. International foods—a growing market in the U.S. *Food Technology* 41:120–134.

Gasser, C.S. and R.T. Fraley. 1989. Genetically engineering plants for crop improvement. *Science* 244:1293–1299.

Glantz, M.H. 1987. Drought in Africa. *Scientific American* 256:34–40.

Grivetti, L.E. 1981. Cultural nutrition: Anthropological and geographical themes. *Annual Reviews of Nutrition* 1:47–68.

Harlander, S. 1989. Introduction to biotechnology. *Food Technology* 43:44–48.

Harper, A.E. 1988. Nutrition: From myth and magic to science. *Nutrition Today* 23:8–17.

Holli, B.B. 1988. Using behavior modification in nutrition counseling. *Journal of the American Dietetic Association* 88:1530–1536.

Institute of Food Technologists' Expert Panel on Food Safety & Nutrition. 1988. Food biotechnology. *Food Technology* 42:133–146.

Jacobson, J.L. 1988. The forgotten resource. *World Watch* 1:35–42.

Jesse, E. and B. Cropp. 1987. Fluid milk reconstitution: Issues and impacts. *Marketing and Policy Briefing Paper*, Department of Agricultural Economics, University of Wisconsin.

Kayman, S. 1989. Applying theory from social psychology and cognitive behavioral psychology to dietary behavior change and assessment. *Journal of the American Dietetic Association* 89:191–202.

Korb, P. and N. Cochrane. 1989. World food expenditures. *National Food Review* 12(no. 4):26–29.

Lappe, F.M. 1982. *Diet for a small planet.* New York: Ballantine Books.

Lappe, F.M. and J. Collins. 1986. *World hunger: Twelve myths.* New York: Grove Press, Inc.

Lecos, C. 1988. We're getting the message about diet–disease links. *FDA Consumer* May, 1988: 6–9.

Martin, R.E. 1988. Seafood products, technology, and research in the U.S. *Food Technology* 42(no. 3):58–62.

Mellor, J.W. 1986. Prediction and prevention of famine. *Federal Proceedings* 45:2427–2431.

Mellor, J.W. and S. Gavian. 1987. Famine: causes, prevention, and relief. *Science* 235:539–545.

Molitor, G.T. 1980. The food system in the 1980s. *Journal of Nutrition Education* 12(no. 2)supplement:103–111.

Myers, N. 1984. *GAIA: An atlas of planet management.* Garden City, NY: Anchor Press, Doubleday and Company Inc.

National Food Review. 1988. Entire Volume 11 Issue 3: July–September, 1988.

Nations, J.D. and D.I. Komer. 1986. Rainforests and the hamburger society. In *The nutrition debate: sorting out some answers,* eds. J.D. Gussow and P.R. Thomas. Palo Alto, CA: The Bull Publishing Company.

Pimintel, D., L.E. Hurd, A.C. Bellotti, M.J. Forster, I.N. Oka, O.D. Sholes, and R.J. Whitman. 1978. Food production and the energy crisis. In *The feeding web,* ed. J.D. Gussow. Palo Alto, CA: The Bull Publishing Company.

Pursel, V.G., C.A. Pinkert, K.F. Miller, D.J. Bolt, R.G. Campbell, R.D. Palmiter, R.L. Brinster, and R.E. Hammer. 1989. Genetic engineering of livestock. *Science* 244:1281–1288.

Redmayne, P.C. 1989. World aquaculture developments. *Food Technology* 43(no. 11):80–81.

Regenstein, J.M. and C.E. Regenstein. 1988. The kosher dietary laws and their implementation in the food industry. *Food Technology* 42:86–94.

Rozin, P. 1988. Cultural approaches to human food preferences. *Nutritional modulation of neural function,* eds. J.E. Morley, M.B. Sterman, J.H. Walsh. Academic Press, Inc.

Rozin, P. and T.A. Vollmecke. 1986. Food likes and dislikes. *Annual Reviews of Nutrition* 6:433–456.

Schutz, H.G., D.S. Judge, and J. Gentry. 1986. The importance of nutrition, brand, cost, and sensory attributes to food purchase and consumption. *Food Technology* 40:79–82.

Smeeding, R.M. and B.B. Torrey. 1988. Poor children in rich countries. *Science* 242:873–877.

Steinhart, J.S. and C.E. Steinhart. 1978. Energy use in the U.S. food system. In *The feeding web,* ed. J.D. Gussow. Palo Alto, CA: The Bull Publishing Company.

Sudman, S., M.G. Sirken, C.D. Cowan. 1988. Sampling rare and elusive populations. *Science* 240:991–996.

Sun, M. 1989. Market sours on milk hormone. *Science* 246:876–877.

Thompson, F.E., D.L. Taren, E. Andersen, G. Casella, J.K. Lambert, C.C. Campbell, E.A. Frongillo, and D. Spicer. 1988. Within month variability in use of soup kitchens in New York state. *American Journal of Public Health* 78:1298–1301.

Trostle, R.G. 1989. Food aid needs during the 1990's. *National Food Review* 12:31–33.

Twaigery, S. and D. Spillman. 1989. An introduction to Moslem dietary laws. *Food Technology* 43:88–90.

UNICEF. 1988. *UNICEF Annual Report 1988.* New York: UNICEF Headquarters.

World Resources Institute and the International Institute for Environment and Development in collaboration with the United Nations Environment Programme. 1988. *World resources 1988–89.* Washington, DC: World Resources Institute.

10

Energy Balance and the Weight Debate

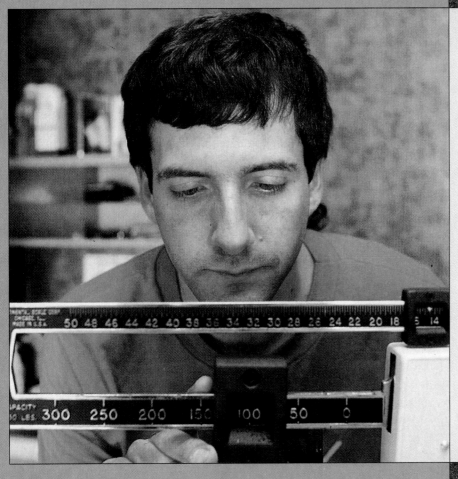

T hin is in. Who could believe otherwise?

Look at the number of articles about how to lose weight in popular magazines and tabloids. Look at the number of people who say they are trying to lose weight—approximately half of the women and one-fourth of the men surveyed in the United States. And look at the support services that abound to aid people in North America in their quest for thinness—diet businesses, restaurants that specialize in low-kcalorie fare, exercise spas, even hypnosis and acupuncture treatments. We also have access to low-kcalorie convenience foods, so-called weight-loss drugs, exercise equipment, and computerized diet scales that give digital readouts of kcalories in foods. Such products and services add up to a $33 billion industry annually in the United States.

Although the attention our culture devotes to the cosmetic aspect of body weight may seem excessive, it is not inappropriate for us to be concerned about body weight from a health perspective. Some experts regard overweight as our number one nutrition problem. It has been linked to the development of chronic conditions—such as heart disease and diabetes—that complicate life and make it less pleasant; and extreme overweight is associated with early death. We will have more to say about the health hazards of overweight in this chapter.

Why do so many people have trouble controlling body weight, when much of the animal kingdom regulates body weight automatically? There are several scientific theories about why people become overweight, which we will look at shortly. We will also open a Pandora's box by asking the question of *what ideal weight is.* (To paraphrase that familiar adage about the weather: everybody talks about ideal body weight, but nobody knows exactly what it is.) And of course we'll discuss techniques—both healthy and unhealthy—that have been used for weight reduction.

All this emphasis on overweight seems to ignore those people with the opposite problem: extreme thinness. People who would like to be heavier but consistently lose the weight gains they have made feel just as frustrated as overweight people who cannot achieve their desired body weights. It is hard for either group to appreciate the other's problem.

What can we say to you who are unhappily underweight? The truth is that there has been very little research directed at moderately underweight individuals in the developed countries. There is some information that can be gleaned from epidemiological studies, though. We will use such materials to address your concerns, but we admit openly that we do not have as much data to work with regarding this problem. We can only hope that the implications of low body weight will become a more thoroughly studied topic in the future.

The only manifestations of underweight that have received intensive scientific scrutiny in the developed countries are eating disorders such as anorexia nervosa and bulimia. These conditions are complex, and we will discuss them in a separate chapter following this one.

Although this entire chapter deals with overweight and underweight in some detail, keep in mind that *the majority of college students do not have either problem*. If you are in that fortunate situation, this chapter has a message for you anyway: why it is important to stay at your ideal weight. It may also improve your understanding of how difficult it is to make a deliberate change in body weight—a fact that is known by anybody who has tried.

Let's begin by discussing what's unhealthy about extremes in body fat.

Too Much or Too Little Fat Interferes with Healthy Living

Before we begin this discussion, we should define some common terms as they are used in the technical literature: **overweight** is often used to mean 10–20% above ideal body weight; **obese** means more than 20% above ideal body weight. In this book we will often use the term **overfat** to include both. We favor this term because it indicates that the concern is about people who have surplus *fat*, not about those who are heavier than average because they have a large frame or an unusually large amount of muscle. The term **underweight** is usually defined in context, such as "10% less than recommended."

People who are overly fat or excessively thin encounter problems in almost every aspect of living. Some of these problems are severe enough to be life-threatening; others may not shorten life but may make it more limited and less enjoyable.

overweight—usually 10–20% in excess of recommended body weight

obese—usually 20% or more in excess of recommended body weight

overfat—term used in this book to refer to surplus fat in any amount

underweight—less than recommended body weight; extent usually defined in context

Effects of Too Much Body Fat

In the United States, approximately 24% of adult males and 27% of adult females are overweight or obese (National Center for Health Statistics, 1987). Overfatness has increased markedly in U.S. children in the last couple of decades; it is estimated that 20–23% of all school-age children are overweight or obese (Dietz, 1988). Females of all ages are more likely to be overweight or obese than are males, and people of lower socioeconomic status are more likely to be heavier.

Health Risks   The likelihood of developing certain health problems is statistically greater in people who are overfat than in the general population. *The Surgeon General's Report on Nutrition and Health* (1988) and the National Research Council's report *Diet and Health* (1989) link the following conditions with obesity:

- high blood pressure (hypertension)
- stroke
- high blood LDL cholesterol
- coronary artery heart disease

- diabetes
- cancer (in women, cancer of the gallbladder, breast, cervix, uterus, and ovaries; in men, cancer of the colon and prostate)
- gallbladder disease
- upper respiratory problems
- arthritis and gout
- skin disorders
- menstrual irregularities, ovarian abnormalities, and complications of pregnancy
- early death, if overweight is extreme

Figure 10.1 illustrates the last point: that overfatness, if severe, can cut your life shorter. The most marked increase in the death rate is seen in people who are approximately 30% above average weight. Notice that both extremes in body weight are related to the ultimate penalty: at extreme *underweight*, the death rate also increases.

People do not have to be 30% above average weight to experience related health problems; they start at more moderate levels of overfatness. Remember, though, that statistical association is not proof of causation. For example, scientists may debate whether overfatness per se causes heart disease or whether the high blood pressure that is often associated with excess body weight causes it.

The relationship between overfatness and risk of disease is considerably more complicated than simply whether or not a person is overfat. For one thing, the *magnitude* of overweight makes a difference: the heaviest people are at greatest risk. (This means that for a person who is *extremely* overfat, there is benefit in losing even *some* of the surplus.) For another, *when* the

Figure 10.1 Body weight and mortality. The death rate is higher among U.S. men and women who weigh substantially more or less than average. In these data, collected over more than a decade by a health care organization, the average weights are between deciles 4 and 5. (Reproduced from Sidney, S., G.D. Friedman, and A.B. Siegelaub. 1987. Thinness and mortality. *American Journal of Public Health* 77:317–322.)

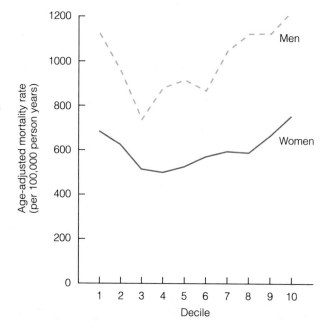

excess weight was gained may be significant: in adults, gaining surplus fat before age 50 carries more risk than adding it later (Hubert, 1988).

An issue that has sparked a great deal of interest recently is the *distribution* of body fat. In the last decade, many scientists have become convinced that excess fat at the waist and abdomen (called *upper body, central, truncal,* or *android obesity*) is more dangerous than a surplus in the thighs and buttocks (called *lower body, peripheral,* or *gynoid obesity*) (Greenwood and Pittman-Waller, 1988; National Research Council, 1989). The former distribution is related to a higher risk of hypertension, cardiovascular disease, and diabetes. However, it is not always possible to identify a clear pattern in a given individual (Garn et al., 1988); many people have fat that is fairly evenly distributed.

Psychosocial Problems   People who are severely overfat experience both psychological and social penalties as a result; research confirms this (Czajka-Narins and Parham, 1990). Obese people have experienced discrimination in all settings, including at school and in the job market. Such treatment often results in a negative self-image, feelings of loneliness, and a sense of not being able to lead a fulfilling life. Discrimination against overfat women is greater than that against overfat men.

In the opinion of many experts, the psychosocial problems can be an even greater handicap than the physical problems. A consensus panel assembled by the National Institutes of Health to consider health implications of obesity stated in its final report: "Obesity creates an enormous psychological burden. In fact, in terms of suffering, this burden may be the greatest adverse effect of obesity" (1985).

Practical Problems   Besides leading to health and psychosocial problems, being very overfat brings with it many inconveniences in living, because so much of our environment is scaled for people of average size. Furniture may not be big enough or strong enough for the very fat person; he or she may find it difficult to get behind the wheel of a car; and attractive clothes that fit may be expensive and hard to find. Even people who carry just 20 pounds of surplus fat can sometimes identify with these problems, although they experience them to a much lesser degree.

Effects of Too Little Body Fat

There is less information available on the consequences of underweight in the developed countries. This, in part, reflects the fact that underweight is found in far fewer people in the industrialized nations than is overfatness, making such research less likely to be funded. Nonetheless, we know of a number of ill effects.

Health Risks   Epidemiological studies done in the more developed countries show that the relationship between mortality and body weight is

J-shaped, with the short end of the J applying to the underweight. That is, both underweight and overweight people are at greater risk of death, particularly the 5–10% at each end of the scale (Brunzell, 1983).

Normal functioning of the immune system can also be influenced by underweight. Although people who are normally lean do not have a hampered immune response, in prolonged, severe protein–energy malnutrition the body is less able to defend itself against infection (Myrvik, 1988).

Low body fatness in females is associated with delay or loss of menstrual function, which may lead to reproductive problems and general deterioration of health. This phenomenon occurs in an estimated 5–20% of female athletes (including dancers) who train vigorously (Mann, 1981). There may not be a direct cause-and-effect relationship, however, since menstruation does not cease at the same percentage of body fat in all individuals.

Menstruation also stops in those who lose a great deal of body fat for other reasons, such as in the eating disorder anorexia nervosa. Here, the *rate* of fat loss seems to have an influence: menstruation may cease even before body fat stores drop to low levels. This fact suggests that hormonal activity may be involved as well. In women who are dieting, menses may stop when 10–15% of normal weight has been lost (Frisch, 1987).

 Impact on Fitness and Sense of Well-Being The Minnesota Starvation Studies, done during World War II using conscientious objectors or military volunteers as subjects, point out other effects of lower-than-normal body weight (Brozek, 1982). For six months, men were fed diets containing approximately half the number of kcalories needed for maintenance of their weight; the result was that they dropped to about 76% of their prestarvation weights.

From 10% weight loss and downward, they had less strength than formerly. The effect on endurance was even more marked: their capacity for aerobic work, indicated by oxygen consumption, also began to deteriorate rapidly after 10% weight loss (Taylor et al., 1957). Both effects are shown in Figure 10.2.

Roughly two-thirds of these subjects reported losses in their feeling of well-being. They had a hard time concentrating, frequently felt "downhearted" and listless, and lost interest in interacting with other people. These effects eventually reversed as the men regained their original weights.

Kcaloric Intake Is One Side of the Energy-Balance Equation

How do people come to weigh what they do? Why do people gain or lose body fat? These questions can be answered on two different levels.

On one level, the answer is simple. *People gain fat because they consume more energy than they expend*—approximately 3500 kcalories more to gain one pound of fat. Conversely, they lose a pound of fat if they expend approximately 3500 kcalories more than they consume. Their long-term experiences with fat gains and losses (plus normal growth) bring people to their current body weights.

However, the matter of *why* there may be, at times, imbalances between energy intake and output becomes considerably more complicated. We need to look at both sides of the energy equation to explore this matter.

In this section, we consider intake. A number of factors influence energy consumption. Some of these are thought to be prompted by regulators within the body (physiological factors); others are sparked by a variety of other circumstances.

Physiological Factors

Humans, along with much of the rest of the animal kingdom, have an inborn mechanism called **hunger** that prompts energy intake sufficient to make up for recent energy output. Eating in response to hunger is referred to as *internal regulation of eating*. But what causes you to experience hunger at one time and the opposite state—**satiety** (satisfaction)—at another?

Scientists have studied a number of factors that may affect hunger and satiety; some are relatively short-term effects, while others have a long-lasting impact. Several theories are described below. [A special 1985 edition of the *American Journal of Clinical Nutrition (AJCN)* was devoted entirely to this complicated topic. Instead of citing those papers individually in the paragraphs that follow, we suggest that people interested in references obtain a copy of *AJCN* volume 42 in addition to other sources we have cited.]

Sense of Fullness in the Gastrointestinal Tract   When your stomach feels full, you are less likely to want to eat more; nerves at the upper part of the stomach sense pressure, which makes you feel uncomfortable and disinclined to eat. Fullness in the small intestine may produce this effect as well (Vasselli and Maggio, 1988).

Levels of Circulating Chemicals   A theory that has been generally accepted for many years is that levels of chemicals circulating in the blood stimulate a hunger or satiety response from particular organs; but scientists are uncertain about which chemicals are most influential and what organs they primarily affect.

Some scientists believe that two centers in the brain—one that controls hunger, the other satiety—respond to levels of circulating fat, amino acids or peptides, hormones, and/or neurotransmitters (Anderson, 1988). Other scientists believe that the liver may take a primary role in intake regulation by sensing levels of circulating macronutrients and metabolites and by initiating nerve messages to start or stop eating.

The effect of hormones on hunger is noticed by many women in relation to their menstrual cycle, and studies show variations in energy intake from one phase to another. One study documented that in the 10 days before

hunger—physiological drive to consume energy in roughly the amounts expended

satiety—satisfaction of hunger

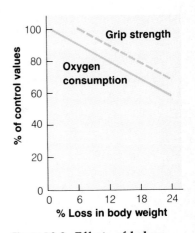

Figure 10.2 Effects of below-normal body weight on strength and work capacity. When men lost more than 10% of their normal body weights, their grip strength decreased. Their capacity for aerobic work also fell, as indicated by oxygen consumption. (Adapted from Taylor et al., 1957. Performance capacity and effects of caloric restriction with hard physical work on young men. *Journal of Applied Physiology* 10:421–429.)

menstruation begins, women increase their intakes on an average of 90 kcalories per day over their energy consumption in the 10 days after menstruation has begun (Lissner et al., 1988); another study showed an average daily premenstrual increase of 215 kcalories (Gong et al., 1989), and even greater increases have been documented. Such increased intakes may be offset by increases in resting metabolic rate, which have also been observed in the premenstrual phase (Solomon et al., 1982).

Levels of circulating chemicals may even influence which *sources* of energy we prefer in some instances. After low levels of protein intake, laboratory animals select a higher protein mixture at the next meal (Pi-Sunyer, 1988a); and some humans seem to crave high carbohydrate foods after unusually low carbohydrate intakes (Wurtman, 1988). Therefore, rather than regulating for overall energy needs, our bodies may regulate our intake of individual macronutrients separately (Bray, 1987).

The "Two-Bin" System A comprehensive model proposed by Van Itallie and Kissileff (1985) acknowledges the impact of many simultaneous influences on regulation of intake. They borrowed concepts from business to create the two-bin theory, which suggests that hunger sensations occur when the volume in the gut (bin 1) becomes depleted and/or when body fat stores (bin 2) decrease. A complex of feedback systems, including chemicals such as those mentioned above, are among the regulators that communicate the status of the bins to the nervous system. Whether or not scientists use this terminology, they have long accepted the existence of a short-term and long-term component to hunger (Vasselli and Maggio, 1988). Figure 10.3 suggests the relationship between these different types of regulators.

Size of Fat Cells Another theory about hunger regulation has to do with the size of a person's fat cells (Kolata, 1985). A group of researchers working with Jules Hirsch at Rockefeller University has found that normal-weight people usually have body fat cells of approximately the same size from one person to the next and that their biochemical "deck is stacked" to defend this size of fat cell.

If this normal person gains weight, the fat cells get larger to accommodate the extra fat, but this "overfill" situation prompts the person to experience less hunger—which typically results in eating less, losing the surplus fat, and reducing the fat cells to their former size. Conversely, if a person's weight falls below what is normal for him or her, the shrunken fat cells stimulate hunger sensations designed to make the person eat more until normal fat cell size is restored.

Hirsch and his colleagues have taken fat cell samples from normal-weight and overweight individuals and have found that many overweight people have fat cells that are 2 to $2\frac{1}{2}$ times larger than normal. From the theory stated above, you would expect that these people with larger-than-normal fat cells would experience reduced appetite, but they don't. Hirsch suspects that these fat people may have "perturbed" regulatory systems that are set to maintain larger fat cells. When these people diet to lose weight and reduce their fat cells to the size of normal-weight people's, they feel as though they are starving.

These researchers also believe that there is a limit to how large fat cells can become. After cells reach a certain maximal size, they divide, thereby increasing the number of fat cells eager to be filled. Although this is most likely to occur during growth periods when body cells of many types are increasing in number, fat cells can divide whenever their size reaches the maximum. Once a fat cell exists in the body, it is there permanently.

We will discuss other aspects of this interesting theory in a later section.

Set-Point   Another theory about hunger and body weight regulation is called the **set-point theory** (Keesey, 1988). This theory states that each person has a particular weight, or set-point, that he or she tends to maintain and at which the body handles energy intake in a metabolically normal way. Although it may be possible to temporarily gain or lose weight by deliberate changes in food intake, body weight will return to the set-point after the person resumes eating in response to hunger. In other words, if you force your body weight below your set-point, you will feel hungry until you eventually eat enough to gain back to your set-point. But if you gain weight so

set-point theory—theory that each person tends to maintain a fairly stable, appropriate body weight by eating in response to hunger

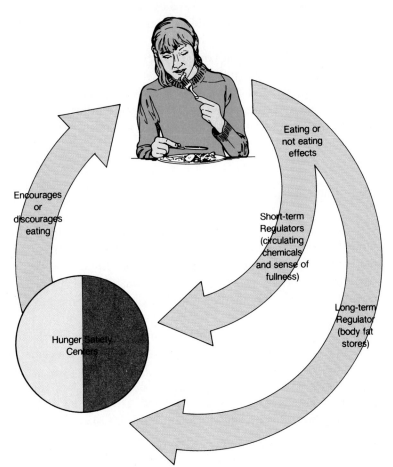

Figure 10.3 Physiological effects on hunger. Hunger and satiety seem to be influenced by short-term and long-term regulating mechanisms working together.

that you weigh more than your set-point, you will experience less hunger. Then if you eat less, you will lose weight to your set-point.

Exercise   Studies to demonstrate the relationship between physical activity, food intake, and body weight were done in the mid-1950s in a mill in India, where different jobs called for very different amounts of physical effort (Mayer et al., 1956). This study revealed that the moderately active and very active workers took in the appropriate number of kcalories to meet their energy needs and keep their body weights at normal levels; but the least active workers ate as much as the most active and were much heavier. The researchers believe their study demonstrates that at least a moderate amount of physical activity is necessary for appetite regulation to work as it should.

But this research has its critics. Although various animal studies and some later human studies support these findings (Sims, 1988), there is still a lot of debate about the role of exercise in energy intake regulation (National Dairy Council, 1989).

Other ways in which exercise functions in body weight control will be mentioned shortly.

What the Theories Share   These theories about regulation of hunger and satiety have been partially validated, although no theory has been conclusively proved, if that is even possible. Although the theories are different, they are not necessarily in conflict with each other.

There are, actually, important points of agreement between all of them: they all acknowledge (1) that most individuals maintain a remarkably constant body weight over many years, and (2) that there are strong biological influences that govern a person's drive to eat and thereby influence the individual's body weight.

Psychological Factors

As you were reading about the hunger theories, you may have been reminded that you sometimes eat when you are not particularly hungry or that there are times when you are hungry but do not eat. This demonstrates that it is possible to override internal signals and eat by *external regulation*, the influence of factors that are not physiological in origin; many of these are psychological. (Of course, it is also possible that you do not eat at times because there is no food available to you; but for most North Americans, this would usually be only a temporary situation when it occurs.)

Psychologists C. Peter Herman and Janet Polivy suggest that there are four categories of psychological influences: stress, palatability of food, social influences, and perceptual salience (1988). This section utilizes their organization and includes input from many other experts.

Stress Emotional factors and psychological states can affect eating behaviors. People who suffer from clinical depression, for example, lose their appetites along with their interest in other aspects of living.

On the other hand, there are people who consume extra food when they are experiencing negative emotions such as anger, loneliness, boredom, and depression; these people claim that eating temporarily reduces the extent of their discomfort. This emotional eating is typically *episodic;* that is, it involves binging during unusually stressful times rather than overeating consistently. Stress-related binging is more likely to be a snack-time (rather than mealtime) behavior, is often done in private, and is done more often by women than by men. Although some people of normal weight may also be emotional eaters (some studies suggest one in ten normal-weight people are), the incidence of emotional eating among overweight people is much higher (three out of four people in some studies) (Ganley, 1989).

Although little research has been done on how *positive emotions* influence eating, it is generally recognized that happy occasions include food as part of the celebration. In fact, this is probably the most universal connection between emotions and eating.

Palatability In Chapter 9, we discussed that sensory characteristics of food (especially taste) are important to making food choices. There is no doubt that your experience with the palatability of a given food also influences your decision about *whether to eat it at all* or *how much* of it to eat. Some psychologists suggest that just as we experience satiety from an adequate energy intake, some people may also have need for a certain *sensory satiety* as well. In other words, they may need adequate sensory experience from the food to feel satisfied, or they will continue eating until they reach it (Herman and Polivy, 1988). Some researchers have found that overweight people seek to experience these sensations to a greater intensity than leaner people do (Schiffman, 1986).

Social Influence Social customs have an enormous influence on eating behaviors. For example, customs teach us to eat, even if we are not hungry, when a host or hostess offers us something. To refuse would be to reject the person's hospitality, which is sometimes interpreted as a personal rejection of *him or her.*

Our choices—at least our public selections of food—may also be affected by a society's determination of what constitutes a beautiful body image. In the United States at this time, leanness is highly prized, especially in women; this influences some women to choose foods they believe to be of lower kcalorie value and to eat less food in public than they might eat in private. Men, because of public admiration of the muscular male physique, may be encouraged to order large servings of meat if they think that it enhances muscle development. Chapter 9 described social influences on our eating behaviors in more detail.

Perceptual Salience Foods are considered to have perceptual salience when they are made more noticeable in some way; you are therefore more likely to choose them. When restaurants and cafeterias want to sell a high volume of a particular food, they will prominently display that item or call particular attention to it on the menu. Of the four psychological influences on our eating behavior discussed in this section, though, Herman and Polivy regard this as the least powerful.

Energy Output Is the Other Contributor to Energy Balance

Let's go back to the basic ways people use energy—for basal metabolism, physical activity, internal food processing, and perhaps for responding to extreme environmental conditions. Here, we will consider how each of these factors might vary in people who are overweight or underweight.

Basal or Resting Metabolic Rate

In Chapter 5 (on energy) we described a few different methods for estimating your basal metabolic rate (BMR). However, a few people may have BMRs or RMRs (resting metabolic rates) that differ by as much as 30% in either direction from those of most people of the same surface area, age, and sex (Pi-Sunyer, 1988a). Therefore, BMR or RMR can account for either a smaller or larger energy use than the estimates suggest. In a study of Pima Indians in the Southwest, RMRs deviated from expected levels by as much as 300 kcalories in either direction. Those with the lower RMRs were much more likely to gain weight during the four years of follow-up (Ravussin et al., 1988).

We do not know the real causes of these differences. One variable may be the amount of thyroid hormone people produce, which affects the rate at which their metabolism functions. *Hyper*thyroid individuals use more energy than those with normal thyroid activity, and *hypo*thyroid people use less. (However, hypothyroidism is more often an excuse for obesity than its actual cause.)

Another hypothesis some researchers are testing is that the body's processes in obese people may use less than normal amounts of energy transporting sodium out of cells and back into the interstitial fluid. If this abnormality occurred in all the cells of the body, energy output would be significantly lower. Some studies of obese animals have shown that sodium transport in their liver and skeletal muscle cells uses less energy than in normal-weight animals. It is not yet known whether a similar condition may cause energy conservation with consequent overfatness in some humans (Bray, 1983).

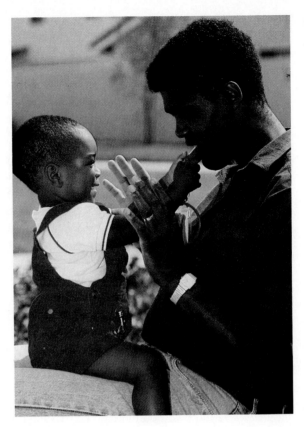

Physical activity and body fatness. At an early age, babies show a difference in the amount of energy they expend for physical activity. A study showed that babies who used less energy for activity at 3 months weighed more at their first birthday than infants who used less.

Thermic Effect of Exercise (TEE)

It might seem logical that people who get fat do so because they exercise less than other people; indeed, studies on some groups of overfat people have shown that they are less physically active than their peers of normal fatness. Still, researchers question which is cause and which is effect. It is plausible that once a person becomes fat, he or she may find exercise uncomfortable and therefore do less of it.

A study of infants shed some interesting light on this topic. The energy usage of newborns (who were of normal weight at birth) was assessed a few days after birth and again after three months. Although the energy intakes and resting metabolic rates of the infants were similar, their use of energy for physical activity was not: some infants used approximately 20% less energy. By one year of age, the infants who expended less energy for activity had become overweight; the others were of normal weight. It is interesting to note that the babies who were overweight at one year all had overweight mothers (Roberts et al., 1988).

Another question for researchers is whether a bout of exercise, after it is completed, causes a person's metabolic rate to stay elevated for a period of time or causes a person to expend more energy for the thermic effect of food (TEF). There is considerable debate about this question, because studies

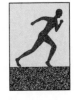

have yielded differing results. A recent review suggests that only exercise of high intensity and long duration has an extended effect on metabolic rate; this effect would be most noticeable in the first 12 hours after exercise (Poehlman and Horton, 1989).

Thermic Effect of Food (TEF)

As you have learned, the thermic effect of food includes heat produced during digestion, absorption, transport, and storage of food. Although TEF is thought to utilize a fairly constant percentage of kcalories consumed, some studies show that less energy is used for this purpose by obese people than by lean people (Pi-Sunyer, 1988a). Those who have achieved moderate levels of fitness may expend more energy for this function than either untrained people or highly trained athletes (Poehlman and Horton, 1989).

Some research has shown that the energy cost of making body fat differs depending on which macronutrients provide the energy. Producing fat from carbohydrate is more metabolically energy-intensive and wasteful than reassembling fat from absorbed dietary fat components; therefore, 100 kcalories of fat may be slightly more fattening than 100 kcalories of carbohydrate. Experts postulate that over the course of a year, when hundreds of thousands of kcalories are consumed, these differences can have a noticeable effect. It is interesting that some studies have shown a closer correlation between fat intake and body fat status than between total kcalorie intake and body fat status (Dreon et al., 1988; Romieu et al., 1988).

Adaptive Thermogenesis

When some people overeat, their bodies produce extra heat and lose it to the environment. Studies done with prison volunteers in the 1960s showed that when people of average body fatness deliberately ate much more food than they normally would, they did gain weight—but not nearly as much as they "should have" according to the standard of one pound for every 3500 surplus kcalories (Sims et al., 1973). However, some studies suggest that obese people have only a very small thermic response to overfeeding (Danforth and Landsberg, 1983). Presumably, they convert more of the extra kcalories to fat than their normal-weight peers do.

Finally, even the body's ability to use energy for nonshivering thermogenesis may differ between fat and lean people, if animal experiments are an accurate model. Some obese strains of laboratory animals do not produce sufficient heat to stay alive when their environment becomes cold (Himms-Hagen, 1983). Although human experiments have not yet been done, it is possible that some people may be similarly unable to produce extra heat in the cold.

In animals, adaptive thermogenesis is mediated mainly by brown fat—fat cells that have a much higher than normal number of mitochondria, the organelles in which energy is produced. It is not known for sure whether brown fat plays a role in adaptive thermogenesis in humans, but there is reason to suspect that it may: a study in Finland showed that outdoor workers had more brown fat than people who worked at office jobs (Sims, 1988).

Why are some people fat, others thin, and others "just right"? Why do some people gain weight easily, while others cannot gain, even when they try? No single explanation applies to all cases: there are likely to be different reasons—genetic and/or environmental—why some people store more or less body fat than the average person.

The next section summarizes some of these possibilities.

Fat Status and Body Weight Depend on How Intake and Output Compare

Earlier we stated that people gain fat when they consume more energy than they expend—to the tune of ~3500 kcalories per pound. To lose a pound, ~3500 more kcalories must be expended than consumed. Nothing we have said in the discussion of energy intake and output changes that. But you have seen that there are many different circumstances that could cause intake and output to deviate from expected levels and bring about an imbalance between energy intake and expenditure. This section suggests some, but does not exhaust the possibilities; furthermore, many combinations of the factors below are possible.

Because more people in our society are overweight than underweight, our listing deals with the possible reasons for weight gain and higher-than-normal body weight.

You will gain fat *if you have a higher than normal energy intake* (and a normal energy expenditure) for any of the following reasons:

- You eat an excessive amount of food because physiological factors cause extreme hunger.
- You eat an excessive amount of food for psychological reasons such as stress or sensory pleasure.
- You eat a high proportion of foods that are high in fat.

Or, looking at the output side of the energy equation, you will gain fat *if you have a lower-than-normal energy expenditure* (and energy intake is normal) for any of the following reasons:

- You have a low basal metabolic rate.
- You are less physically active than normal.
- You expend fewer kcalories as thermic effect of food.
- You are unable to throw off part of unneeded energy intake as heat (adaptive thermogenesis).

Of course, if both intake is high *and* output is low, fat gain is also assured. The greater the discrepancy between intake and output, the more rapid and pronounced the gain will be.

Keep in mind that it is the *discrepancy* between intake and output that leads to fat gain. People even gain fat when their energy intake is *lower than normal*—that is, if their energy output is still lower than their intake. Studies have documented that many overweight people actually eat less than their normal-weight peers (National Research Council, 1989).

Some scientists have attempted to determine whether the various factors that influence energy intake and output are genetically determined or whether they have their origins in the culture (environment) or in an individual's psyche (one's response to the environment). Much research has been done on these issues; however, it can be difficult to separate the causes from one another, and the literature is awash with theories and mathematical models that cannot accurately predict body weights of individuals in practical situations.

There is no question, however, that particular levels of body fatness tend to run in families (Figure 10.4). *This in itself does not prove that you inherit* the predisposition to a certain body weight; since family members often share a similar environment, environment may also affect the fatness of a family. Attempts have been made to separate the two factors. Studies of identical twins who were reared apart show considerable similarity in the weights of the twins, pointing to inheritance as a strong influence (Stunkard, 1988). In addition, studies have been done with people who were adopted as infants; when their adult weights were compared with those of their biological parents and those of their adoptive parents, the weights of the children were more similar to those of their biological parents (Stunkard et al., 1986).

Figure 10.4 Body weight runs in families. If both of your biological parents have a similar level of fatness, the odds are that you will too. Is this the effect of genetics or environment? Studies suggest that both factors play a role. (Garn, S.M., 1985. Continuities and changes in fatness from infancy through adulthood. *Current Problems in Pediatrics* 15:1–47.)

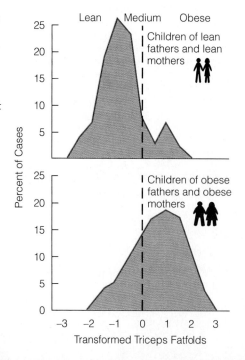

Some recent research has compared the effects of genetics to those of the environment. One research group concluded that *energy intake* is more influenced by cultural rather than genetic factors (Perusse et al., 1988). Other studies suggest that *energy output* may be substantially affected by genetics (Roberts et al., 1988; Ravussin et al., 1988). Professor Albert Stunkard, distinguished for his research on body weight, suggests that various genetic and environmental factors may need to *interact* in order for obesity to develop; this could explain why people living in a given environment can have very different body weights (1988).

Of what practical importance is this area of research? If we have a better understanding of the causes of overweight in a given population, it may be possible to plan better public health programs to help people reduce high-risk levels of body fatness. Additionally, if this research can uncover ways of determining which factors are most responsible for an *individual's* excess body fat, it should be possible to design more effective weight loss programs for individuals as well. For some people of extremely high or low body weights, simply *knowing* the cause(s) of their distress may help them deal more effectively with their situations.

What Sets the Standard for a Healthy Level of Body Fatness?

It's easy to recognize extremes in body fatness such as those pictured in Figure 10.5, which are far from ideal. However, it's not as easy to identify what *is* ideal.

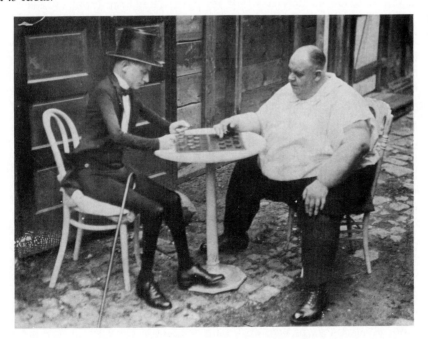

Figure 10.5 Body weight extremes. It is obvious that the sideshow attractions in this picture are underfat and overfat. It is not so easy to determine what weights would be ideal for them, although there are several ways to estimate.

Our culture has the greatest influence on our perception of what the ideal body image is for ourselves. On the other hand, data on what levels of fatness favor the best health and longest life are not well developed: as our means of assessing body fatness improve and become easier to use, better data on their relationship to health will be collected.

In the absence of good data on fatness, researchers and clinicians have commonly used standards based on heights and weights. These have some validity because a high body weight is often caused by excess body fat, but this is not always the case. In recent years, much more consideration has been given to characteristics of the individual in addition to height and weight in setting goals. The upcoming section will discuss the usefulness of these standards and suggest how you can establish your own weight goals.

Cultural Standards (Not Recommended)

Cultures in different times and places prefer different levels of body fatness. What prompts these attitudes in a society is a complex matter, involving not only aesthetics but also economic and political considerations as well as other factors. For example, in some very poor societies it is considered desirable to be fat, because it demonstrates the relative wealth (and probably power) of the person who can afford enough food to become overfat. In more affluent societies, leanness may be regarded as admirable because it indicates self-control in the midst of plenty.

You can trace changes in attitudes about body fatness in the United States by studying popular magazines. One group of researchers studied photographs of women that appeared in the trend-setting magazines *Vogue* and *Ladies Home Journal* between 1901 and 1981. They found that a high degree of curvaceousness was admired early in the century. After 1910, the ideal became increasingly flattened until 1925, when the preferred silhouette appeared to be almost a straight line (minimal body fat). Interest in curves increased again through the 1940s but again declined steadily until the end of the study in 1981 (Silverstein et al., 1986). Late in the 1980s, some magazines suggested that the curvy look was returning to popularity, but it is too soon to know whether this represents a trend.

The 1980s also saw the introduction of a new category of magazine to the newsstand—magazines that maintain that it is all right to be fat (Czajka-Narins and Parham, 1990). These publications feature articles about overweight people who are professionally successful, and they carry advertisements for fashions and other products produced for people of large body size. These magazines are not likely to influence the attitudes of the general public as much as they may have a positive effect on the self-concept and coping mechanisms of the overweight people who read them.

Much (but not all) of the current focus on leanness seems to be directed toward females, and studies reflect this pressure on women to be slim. The pressure affects people of all ages. A survey of U.S. adults in the mid-1980s reported that 46% of women and 27% of men were trying to lose weight

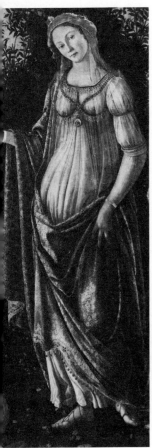
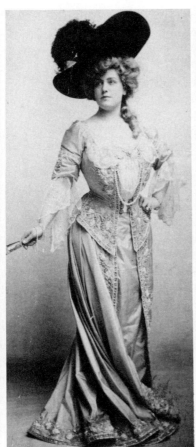
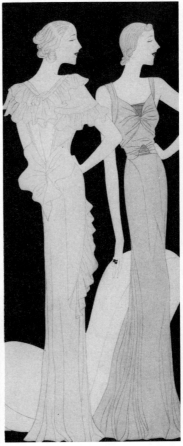
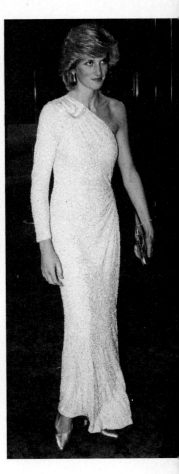

(National Dairy Council, 1988). A study on a college campus regarding weight and dieting found that 37% of female and 17% of male participants stated that gaining weight was *the most powerful fear in their lives* (Collier et al., 1990). A survey of girls in an upper middle-class parochial high school found that 72% had made recent attempts to lose weight, although 47% were of normal weight, 36% were underweight, and only 17% were overweight (Moses et al., 1989).

Women seem to set standards for their own weight that are lower than health standards (height/weight tables) and also lower than apparent cultural standards. When various groups of women on one campus were studied, their weights averaged 94% of recommendations based on height and weight standards; yet, the weights they aspired to averaged only 87% of the standard (Kurtzman et al., 1989). In another study, 44% of the women and 16% of the men stated that they "felt fat" although their friends told them they were thin (Collier, 1990).

In a 1985 study, hundreds of male and female college undergraduates were given a set of nine figure drawings of their sex arranged from very thin to very heavy. They were asked to identify their current figure, their ideal figure, and the figure they thought would be most attractive to the opposite sex. For men, the figures they chose to match these three descriptions were

Various cultural ideals of body fatness for women. Attitudes about ideal body weight vary from time to time and from culture to culture. Curves were "in" and some body fat was considered beautiful when Boticelli painted *Primavera* (c. 1478), and 186-pound soprano Lillian Russell was a popular entertainer around the turn of the century. The Art Nouveau fashion drawing from the 1920s and the recent photo of Princess Diana demonstrate that extreme thinness has enjoyed popularity at other times and places. Cultural attitudes can affect people's food choices and satisfaction with their bodies but may have little to do with physical health.

almost identical; but most women saw themselves as being heavier than they regarded as ideal or attractive. The study's summary makes the succinct statement: "Overall, men's perceptions serve to keep them satisfied with their figures, whereas women's perceptions place pressure on them to lose weight" (Fallon and Rozin, 1985).

In general, current cultural standards, especially for women, do not match well with height/weight standards and are therefore unhealthy. Nevertheless, it appears that many women have converted the societal standard to be thin into a personal one.

Amount of Body Fat

Practically speaking, the best method of estimating body fat is *underwater weighing*, in which the overall mass and density of the body is determined. Because the densities of lean and fatty tissues are different, knowing the overall density makes it possible to determine what proportions of body mass are lean and fat.

Whole body counting measures the total amount of K-40, a naturally occurring form of potassium present in the body. Since it occurs primarily in lean tissue, and since it is present in such tissues in known concentration, the total K-40 value is used as a basis for calculating lean body mass.

Other methods of assessment involve introducing particular chemicals into the body, determining their concentrations in body tissues, and calculating from this the amount of fat and lean tissue. For example, if the chemical that was used is water-soluble, then it will be distributed mainly in lean body mass, not in fat. The more lean body mass a person has, the more dilute the concentration of the substance in the tissues will become.

Various imaging methods, such as computed tomography (CT) and magnetic resonance imaging (MRI), are effective but are so costly that they are rarely used (Meredith, 1989). Obviously, all of these methods involve extensive special equipment and expertise; they are more likely to be used for research than in the clinical setting.

A much easier but less accurate method of assessing fatness is to use skinfold calipers to measure the thickness of the fat layer beneath the skin at various body sites, and then to use tables to convert the measurements into body fat percentages. Because this procedure can be done quickly and with less expensive equipment (good calipers can be purchased for approximately $200), measuring of skinfolds has become increasingly popular among dietitians, doctors, athletic coaches, and trainers. Appropriately used in expert hands, skinfold measurements can show comparisons in fatness between people, or in the same person from one time to another. However, the accuracy of estimating the absolute percentage of body fat from skinfolds is questioned.

Because of differences in technique and/or equipment, individual practitioners can get varying measurements on the same person. The locations (and the number of locations) that are measured also affect results: generally, the more sites that are measured, the more reliable the results will be. Then, depending on which of several available tables are used for converting the skinfold measurements into body fat percentages, the values can differ. A 1984 study points out how large the variation in results can be. When investigators evaluated 16 female athletes, the mean percentage of body fat for the group varied from approximately 14% to 28%, depending on the brand of calipers used, the practitioner doing the measuring, and the conversion tables used (Lohman et al., 1984).

However, we do endorse this application of skinfold measurements: done at intervals with the same caliper by a person who is highly skilled in using the method, it can be determined whether fat deposits are increasing or decreasing. This can be particularly valuable to a person who is both dieting and exercising: the person's body weight may not be changing at all, but fat may be decreasing while muscle is being added. Without skinfold testing, the person who sees no change in the weight shown on the scale might be inclined to say, "This program's not working," and abandon what might actually be a very successful fat-loss program.

Two innovative approaches that have been tried for measuring body fatness are *ultrasonography* and *bioelectrical impedance assessment (BIA)*. They are beginning to be used frequently in research with human subjects. Ultrasonography can measure the fat layer with less likelihood of error than when using skin calipers, although some judgment by the operator is necessary in interpreting results (Yang, 1988). The probe of the ultrasound meter is placed on the skin surface. It emits pulses of high-frequency sound waves that penetrate the skin and fat layer but are reflected from the fat-muscle interface. The echoes that return to the meter are converted to a distance score.

BIA involves the measurement of the resistance of the body to the flow of an alternating electric current (Baumgartner et al., 1989). Lean body mass can be calculated from measurements of the amount of resistance encountered over specific distances in the body. The process itself is simple and painless; the operator attaches terminals to specific locations on the subject's wrist and hand, and ankle and foot. Electric current travels the *two short distances on wrist to hand and ankle to foot*. Initial reports find the accuracy of bioelectrical impedance to compare closely with results from underwater weighing, except when people's hydration status is abnormal and in very obese individuals (Gray et al., 1989). Since these two methods are safe, portable, and relatively inexpensive compared with some of the research methods described above, they hold promise for more general use in the future if continued testing confirms their reliability. Another method about which we are likely to hear more in the future is *infrared spectroscopy*.

When you and I have accurate information about our percentage of body fat, what will it tell us? At present, we have data regarding what percentage of body fat is *typical*, but we do not know what is *ideal*. Once it is easier to collect body fatness data, researchers will begin to identify correlations between body fatness and health and longevity. Until then, we can compare our body fatness with *typical* values for our population. One expert says 15% is typical for men and 27% for women (Lohman, 1981); another suggests ranges of 12–16% for men and 22–26% for women (Williams, 1985).

Values Based on Height and Weight

For practical reasons, most of us have used standard height and weight data to assess our body fatness. For most people, these data work because there is a general correlation between sex, height and weight, and the percentage of body fat. There are a number of possible exceptions; for example, it is possible that a person who has an unusually large muscle mass, bone structure, or even water content, could weigh more than a fat person but have less fat (Frisancho, 1988).

In the United States, members of the insurance industry took the lead in developing tables of suggested weight for height. They compiled the tables from information routinely obtained from clients: age and body weight at the time a policy is purchased (usually in early adulthood) and subsequent age at death. The Metropolitan Life Insurance Company has published these tables, which indicate the weights of people who live the longest. The most recent version, published in 1983, is given in Table 10.1. Separate weights are given depending on sex, height, and frame size.

Although the Metropolitan Height and Weight Tables have been widely accepted as authoritative by the general public, health experts have criticized the insurance company tables on several grounds. For one, the tables are based on a limited segment of the population rather than a cross-section of the entire population. Also, the designations of body frame size were not established by measuring the insured population, from which the data about weight and age at death were obtained; therefore, the data do not really relate to one another (Frisancho, 1988).

These criticisms notwithstanding, the tables serve as a readily available, easy-to-use, rough guideline: despite their many flaws, they are better than nothing. Anybody who is markedly outside the weight range for his or her height should check with a physician for individualized evaluation. The National Institutes of Health Consensus Report on Obesity (1985) recommended that anybody who weighs 20% or more above the midpoint of the medium weight range for height should lose weight.

body mass index (BMI)—body weight (in kilograms) divided by height (in meters) squared; a standard some experts have proposed for ideal weight determination

Another standard that uses height and weight data is **body mass index (BMI),** which is body weight (in kilograms) divided by height (in meters) squared. Many experts in obesity research believe that this number provides a more reliable basis on which to judge overfatness than the height/weight table ranges.

BMI can be determined without doing any calculation. You can use the special chart (called a *nomogram*) in Figure 10.6 to convert your height and weight to BMI and to see whether it is within the acceptable, underweight, or obese range. Since the ranges were originally drawn, suggestions have

Table 10.1 1983 Metropolitan Height and Weight Tables

Men

Height Feet	Inches	Small Frame Weight (pounds)	Medium Frame Weight (pounds)	Large Frame Weight (pounds)
5	1	123–129	126–136	133–145
5	2	125–131	128–138	135–148
5	3	127–133	130–140	137–151
5	4	129–135	132–143	139–155
5	5	131–137	134–146	141–159
5	6	133–140	137–149	144–163
5	7	135–143	140–152	147–167
5	8	137–146	143–155	150–171
5	9	139–149	146–158	153–175
5	10	141–152	149–161	156–179
5	11	144–155	152–165	159–183
6	0	147–159	155–169	163–187
6	1	150–163	159–173	167–192
6	2	153–167	162–177	171–197
6	3	157–171	166–182	176–202

Women

Height Feet	Inches	Small Frame Weight (pounds)	Medium Frame Weight (pounds)	Large Frame Weight (pounds)
4	9	98–108	106–118	115–128
4	10	100–110	108–120	117–131
4	11	101–112	110–123	119–134
5	0	103–115	112–126	122–137
5	1	105–118	115–129	125–140
5	2	108–121	118–132	128–144
5	3	111–124	121–135	131–148
5	4	114–127	124–138	134–152
5	5	117–130	127–141	137–156
5	6	120–133	130–144	140–160
5	7	123–136	133–147	143–164
5	8	126–139	136–150	146–167
5	9	129–142	139–153	149–170
5	10	132–145	142–156	152–173
5	11	135–148	145–159	155–176

These weight ranges show weights in pounds at ages 25–59 that resulted in the lowest mortality. Tables have been adjusted to represent weights without clothes and heights without shoes.

How to Determine Your Body Frame Size by Elbow Breadth

To make a simple approximation of your frame size, extend your arm and bend the forearm upwards at a 90 degree angle. Keep the fingers straight and turn the inside of your wrist away from your body. Place the thumb and index finger of your other hand on the two prominent bones on *either side* of your elbow. Measure the space between your fingers against a ruler or a tape measure. Compare the measurements on the tables on the top of page 328.

Table 10.1 continued

These tables list the elbow measurements[a] for medium-framed men and women of various heights. Measurements lower than those listed indicate that you have a small frame, and higher measurements indicate a large frame.

Men	
Height	Medium Frame Elbow Breadth
5'1"–5'2"	$2\frac{1}{2}''$–$2\frac{7}{8}''$
5'3"–5'6"	$2\frac{5}{8}''$–$2\frac{7}{8}''$
5'7"–5'10"	$2\frac{3}{4}''$–$3''$
5'11"–6'2"	$2\frac{3}{4}''$–$3\frac{1}{8}''$
6'3"	$2\frac{7}{8}''$–$3\frac{1}{4}''$

Women	
Height	Medium Frame Elbow Breadth
4'9"–4'10"	$2\frac{1}{4}''$–$2\frac{1}{2}''$
4'11"–5'2"	$2\frac{1}{4}''$–$2\frac{1}{2}''$
5'3"–5'6"	$2\frac{3}{8}''$–$2\frac{5}{8}''$
5'7"–5'10"	$2\frac{3}{8}''$–$2\frac{5}{8}''$
5'11"	$2\frac{1}{2}''$–$2\frac{3}{4}''$

[a] For the most accurate measurement, have your physician measure your elbow breadth with a caliper.
Adapted from 1983 Metropolitan Height and Weight Tables. Reprinted courtesy of the Metropolitan Life Insurance Company.

been made for slightly different ranges based on age; these are found in Table 10.2.

Presence of Other Risk Factors

If a physician is undecided about whether or not to recommend that a patient lose weight, the presence or absence of other risk factors can help to make the determination (Greenwood and Pittman-Waller, 1988). If an overweight person has high blood pressure, elevated blood cholesterol, or type II diabetes, for example, weight loss should be recommended. When overweight people lose weight, these risk factors are often reduced without using any other means of intervention.

Another criterion the physician can consider is the person's body fat distribution. As we mentioned early in the chapter, a preponderance of upper body fat (at the waist) has been found to correlate with higher risk of high blood pressure, cardiovascular disease, and diabetes (National Research Council, 1989). A nomogram using two measurements—waist and hip—has been developed from which relative risk at various ages can be assessed (Figure 10.7 and Figure 10.8).

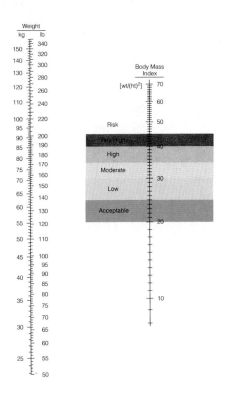

Figure 10.6 Nomogram for determining body mass index (BMI). To use this nomogram, place a straightedge between your body weight (without clothes) on the left and your height (without shoes) on the right. Your BMI is at the point where the line crosses the middle column. (Source: National Research Council, 1989. *Diet and Health,* Washington, D.C.: National Academy Press.)

Best Functional and Maintainable Weight

There is a subjective standard that may be useful: ask yourself at what weight you function best both physically and mentally. If you give similar answers to all of the following questions, this method may help you to zero in on your own best body weight.

At what weight do you:

• Have enough stamina to live through each day with reasonable vitality?
• Have the ability to concentrate well on the task at hand?
• Keep from feeling hungry or being obsessed with food until shortly before the next mealtime?

Table 10.2 Desirable Body Mass Index in Relation to Age

Age Group (years)	BMI (kg/m^2)
19–24	19–24
25–34	20–25
35–44	21–26
45–54	22–27
55–65	23–28
>65	24–29

Source: National Research Council. 1989. *Diet and health.* Washington, DC: National Academy Press.

Figure 10.7 Nomogram for determining waist-to-hip ratio (WHR). To use this nomogram, place a straight-edge between your waist circumference on the left and your hip circumference on the right. The point at which the line crosses the center column is your WHR. To interpret your level of risk, see Figure 10.8. (From Bray, G.A. and D.S. Gray. 1988. Obesity: Part I: Pathogenesis. *Western Journal of Medicine* 149: 429–441.)

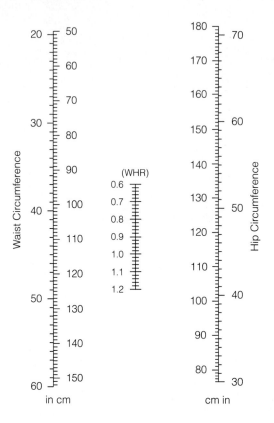

These questions are admittedly far from objective; besides, your answers could be influenced by other factors. But under normal circumstances, they may help you come to an individually determined ideal weight in a way that the other external standards cannot.

Your Status

You have just read your way through several criteria that are used for suggesting what levels of body fatness are acceptable from a health perspective: indirect assessments of amounts of body fat, standards based on height and weight, presence of other risk factors, and best functional and maintainable weight. You have probably applied some of these standards to yourself already. The different methods may have yielded slightly different recommendations about what is ideal for you, but that should not be surprising—all of these methods are imperfect. Nonetheless, most of you have probably found that your body fat status is within the appropriate range for you.

Some of you, however, will find that your current weight or measures of fatness do not fall within the recommended ranges. Yet you may say, "This is the weight at which I function best. Besides, whenever I intentionally lose or gain, I always return to this weight afterwards." In this case, if your food intake meets your nutritional needs; if you get at least a moderate amount of exercise; and if you have no weight-related risk factors such as high blood

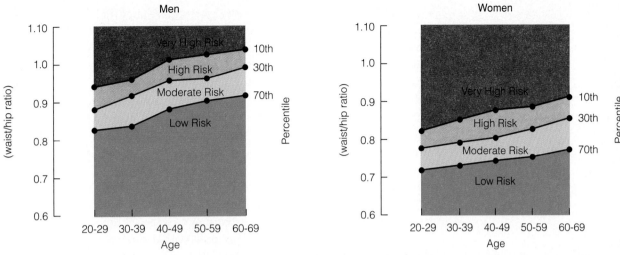

pressure, high blood cholesterol, or obvious upper body obesity, then it may be wisest for you to accept your current body weight and get on with other important aspects of living. Increasingly, physicians consider the presence of other risk factors before recommending weight change.

If you are above the weight ranges, have other risk factors, and seldom exercise; or if you are below the ranges and eat erratically or exercise excessively, some changes are probably in order. You should ask your doctor's advice about whether to attempt to gain or lose fat.

You should be forewarned that it is not easy to modify body fat stores. In the next section, we will discuss the physiological and psychological factors that come into play in response to energy deficit or surplus—especially when the discrepancy is drastic.

Figure 10.8 Relative risk from waist-to-hip ratio (WHR) for men and women. Identify your risk range on the graph for your gender by locating the meeting point of lines drawn from your WHR and age range. (Reprinted by permission of the *Western Journal of Medicine.* Bray and Gray: Obesity: Part 1; Pathogenesis 149:429–441).

Our Bodies Resist Changes in Weight

If you have decided that you should change your weight, it is only fair to let you know what you are up against: we have inborn mechanisms to resist weight change that are especially evident under certain circumstances.

One instance in which the body rebels against weight loss is when a person tries to lose a great deal of weight quickly, as the next section explains.

The Body's Overall Reaction to Extreme Weight-Loss Attempts

If you try to lose more than 1 or 2 pounds of fat per week, your body makes certain changes to help defend its weight. Here are some things that happen in a person's body when it experiences a severe shortage of energy:

- At first, weight drops quickly; but only about one-fourth of the lost weight is fat—almost three-fourths is water and the remainder is protein.

• If the diet is very low in carbohydrate, there may not be a sufficient amount of it to promote complete metabolism of the fat being broken down, and fat fragments called *ketone bodies* or *ketoacids* are produced. These are removed from the body with large amounts of water, which causes further fluid loss but not significantly greater fat loss. In some instances, an accumulation of ketone bodies (a condition called *ketosis*) is evident. This condition has been extreme in people who died while on severe weight-reduction diets. Such deaths are likely to be the result of a combination of factors including uncontrolled ketosis and mineral imbalance.

• Basal metabolic rate may slow down—in some people by as much as 30% below what is normal (Pi-Sunyer, 1988a). This problem is evidenced by a slowing pulse rate and the tendency to feel chilly at temperatures that were comfortable before. This means that energy expenditure has decreased, which results in less weight loss.

• A person tends to cut down on physical activity; for example, even though she may run as far, she may not raise her feet as high or move her arms as much; her body automatically tries to conserve some energy. This is an additional factor in decreasing energy expenditure.

Psychological reactions to extreme weight-loss attempts include:

• craving for food
• preoccupation with thoughts of food and decreased ability to concentrate on the tasks at hand
• feeling stressed
• feeling "down" (all studies do not agree on this [Buckmaster and Brownell, 1988])
• hyperemotionalism, including increased irritability
• feelings of stress.

The normal reaction to these combined physical and psychological forces is to go off the diet and make up for the earlier food deprivation by rebound eating (Callaway, 1988). People who have experienced this often criticize themselves for being "weak" because they could not stay on the diet. But considering how strong these pressures are, it is no wonder that the person gives up the diet.

The more severe the diet a person has been on, the greater the reaction to it may be. People who try to subsist on just a few hundred kcalories per day may be setting themselves up for colossal overeating later. They will experience rapid weight regain (maybe to a greater weight than before), probably a sense of disgust and shame, and possibly a renewed determination to "diet better the next time." If this occurs, the result is a vicious cycle of dieting and overeating that is counterproductive and makes a person feel quite helpless and miserable. The experts call this *weight cycling* or *chronic dieting;* the popular press calls it *yo-yo dieting.*

Figure 10.9 summarizes this phenomenon of chronic dieting.

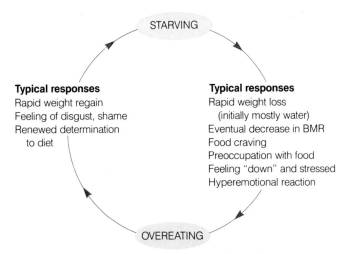

STARVING

Typical responses
Rapid weight regain
Feeling of disgust, shame
Renewed determination
   to diet

Typical responses
Rapid weight loss
   (initially mostly water)
Eventual decrease in BMR
Food craving
Preoccupation with food
Feeling "down" and stressed
Hyperemotional reaction

OVEREATING

Figure 10.9 The vicious cycle of chronic dieting and overeating. If a person uses a weight-loss diet that is very low in kcalories, the body and mind react against the severe deprivation, and rebound eating is likely to occur. This results in weight regain and often self-criticism, which may lead to another and yet another trip around the circle. A moderate approach that is more likely to succeed is described in the text.

This is an eating style seen in girls and women who feel generally pressured to try to be thinner than they are. It also occurs in people with specific reasons to maintain a lower-than-natural body weight, such as wrestlers, gymnasts, dancers, cheerleaders, and models. It is sometimes difficult to know where the dividing line is between this pattern and a full-blown eating disorder, the topic of the next chapter.

Some researchers believe that *the chronic dieter is likely to eat more (eventually and overall) than the same person would eat in response to genuine hunger.* In this way, *severe dieting may cause people to gain weight rather than to lose it* (Polivy and Herman, 1983). Another possible explanation of why "weight cyclers" regain weight is that their bodies may respond to the reduced energy intake by expending fewer kcalories for RMR (Van Dale and Saris, 1989); also, various metabolic alterations favor fat storage after people stop dieting (Callaway, 1988).

An animal study provided dramatic evidence of this theory. Rats were cycled between diets allowing either free access to a high-fat diet that resulted in weight gain OR restricted access to a low-fat diet with half the kcalories that resulted in weight loss. As the animals were cycled through the weight-loss phase for the second time, it took them *twice as long to lose the weight;* and when they were switched to the weight-gain diet again, they *regained the weight three times as fast* as they had with the first regain (Brownell et al., 1986). At the end of the study, after two complete periods of weight loss and regain, the weight-cycled animals weighed almost as much as control animals who had been allowed free access to the high-fat diet throughout the study. If this same phenomenon occurs in humans, it provides strong evidence of the futility of severe dieting.

There is reason to believe that the phenomenon may hold true for us too, but the data are inconsistent among studies. In a small study, Dutch investigators were unable to demonstrate that RMR differed between frequent dieters and women without such a history when they were compared before and after a 14-week period of weight loss (van Dale and Saris, 1989). Other investigators have noted differences in energy expenditure of people who chronically weight-cycled. One study involved people with eating disorders who had binged and purged, and some had a history of low body weight due to self-starvation; they were found to have lower RMRs than normal controls whose weights had been quite consistent (Gwirtsman, 1989). Another study measured the RMRs of wrestlers who practiced a pattern of severe dieting to "cut weight" before matches and rapid regaining afterwards; the weight cyclers were found to have RMRs that averaged 14% lower than their teammates who had not weight-cycled (Steen et al., 1988). Of course, since RMRs had not been determined in the weight cyclers before they began the practice, it could be argued that the lower RMRs may have existed prior to the weight cycling; however, the animal data make this explanation less plausible.

What happens to people whose RMRs drop after weight cycling? Can a person's RMR be made to go up again? Most studies are not very encouraging in this regard. In one study, a severe weight reduction program (allowing only 500 kcalories per day) produced a 22% decrease in RMRs; during a subsequent 8-week weight maintenance phase, the RMR stayed depressed (Elliott et al., 1988). This study lasted only for the 8 weeks, so we don't know whether the effect persisted for longer; but there is other evidence that total daily energy usage can be depressed during 6 years of weight maintenance following weight loss (Pi-Sunyer, 1988a).

The previous studies did not consider the potential importance of the type of weight loss regimens that were used. One group has reported that if a person exercises during weight loss, the reductions in RMR are not as large (van Dale and Saris, 1989). Other research refutes this (Hill et al., 1987; Hammer et al., 1989). Variables such as the nature and duration of the exercise and the severity of the diet may need to be considered as well.

Keep in mind that this discussion refers to what happens when people go on *diets that are very severe.* Moderate weight-reduction approaches do not lead to the extreme physical and psychological consequences listed above, nor are they as likely to result in entrapment. Most important, moderate approaches can be successful.

In this section, where we are dealing with the body's natural resistance to weight change, we should also discuss a theory about what happens at the cellular level to affect changes in body fat.

A Fat Cell's Response to Weight-Change Attempts   Remember our reference earlier in this chapter to the work of Jules Hirsch and his colleagues, who studied fat cell size? Their theories, although quite controversial, provide some interesting perspectives.

Their research suggests that as a body gains fat, it does so by enlarging existing fat cells **(hypertrophy),** by producing additional fat cells **(hyperplasia),** or by doing a combination of the two. According to studies done on both laboratory animals and humans (Hirsch and Knittle, 1970), hyperplasia of fat cells usually starts in childhood, whereas hypertrophy generally is

hypertrophy—enlargement of cells already present (here, fat cells)

hyperplasia—an increase in the number of cells (in this case, fat cells)

seen during adulthood. Other findings suggest that although the above generalizations usually hold true, *new fat cells can be created at any age if existing fat cells reach a certain critical size and there is still more fat to deposit* (Bjorntorp, 1983).

According to these researchers, when weight is lost, fat cells shrink but never disappear entirely. Furthermore, the fat cells endeavor to maintain a certain minimal size: if they become smaller than that size, body mechanisms work to restore their lost mass.

Consider the person with normal-sized cells but an above-normal number of them. When that person loses weight, the fat cells shrink to less-than-normal size, and forever after hunger to be refilled. This person, say some researchers, is likely to regain weight quickly when dieting is stopped. On the other hand, the person with large-sized fat cells but a normal number of them theoretically has an easier time of it: when he or she diets, the large cells are reduced to normal size, and are more likely to stay that way. (Table 10.3 summarizes this information.)

For reasons as yet unknown, metabolic disorders such as diabetes, hypertension, and high blood cholesterol occur more often in people who have large fat cells. Fortunately, such people often have better success at weight loss, and the accompanying health problems are often reversed simultaneously (Bjorntorp, 1983).

As we noted earlier, these theories are quite controversial, and they have sparked much research that proposes interesting answers about why people vary in body weight and their ability to change weight.

Another path that fat cell research has taken is to look into why it is that when people lose weight, one person loses it fairly evenly over the whole body, whereas another loses it in some locations but not others. Researcher Rudolph Leibel has found that fat cells have two types of receptors on their surfaces: alpha receptors (which stimulate fat accumulation) and beta receptors (which stimulate fat breakdown). Fat cells vary in which type of receptor is predominant, and this determines whether the cells will be resistant to giving up their fat (Kolata, 1985).

Table 10.3 Types of Obesity As Proposed by Hirsch and Knittle

Type of Obesity	Description	Consequences
Hyperplastic	Person has a large number of fat cells that are normal in size; the condition is usually established during childhood	If weight is lost, regain is likely
Hypertrophic	Person has a normal number of fat cells that are large in size; the condition is usually established during adulthood	If weight is lost, it is less likely to be regained. Diabetes and/or high blood lipids may occur with overweight; reversal is likely with weight loss
Combination	Person has a large number of fat cells that are large in size; the condition is usually established during childhood, but may occur at any age	Combination of the above consequences

Leibel has found that women tend to have fat cells with more alpha (accumulating) receptors on their hips and thighs, whereas men tend to have more of that type around their waists. Recall that this latter pattern of fat distribution—upper body obesity—is statistically related to a higher risk of certain diseases.

Now let's move on to take a look at different techniques that have been tried for losing body weight.

People Have Tried Thousands of Techniques for Losing Body Fat

It is amazing how many claims, theories, and treatments for losing weight have been developed: information about 30,000 of them has been collected at Johns Hopkins University! Some focus on regulating food intake, others emphasize increasing energy output, and a few include both. There are even some that do neither of these, relying on measures such as temporary water loss to fool a person into thinking that some fat has been lost. Such programs are not only deceptive but may be dangerous as well.

All weight-loss methods are successful in the short run for some people but unsuccessful for others. When the *long-term* results of various methods have been evaluated, 80% or more of those people who lost weight are found to have regained their losses (Pi-Sunyer, 1988a). Even people who had so much success in commercial programs that their "before" and "after" pictures were used in newspaper advertisements have been found to backslide; in one study, 20 months later, 72% who had given this public testimony had regained 5 pounds or more (Fatis et al., 1989). The data seem so overwhelming against long-term success that the Council on Scientific Affairs of the American Medical Association pronounced, ". . . it is more likely that a person will be cured of most forms of cancer than of obesity" (1988). (Although many experts may prefer to think in terms of "sustained remission" rather than "cure" of obesity, the Council statement makes its point effectively.)

If you have excess body fat, should you give up trying to lose it? Not at all. Achieving and maintaining your individualized best body weight is an important health goal—and weight loss *is* possible if a person goes about it in a way that favors success.

In this section, we will begin by discussing the best way to lose fat and keep it off. Following that, we will comment on methods that have been used but that are not as effective or are suitable only for very limited use.

The Best Way to Lose Fat and Keep It Off

How can you beat the odds? First of all, realize that excess body weight is usually a multifactorial condition; like other health problems that have a number of contributing factors, it is likely to take a combination of approaches to deal with. Since it is not yet possible to analyze to what extent an overweight person's problem is caused by the various factors that affect body weight, the best approach is to use a program that is comprehensive. Be aware that some of the dismal data collected on weight-loss programs of the past have involved a single approach—such as *just* going on a diet, *just* controlling certain eating behaviors, or *just* exercising regularly. Recently, the overwhelming trend in professionally developed weight-loss programs is to deal simultaneously with nutrition, exercise, and support systems.

Another feature many recent professionally developed programs share is that before people begin a program, they are urged to think carefully about whether they are prepared to make permanent lifestyle changes. If not—if what they really want is a "quick fix" and then go back to their current lifestyle—they are advised that it would be counterproductive to start; it would simply lead to another failure and may make it harder yet to lose weight in the future. A number of programs actually turn away prospective clients who do not seem committed to making enduring changes.

For long-term effectiveness, people should not try to lose more than 1 or 2 pounds per week; people who lose fat at this rate have a far better likelihood of sustaining their losses. The best way to lose 1 to 2 pounds per week is to moderately reduce kcalorie intake and moderately increase energy output through exercise. Since a pound of body fat has the energy potential of approximately 3500 kcalories, you must create a discrepancy between energy intake and output of 500 kcalories per day to lose 1 pound of fat per week; to lose 2 pounds per week, a deficit of 1000 kcalories per day is necessary.

Now let's discuss more thoroughly the three program components: nutrition, exercise, and support.

Successful Program Component #1: NUTRITION The nutrition part of a weight-loss program should satisfy all of the following (American Dietetic Association, 1987; Rock and Coulston, 1988):

1. Provide all the nutrients your body needs without as many kcalories as you have been eating; it should contain *at least* 1200 kcalories per day for women and 1500 kcalories per day for men, since it is very difficult to meet the RDA for many nutrients at lower energy levels.
2. Be as close as possible to your own tastes and eating habits.
3. Keep you from being hungry or unusually tired.
4. Consist of foods that are readily obtainable and allow you to eat away from home without feeling like a social outcast.
5. Offer changes in eating habits that you can use from now on.
6. Be conducive to improvement in overall health.

Develop your own eating plan that meets the above criteria; this way you can be sure it incorporates your individual preferences. Using the Basic Food Guide, analyze your current diet to make sure it meets your nutritional needs. Then consider ways in which you could moderately lower your kcalorie intake without substantially affecting the aspects of your eating style that you most enjoy. Assessment 10.1 on pages 344–345 provides one format for this process; it also incorporates the second successful program component—exercise.

Some experts believe that it is best not to think of this new way of eating as "a diet," because this term suggests a temporary eating pattern. Dieting may also suggest having to adhere to a plan that is rigid, full of self-denial, and lacking in taste satisfaction. Rather, some weight-control counselors prefer to teach *eating management,* in which a person identifies and reinforces the aspects of his or her current eating style that are consistent with good nutrition and weight control; introduces carefully selected new foods and eating behaviors to replace some counterproductive current practices; and reduces (but does not necessarily totally extinguish) food practices involving so-called "junk" or "guilt" foods (Dalton, 1988).

There are more and more products available—from entrees to desserts—that can help people get the tastes they enjoy without eating as many kcalories. For example, there are several product lines of single-serving, low-fat, kcalorie-controlled frozen entrees that offer a variety of flavors and cuisines along with considerable convenience. Salad dressings, ordinarily high in fat, are now available with less fat or almost no fat. Even desserts, often a source of guilt for would-be weight-losers, are now available in reduced-kcalorie forms. Some of these products have been made possible by the development of palatable fat and sugar substitutes; many that are used commercially or can be purchased for home use are described in Table 6.2 (in the carbohydrate chapter) and Table 7.2 (in the lipid chapter).

Two artificial fats have been developed. One, *Simplesse,* was approved for limited use early in 1990. It is made from protein, can be used only in unheated foods, and provides between 1 and 2 kcalories per gram. The other, *sucrose polyester,* is currently being tested. It looks and tastes like fat but cannot be digested or absorbed by humans. Although early tests look promising, it remains to be seen whether these substances will actually aid in weight loss.

If you do not want to develop your own lower-kcalorie way of eating, there are hundreds of different types of preplanned diets around. Be forewarned that their quality varies substantially, ranging from those that are safe and could be successful to those that are very hazardous. Table 10.4 describes various types of diets, gives some examples, and states their possible effects.

Because of its high kcaloric density, fat is the most restricted nutrient in most diets. One effective way to limit fat is to restrict certain animal products while allowing more liberal use of many plant foods. Some diets therefore resemble semivegetarian or vegan eating styles. Experience shows that this approach has merit. A review of the health aspects of vegetarian eating styles points out that vegetarians in general (who are not necessarily trying to lose weight) are leaner and closer to their recommended weights than omnivores are (Dwyer, 1988).

Table 10.4 Summary of Popular Dietary Approaches to Weight Control
The only method likely to lead to healthy, maintainable fat loss is the first one.

Approach	Characteristics	Potential Problems	Examples[a]
Moderate kcaloric restriction	Usually 1200–1800 kcal per day Reasonable balance of macronutrients Encourages exercise May employ behavioral approach	Loss of motivation because there are no dramatic, immediate results	The Setpoint Diet Slim Chance in a Fat World Weight Watcher's Diet The American Heart Association Diet Mary Ellen's Help Yourself Diet Plan
Extremely low carbohydrate	Less than 100 gm carbohydrate per day	Initial loss of water weight primarily—which is often quickly regained Fatigue Headaches May predispose to subsequent binging	Atkin's Diet Revolution Calories Don't Count Drinking Man's Diet Woman Doctor's Diet for Women The Doctor's Quick Weight Loss Diet (Stillman's) The Complete Scarsdale Medical Diet
Extremely low fat	Less than 20% of calories from fat Limited (or elimination of) animal protein sources, all fats, nuts, seeds	May be inadequate in protein and certain minerals May decrease absorption of fat-soluble vitamins Low satiety value	The Rice Diet Report The Macrobiotic Diet The Pritikin Diet
Novelty diets	Promote certain nutrients, foods, or combination of foods as having unique, magical, or previously undiscovered qualities	Usually severely limit or eliminate certain food groups, thereby making diet nutritionally inadequate Difficult to adapt to normal lifestyle	Dr. Berger's Immune Power Diet Fit for Life Diet The Rotation Diet The Beverly Hills Diet
Very low-kcalorie diets	Less than 800 kcal per day Also known as protein-sparing modified fasts	Likely to result in body protein losses if used by other than severely obese Requires close medical supervision Usually weight is regained after program is ended Difficult to adapt to normal lifestyles May cause dry skin, thinning hair, constipation	Optifast Cambridge Diet The Rotation Diet Genesis

Continues

Table 10.4 continued

Approach	Characteristics	Potential Problems	Examples[a]
Formula diets	Based on formulated or packaged products Many are very low calorie diet regimens (see above)	Weight regain when person resumes eating regular food Often very low in kcalories, potentially leading to additional problems described above, including electrolyte imbalance	U.S.A. (United Sciences of America), Inc. Optifast Genesis Cambridge Diet Herbalife Slimfast

[a]Diets may be listed in more than one category if multiple characteristics apply.

Adapted from: 1) American Dietetic Association. 1987. *Weighty issues/Evaluating diets.* Chicago: The American Dietetic Association. 2) Rock, C.L. and A.M. Coulston. 1988. Weight-control approaches: A review by the California Dietetic Association. *Journal of the American Dietetic Association* 88:44–48.

Be aware that of all the types of diets, the balanced diets with moderate kcaloric restriction—the first listing in Table 10.4—are the only ones that earn the support of most professional nutritionists and physicians; most experts have reservations about all of the others.

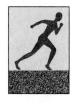

Successful Program Component #2: EXERCISE The benefits of exercise already have been mentioned many times in this chapter: exercise increases energy output; it may help regulate hunger; if exercise helps retain or even increase lean body mass, it may help keep the metabolic rate elevated beyond the time of the activity; and it may increase kcalories expended for the thermic effect of food. Exercise can also reduce stress, improve cardiovascular health, and help maintain strength and flexibility. Although the extent to which some of these effects occur is controversial, one thing that is *not* controversial is that exercise is an effective component of a weight-loss and maintenance program (Grinker et al., 1985; Stern and Lowney, 1986; Sims, 1988; Pi-Sunyer, 1988b).

Before beginning an exercise program, it is a good idea to have a medical examination. This is especially true if the person is more than 130% of recommended weight, smokes, or has any other risk factors for heart disease. Certain health problems may make it advisable to get professional help in planning the exercise program and to exercise in a supervised setting.

The exercise component of a weight-loss program should satisfy all of the following (McArdle and Toner, 1988):

1. Be a type of exercise that uses a large muscle mass in rhythmic, sustainable activity.
2. Be safe and adaptable to any physical limitations you may have.
3. Provide pleasure and be relatively convenient for you.
4. Be done at sufficient intensity, frequency, and duration to achieve results.

Some of the types of activities that fit the first criterion are walking, jogging, running, bicycling, swimming, water walking, cross-country skiing, aerobic dancing, and circuit weight training. Choose an activity that you enjoy, because then you are more likely to do it often enough for it to be of benefit. Another important factor is that it should be relatively convenient for you; no matter how much you like swimming, if it takes you 45 minutes to get to the nearest pool, swimming is not a practical choice. Probably the best situation of all is to have several activities that you enjoy and have access to, so that you can have some variety.

There are other things to consider. Do you prefer to work out alone, or would you enjoy being with a group? There are organized programs for many of the activities mentioned above; they offer camaraderie, encourage regular participation, and provide help with monitoring your progress and modifying your program as your training state improves (Sims, 1988). On the other hand, if you like to be independent, being on your own allows you more flexibility regarding when and where you exercise.

In order to be of benefit, your exercise program needs to meet criteria for intensity, frequency, and duration. Your workout should be at an intensity that brings your heart rate into the recommended training range for your age, as shown in Figure 10.10. If you exercise within your range, you will experience various physiological effects over time such as improved heart and lung function and greater metabolism of fat during exercise. Figure 10.11 illustrates how to take your pulse.

How often do you need to exercise to help lose weight? Studies have shown that you should work out at least three times per week to affect your

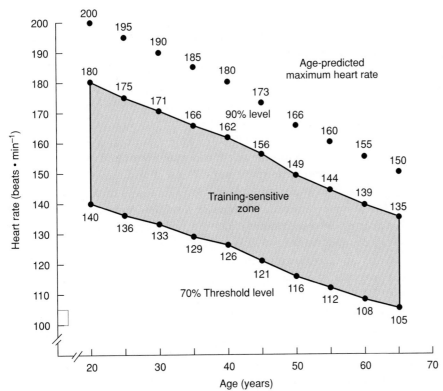

Figure 10.10 Recommended training heart rate ranges for age. To get weight-loss and cardiovascular benefits from physical activity, the intensity should bring your pulse within the training-sensitive zone for your age. (McArdle et al., 1986. *Exercise physiology: Energy, nutrition and human performance.* Philadelphia: Lea and Febiger.)

Figure 10.11 How to determine your heart rate. Immediately as you stop exercising, place the middle fingers of your right hand over your carotid artery at the left side of your neck where you can easily feel the pulse, usually about an inch below your jaw. Do not press hard; this can slow the rate. Count your pulse for 10 seconds and multiply by 6 to get your heart rate per minute. Figure 10.10 shows training heart rates at various age ranges.

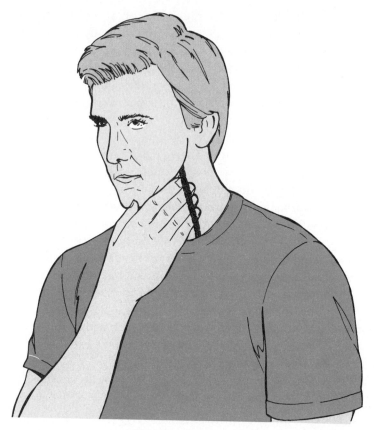

body weight and/or skinfold thickness (McArdle and Toner, 1988). Many programs recommend three to five exercise sessions per week. People often find that if they take an occasional day off from programmed exercising, they are eager to get back to it again the next day.

As far as duration is concerned, the experts suggest that a workout should be long enough for you to expend about 300 kcalories. Since energy expenditure during activity is a function of the type and intensity of activity, of your body weight, and of the length of time you do it, it is best to calculate workout times for your chosen sport(s) and your own body weight. Table 5.1 (in the energy chapter) lists the energy costs of various activities based on kcalories per kilogram per minute. In general, a person doing moderate to vigorous activity will need to exercise for 20–30 minutes to burn 300 kcalories; someone exercising at a lower intensity may need to work out for 40–60 minutes (McArdle and Toner, 1988).

If you are unaccustomed to much physical activity and you are starting an exercise program, it is best to begin at a lower intensity and duration (for example, 10–15 minutes), and eventually build up to the levels we have described here. Doing too much too soon puts you at risk of overtiredness, soreness, and injury; it is far better to work up gradually to a full program. For some people, this may take as long as 8–10 weeks.

Deliberate exercise sessions that are set apart from the performance of routine daily activities are not the only way to increase energy usage. You can, for example, walk a greater share of your way to school or work, take stairs during the day instead of elevators, and move around during breaks instead of sitting. Although these activities may be hard to measure and some may be of short duration, if done regularly they can contribute significantly to overall energy expenditure.

Successful Program Component #3: SUPPORT   The support part of a weight-loss program includes all the mental and psychological aspects of developing new eating and exercise behaviors and sticking with them. The support component should do all of the following:

1. Provide cognitive training for setting goals, maintaining motivation, coping with mistakes and reducing their likelihood in the future (relapse prevention).
2. Teach behavioral techniques such as self-monitoring, modifying the environment to control cues that make us eat, and substituting alternate activities.
3. Help to identify people who will support you in your proposed lifestyle changes as well as those who might sabotage your efforts.

These activities are often cumulatively called **behavior modification techniques.** When behavior modification was first applied to weight control in the early 1960s, it primarily involved goal setting, self-monitoring, changing the environment to reduce food cues, breaking the chain of events that lead to inappropriate eating, slowing the pace of eating, and substituting alternative activities. In other words, the focus was on making people aware of their eating habits and on gradually reshaping these behaviors; there was little attention given to nutrition or to exercise.

behavior modification techniques—carefully planned methods for changing living habits

Individuals in early group programs often achieved initial gradual weight loss of approximately 1 pound per week in an 8 or 9 week program. In follow-up studies that were done as much as a year later, average losses for the group as a whole were maintained (Buckmaster and Brownell, 1988). However, there was a great deal of unevenness between individuals at follow-up; some people had continued to lose weight, whereas others had regained it. It became obvious that in its original form, behavior modification had its limits.

In recent years, the scope of many behavior modification programs has been broadened considerably. In addition to the general principles of behavior modification discussed in Assessment 9.1, now *good nutrition* and *increased exercise* are being emphasized in many programs, along with additional cognitive skills and psychological support. An example of the application of these principles is shown in the Slice of Life on page 346.

Part of the additional cognitive training in the newer programs is *relapse prevention*, originally discussed in Assessment 9.1. Without this training, when people overeat on a given occasion, they might feel as though this "failure" proves that they are incapable of maintaining the program, and they may wonder why they should continue to try. With training, people

Planning a One-Pound/Week Weight Loss

The majority of people in college are at a healthy weight, but it is in the years after college graduation that many people find themselves gradually gaining fat. This self-assessment is designed to help you think ahead to how you might modify your eating and exercise habits to achieve a one-pound per week weight loss if necessary.

(If your energy intake and/or body weight are currently very low, change the goal of this assessment to planning a one-pound per week weight *gain*. In this case, it may be advisable to reduce exercise somewhat if you are unnecessarily active now, but continue 3–4 vigorous workouts per week to help maintain general fitness.)

Assessment 10.1

Keep and Evaluate Your Record

1. Keep several days of food records (although just one day is shown in this example).
2. Check the overall adequacy of your nutritional intake against the recommendations of the Basic Food Guide, as you learned to do in Chapter 2. If your diet doesn't measure up satisfactorily, make appropriate modifications under "Changes."
3. Using Appendices E and F or information from food labels, enter the kcalorie value of all items you consumed or put under "Changes."

Plan How to Achieve a 500-Kcalorie per Day Energy Deficit

4. Decide what proportion of the 500-kcalorie per day energy deficit you want to achieve through increased exercise and what proportion from decreased kcaloric intake.
5. Using Table 5.1, consider which activity you will do and the average number of minutes per day you'll do it. You may simply choose to pursue an activity you already enjoy but to do it for a longer time or more times per week. (Be realistic, and remember to allow extra time needed for getting to the exercise facility, changing clothes, and showering later.) In the space below, multiply your weight in kilograms times the kcal/kg/min for the activity by the number of minutes (or additional minutes) you will do it; this will give you the extra number of kcalories per day you will expend.

$$\frac{\text{weight}}{\text{in kg}} \times \frac{\text{kcal/kg/min}}{\text{for activity}} \times \frac{\text{minutes of}}{\text{activity}} = \frac{\text{extra kcal}}{\text{expended}}$$

_____ kg × _____ kcal/kg/min × _____ minutes = _____ kcal

6. Calculate by how many kcalories you will need to decrease your intake to achieve the 500-kcal deficit per day.

500 kcal − _____ activity kcal = _____ needed decrease in intake

7. Evaluate your intake for types of foods that are providing excess kcalories:

a. Check the limited extras column for low-nutrient-density foods.
b. Check food group foods for their relative fat and sugar contents, using the rulers at the bottom of the food group lists in the Basic Food Guide in Chapter 2.
c. Check food group columns for types of foods you consumed at levels considerably above the minimal recommendations—for example, 150% or more of the minimum.

8. Consider behavior modification techniques to help change certain habits. For example, you might be able to forego your evening snack if you had something else to interest you as you watched your favorite TV show at the end of the day. How about having a big puzzle in process near the TV set?

Very likely, your new plan will closely resemble your habitual diet pattern, and that's the point. To succeed over the long term, the changes must be small but constructive. As time goes along, you may want to re-evaluate how much exercise and dietary change you make to better fit your weight control needs and lifestyle.

Sample Assessment 10.1 Planning a one-pound/week weight loss

| Food or Beverage | Amount Eaten | Fruits and Vegetables | | | | Grain Products | Milk and Milk Prod. | Meats and Alternates | Limited Extras | Energy (Kcal) | | Changes and (Kcal) |
		A	C	Other	Total							
Instant oatmeal	1¼ c.					2				145		
Milk, 2%	¾ c.						¾			91	64	skim milk (−27)
Cheeseburger:												
Bun, enriched	1					2				129		
Meat patty	3 oz.							1		230		
Cheese, processed	1 oz.						½			94		
Catsup	1 T.			tr						18		
French fries	20			2						274		
Regular cola	12 oz.								x	151	2	diet pop (−149)
Oatmeal cookies	2 large					2				123		
Milk, 2%	½ pint						1			121	86	skim milk (−35)
Cr. of mushroom soup	1 c.			¼			½	½		205		
Toasted ham sandwich:												
Bread, enriched	2 sl.					2				150		
Ham	2 oz.							1		74		
Butter	2 t.								x	68		
Apple	1 med.			1						80		
Milk, 2%	1 c.						1			121	86	skim milk (−35)
Orange juice	1 c.		2								+31	raw carrot (+31)
Crackers, enriched	12					2						−6 crackers (−75)
Cheddar cheese	3 oz.							2				−1½ oz. cheese (−171)
Subtotals		0+	2+	3¼ =	5¼					2105	1859	−492 + 31 = 461
Group totals					5¼	10½	5¾	2	2			
Standards		1	1		5	6	3	2				
Shortages			1									

Slice of Life

▼ ▲ ▼ ▲ ▼ ▲ ▼ ▲ ▼ ▲ ▼ ▲ ▼ ▲ ▼ ▲ ▼ ▲

Behavior Modification for Weight Control

Diane threw the apple core into the wastebasket, and then remembered, "Better put that on my food diary for today." She took out the form on which she had been recording her intake (see opposite).

She added the information about the apple and glanced over the other entries on the sheet. This had been her fourth day of keeping a food diary. She felt optimistic that this behavior modification method would help her lose the 12 pounds she had gained last semester. She hoped so. The two diets she had read about in magazines and tried on her own hadn't worked; in fact, she now weighed three pounds more than when she had started them.

Later that week, before her behavior modification group meeting, she discussed the week's food diaries she had kept with the dietitian leading the sessions. She could quickly see some habits that had added unneeded kcalories to her intake, such as her liberal consumption of cola and cookies. Other habits were less obvious, such as her use of whole milk instead of a lower-fat milk. With the leader's help, she listed them all, and then put them in order from the easiest to the hardest for her to change.

Time	Minutes Spent Eating	M or S*	H**	Activity While Eating	Place of Eating	Food and Quantity	Others Present	Feeling Before Eating
8:10 a.m.	17	M	1	standing, fixing lunch	Kitchen	1 c. O.J. 1 c. corn flakes ½ c. whole milk 2 t. sugar	—	sleepy
						black coffee		
10:30 a.m.	10	S	1	sitting, taking notes	classroom	12 oz. cola	class	busy
11:45 a.m.	20	M	2	sitting, talking	union	1 sandwich 1 apple	friends	good
2:30 p.m.	15	S	1	sitting, studying	library	12 oz. cola	friend	bored
5:30 p.m.	15	M	3	sitting, talking	kitchen	1 chicken leg 1 baked potato 2 T. butter lettuce 1 oz. dressing 1 c. whole milk	roommate	good
						4 cookies		
8:15 p.m.	10	S	0	sitting, studying	living room	12 oz. cola	—	tired

*M or S: Meal or snack **H: Degree of hunger (0 = none; 3 = maximum)

Her goal for the following week was to make just the easiest change on the list. She chose to limit herself to two colas per day, although the leader suggested that another alternative would be to switch to an artificially sweetened beverage instead. She decided to substitute a short walk for the third cola, making stops at the water fountain to replace the fluids it would have provided.

Diane left the session feeling confident that she could manage this much change—after all, she wasn't giving up colas entirely, and she thought she'd really enjoy the walks.

This self-monitoring and gradual changing of eating behaviors is one aspect of behavior modification for weight control. Other important elements include relapse prevention, social support, and exercise. ▼

gain many advantages. First, they identify which kinds of situations are likely to be high-risk for them; for example, many people find that social situations and negative moods increase temptation to overeat.

Next, they plan ahead for how they might ward off overindulgence when those situations arise (Mayo Clinic Nutrition Letter, 1989). At a social event, they might plan to look carefully over the buffet table and eat only those items that look especially good; or they might commit to getting just one plate of food and no more. They "practice" these situations repeatedly in their mind, so that when they occur, the new behavior will be familiar. Even with this preparation, people sometimes lapse from their intended behavior; the program teaches how to cope immediately after a lapse and get back on course with a more balanced lifestyle.

Another newer aspect of behavior modification programs is increased social support. Some people benefit considerably from having others around them who are aware of their efforts and will provide encouragement and reinforcement; this can come in various forms. Family members can be great allies; a number of studies have shown increased weight losses when a key family member learns how to be supportive (Buckmaster and Brownell, 1988). Others may prefer therapeutic support from a health care professional trained to assist people with weight loss. This can be very useful, especially for the first few months. But for practical reasons, the person eventually must give up relying on the professional. Lastly, some self-help groups can also provide effective support. Those that are extensions of behavior modification programs that were professionally run to begin with have the best records (Buckmaster and Brownell, 1988).

One final thought on the matter of social support: some social relationships can have a negative effect. People who are trying to lose weight should consider whether anybody around them might be eager to sabotage their efforts, such as an overweight friend who might feel their weight loss would put pressure on him or her. If so, it is possible to learn how to get around these negative influences.

Available Programs There are many programs that claim to help people lose fat. Some consist of print materials that can be used either individually or in a group setting. Appendix H lists eight programs published in workbook format and 55 other programs in traditional book form. In addition to indicating what features are part of each program (such as nutrition, exercise, behavior modification, stress management, recipes, etc.), these appendices *rate the quality* of various components.

Table 10.5 lists some weight-reduction services and identifies their features. The fact that we have included this list does not constitute our endorsement of these services. Some of them have been known to promote greater losses of weight than are healthy or sustainable. If you are interested, check on programs in your own area to see what kind of goals they set for their patrons. Talk to your physician and evaluate the programs carefully before you enroll.

Ineffective or Limited Fat Loss Methods

Many other methods have been used to try to help people lose body fat, but they either do not work in the long run or are appropriate for only very few people. Three of these methods, very low kcalorie diets, the use of drugs, and surgery, are discussed below. There are many other methods of unusual nature that come and go; some of these are identified in the *Slice of Life* on page 349.

Very Low Kcalorie Diets A number of weight-loss programs and diet plans have been developed that allow fewer kcalories than the 1200 and 1500

Table 10.5 Features of Some Weight-Loss Programs (Being on this list does not constitute endorsement.)

Program[a]	Eating Plan[b] Determined By:	Exercise Promoted?	Support Structure	Behavioral Change Principles Taught?
Diet Center	Program	Yes	Individual and group	Yes
Nutri/System	Program; requires purchase of their food at additional cost	Yes	Individual	Yes
Overeaters Anonymous	Physician	No	Group	No
Slender Center	Program	Yes	Individual	Yes
Weight Loss Clinic	Program	Yes	Individual	Yes
Weight Watchers	Program	Yes	Group	Yes
TOPS	Physician	No	Group	Yes

Adapted from Rosenblatt, E. 1988. Weight-loss programs. *Postgraduate Medicine* 83:137–148.

[a]Check on programs in your area, and avoid those that attempt greater losses than 2 pounds per week; weight is likely to be regained after ending program when losses are higher. Talk with your physician about any program you are considering.

[b]Avoid any eating plan that reduces kcalorie intake to less than 1200 kcalories per day for women or 1500 kcalories per day for men; these may be nutritionally inadequate.

kcalories/day that should be the minimum for women and men, respectively. In general, very low kcalorie diets are unable to supply adequate levels of nutrients and are therefore not in our best health interests. If they are used by people who are only moderately overweight, they can result in large losses of body protein (Wadden et al., 1990). Furthermore, they often

Slice of Life

Fat Loss Fantasies

Most of us *know* that the only effective way to lose fat is to eat less and exercise more. Yet, hope springs eternal, and many people secretly wish for ways to lose weight without having to make permanent lifestyle changes.

There is no magic bullet. Nonetheless, here are some of the methods people have bought into in hopes of losing fat:

- eyeglasses with two different-colored lenses that were supposed to make food look unappealing and thereby cause weight loss
- a special tea that was supposed to cause weight loss
- a patch to wear on the skin that was supposed to release a chemical that would cause weight loss

Although you may have seen through those particular scams if they hit your area, there are hundreds of others out there waiting for you. You are vulnerable if the product is marketed in ways that appeal to you—with sophistication, or with the insinuation that only the intelligent or affluent are privy to the secret, or with a claim (unproved) of scientific authenticity.

Another ploy is the promise of fast results—but the weight you lose may not be fat. Con-

sider the plastic wraps and various sweat suits guaranteed to make you lose weight. They make you sweat and result in temporary water loss, which registers on the scale as weight loss. Vibrating machines are marketed to wiggle the fat right off of you, but since the only energy you expend is to keep yourself upright and slightly resist the belt while it works, there is almost no benefit. Electrical muscle stimulators supposedly stimulate muscles to expend energy, but the effect is so localized and meager that benefits are negligible.

Skin creams have also been marketed for weight loss. Some of them contain irritants that cause skin to tingle and redden; you may prefer to believe the ad's claim that this is evidence that "it's working to melt away fat."

As long as there are people who want to lose weight, there will be products and services that purport to separate people from their fat. Many are only effective at separating them from their money. Let the buyer beware.

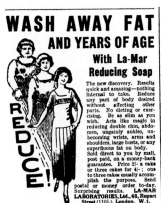

Ineffective products for reducing body fatness. People want to believe that fat can be diminished without dieting or exercising. This phenomenon is not new: half a century ago, the ad shown here undoubtedly sparked wishful thinking in many people— but produced dubious results. Today's media contain hundreds of current examples.

lead to weight regain, weight cycling, and increased subsequent difficulty in losing excess fat.

However, some physicians recommend these programs for patients whose substantial overfatness puts them at increased risk for health problems. The American Dietetic Association (ADA) has published criteria for the use of such programs. They should be administered only by health care professionals who have specialized training in weight loss management (ADA, 1989). The program is not recommended for infants, children, adolescents, pregnant women, or elderly people. Prospective patients for this treatment should be:

1. At least 30% overweight.
2. Free from the following conditions: active cancer, insulin-dependent diabetes mellitus, liver disease, kidney failure, cardiac problems, or severe psychological disturbances.
3. Committed to establishing new eating behaviors that will assist in the maintenance of weight loss.

In a study involving almost 500 people, results were better among the patients who participated in nine additional behavior modification sessions during the year after they achieved their weight loss (Hovell et al., 1988). About half of those patients maintained 60% or more of their weight loss 18 months later; of those who did not attend the sessions, only 11% maintained similar losses.

Drugs Different pharmacological methods have been used to promote weight loss. They are designed to decrease intake and/or to increase energy output. Various types of appetite supressants, substances to prevent absorption, and thermogenesis enhancers have enjoyed popularity for weight reduction (Nauss-Karol and Sullivan, 1988). Each drug has one or more negative effects, such as the potential for addiction, nervousness, rapid heartbeat, insomnia, and central nervous system depression (Sullivan et al., 1988).

Long-term studies using drug therapy for weight loss show poor results. Although pharmacological agents often promote initial weight loss, after the drug is withdrawn, weight regain typically occurs (Figure 10.12). For this reason, and because of the accompanying dangers of drug treatment programs, their general use should be discouraged.

Surgical Interventions Several types of surgery have been developed to bring about weight loss. The most drastic of these is surgery that modifies the gastrointestinal tract to restrict intake or to interfere with absorption. These procedures constitute major surgery; they involve risk, the possibility of serious complications, and substantial expense. Such methods are reserved for people whose obesity puts them at greater health risk than the surgery would, and who have been repeatedly unsuccessful at weight loss by other means (Kral, 1988). In most cases, a surgeon would consider one of these types of surgery only if the person were 100 pounds overweight or

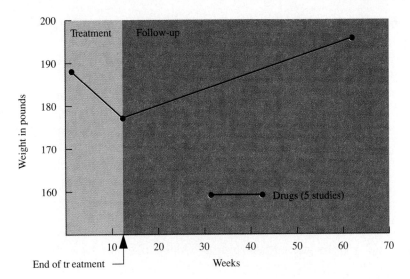

Figure 10.12 Lack of long-term success for weight loss using drug therapy. This illustration shows that drugs are helpful for weight loss only as long as they are being taken. When treatment ends, weight regain begins; weight often increases to higher than pretreatment weight. (Adapted from R.B. Stuart, C. Mitchell, and J.A. Jensen. 1981. Therapeutic options in the management of obesity. In *Medical Psychology: Contributions to Behavioral Medicine*. New York: Academic Press.)

twice normal weight. People who have had such gastrointestinal surgery usually do not lose all of their surplus fat; weight loss averages about 60% of their excess weight, at which point they generally stabilize (Forse et al., 1989).

Other less drastic methods to reduce intake are of dubious long-term benefit. Jaw wiring has been done for periods of time to temporarily limit intake of solid foods; but without behavior modification training, weight regain is assured. Acupuncture has been thought by some to be able to reduce appetite, but no long-term studies support this.

Some methods involve direct removal of fat. With lipectomy, fat tissue is surgically removed. Fat suctioning, on the other hand, involves making only a small incision where the fat is to be reduced, breaking up the excess adipose tissue, and vacuuming it out. These procedures are expensive and of uncertain benefit in the long term. They provide localized, cosmetic fat reduction; overall reduction of body fat by surgical means is not practical. Once again, if people who have had such surgery do not change their eating and exercise habits, they will regain body fat. Also be aware that the fact that these procedures are cosmetic does not mean that they are without risk; a few patients have developed fatal blood clots after fat suctioning. Others from whom lower body fat was removed have later accumulated a greater amount of upper body fat, putting them at increased risk of various health problems.

Opposite Techniques Can Be Used to Add Body Weight

A person who is considerably underweight, or has lost weight without trying to, would be best advised to have a thorough physical exam just to be sure that there is no physical problem responsible for the low weight.

Then, to attempt to tip the energy balance in favor of weight gain, consider these suggestions, many of which are simply the opposite of techniques suggested for fat loss:

- *Consume more energy.* Starting with a nutritionally adequate diet, eat larger meals, eat more often, and/or increase the energy density of the foods chosen. You may have noticed that there are some special supplements available for weight gain, but be wary of those that are mainly fat, because they can increase your fat intake above the recommended levels. You can be more liberal in your intake of limited extras; for you, they are really "not-so-limited" extras. However, your emphasis should still be on high-nutrient-density foods.

- *Modify your eating behaviors.* Set some reasonable goals for slow, gradual weight gain. Make a step-by-step plan for how to accomplish the goals, and implement the easiest change first.

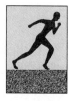

- *Decrease aerobic physical activity if you do much of it.* Sustained aerobic activity is a substantial energy-burner, so hold such exercise to a moderate level that will achieve fitness and no more. For general maintenance of fitness, the American College of Sports Medicine recommends three to five exercise sessions per week of 15–60 minutes each, depending on the intensity of the exercise (1978).

- *Consider body building.* If your muscles need further development, a moderate, progressive program of weight lifting can help you add more "muscle pounds" along with the new "fat pounds" your extra energy intake will produce. (But be wary of the dietary recommendations of body builders; many practice poor eating habits.)

- *Accept your genetically determined limits.* If you find that even when you implement these suggestions you do not achieve your goal weight (or you initially achieve it but then lose it quickly), you may need to accept the fact that your body is regulated at a lower level of fatness. Maintaining a larger amount of fat may require more time, effort, and expense than you consider worthwhile, and you may decide that your resources could be applied more productively to other kinds of goals.

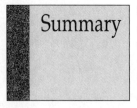

Summary

▶ Although the attention our culture devotes to the cosmetic aspect of body weight seems excessive, it is appropriate to be concerned about weight from a health standpoint. But the issue of what ideal weight means or should be is not at all obvious, and often the wrong people are concerned about their weight.

▶ Certain hazards are associated with being either too fat or too thin. **Overfat** (or **overweight** and **obese**) people have statistically higher risk of developing many types of health problems and have to deal with numerous psychosocial and practical problems as well. People who have too little body fat have less endurance and, in some extreme cases, are more susceptible to infectious diseases. Both extremely overfat and extremely **underweight** people are likely to die younger.

▶ Many factors influence how people arrive at their individual body weights. Changes occur when intake and output are not equal. Energy intake is regulated both by physiological factors (**hunger** and **satiety**) and by psychological factors. The **set-point theory** suggests that each person tends to maintain their unique body weight when they eat primarily in response to physiological factors. Energy output is affected by metabolic rate, activity level, and thermic effect of food. Body weight is affected by both hereditary and environmental influences.

▶ You can estimate your ideal body weight from a combination of guidelines, all of which *approximate* what healthy individuals of a given sex, height, and build should weigh. These guidelines include estimation of body fatness, values based on height and weight such as **body mass index,** and a subjective assessment of your own best functional weight. In the U.S., cultural standards for women are currently lower than generally accepted standards for good health.

▶ There is a theory about what happens at the cellular level during energy imbalance: that the body responds to excess energy by adding more fat cells **(hyperplasia),** enlarging those it already has **(hypertrophy),** or doing both. Energy deficits are thought to result in decreased fat cell size but not cell number.

▶ People have tried thousands of techniques for losing body fat, ranging from very sensible to very dangerous. Approaches that have been tried include dietary restriction, behavior modification, increased physical activity, drugs, surgical interventions, and others. They vary in their safety and effectiveness. The programs that are most safe and effective encourage 1–2 pounds of weight loss per week by using a combination of diet, exercise, and support systems including **behavior modification.**

▶ Severe weight-reduction diets lead to physical and psychological consequences that usually result in failure of the diet and weight regain. Because such diets are often dangerous and unsuccessful in the long run and may lead to a vicious cycle of starving and overeating, they should be avoided.

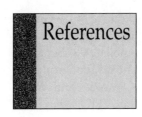

References

American College of Sports Medicine. 1978. Position statement on the recommended quantity and quality of exercise for developing and maintaining fitness in healthy adults. *Medicine and Science in Sports and Exercise* 10(no. 3):vii–x.

American Dietetic Association (ADA). 1987. *Weighty issues/Evaluating diets*. Chicago: The American Dietetic Association.

American Dietetic Association (ADA). 1989. Timely statement of The American Dietetic Association: Very low calorie weight loss diets. *Journal of the American Dietetic Association* 89:975–976.

Anderson, G.H. 1988. Metabolic regulation of food intake. In *Modern nutrition in health and disease,* eds. M.E. Shils and V.R. Young. Philadelphia: Lea & Febiger.

Baumgartner, R.N., W.C. Chumlea, and A.F. Roche. 1989. Estimation of body composition from bioelectric impedance of body segments. *American Journal of Clinical Nutrition* 50:221–226.

Bjorntorp, P. 1983. The role of adipose tissue in human obesity. In *Obesity,* vol. 4, *Contemporary Issues in Clinical Nutrition,* ed. M.R.C. Greenwood. New York: Churchill Livingstone.

Bray, G.A. 1983. The energetics of obesity. *Medicine and Science in Sports and Exercise* 15:32–40.

Bray, G.A. 1987. Obesity—a disease of nutrient or energy balance? *Nutrition Reviews* 45(no. 2):33–42.

Brownell, K.D., M.R.C. Greenwood, E. Stellar, and E.E. Shrager. 1986. The effects of repeated cycles of weight loss and regain in rats. *Physiology and Behavior* 38:459–464.

Brozek, J.M. 1982. *The effects of malnutrition on human behavior.* American Dietetic Association (ADA) audio cassette tape 9, 1982. Chicago, IL: ADA.

Brunzell, J.D. 1983. Obesity and risk for cardiovascular disease. In *Obesity,* vol. 4, *Contemporary*

Issues in Clinical Nutrition, ed. M.R.C. Green-wood. New York: Churchill Livingstone.

Buckmaster, L. and K.D. Brownell. 1988. Behavior modification: The state of the art. In *Obesity and weight control*, eds. R.T. Frankle and M-U. Yang. Rockville, MD: Aspen Publishers, Inc.

Callaway, C.W. 1988. Biologic adaptations to starvation and semistarvation. In *Obesity and weight control*, eds. R.T. Frankle and M-U. Yang. Rockville, MD: Aspen Publishers, Inc.

Collier, S.N., S.F. Stallings, P.G. Wolman, and R.W. Cullen. 1990. Assessment of attitudes about weight and dieting among college-aged individuals. *Journal of the American Dietetic Association* 90:276–278.

Council on Scientific Affairs, American Medical Association. 1988. Treatment of obesity in adults. *Journal of the American Medical Association* 260:2547–2551.

Czajka-Narins, D.M. and E.S. Parham. 1990. Fear of fat: Attitudes toward obesity. *Nutrition Today* 25(no. 1):26–32.

Dalton, S. 1988. Eating management: A tool for the practitioner. In *Obesity and weight control*, eds. R.T. Frankle and M-U. Yang. Rockville, MD: Aspen Publishers, Inc.

Danforth, E., Jr., and L. Landsberg. 1983. Energy expenditure and its regulation. In *Obesity*, vol. 4, *Contemporary Issues in Clinical Nutrition*, ed. M.R.C. Greenwood. New York: Churchill Livingstone.

Dietz, W.H. 1988. Childhood and adolescent obesity. 1988. In *Obesity and weight control*, eds. R.T. Frankle and M-U. Yang. Rockville, MD: Aspen Publishers, Inc.

Dreon, D.M., B. Frey-Hewitt, N. Ellsworth, P.T. Williams, R.B. Terry, and P.D. Wood. 1988. Dietary fat:carbohydrate ratio and obesity in middle-aged men. *American Journal of Clinical Nutrition* 47:995–1000.

Dwyer, J.T. 1988. Health aspects of vegetarian diets. *American Journal of Clinical Nutrition* 48:712–738.

Elliott, D.L., L. Goldberg, K.S. Kuehl, and W.M. Bennett. 1989. Sustained depression of the

resting metabolic rate after massive weight loss. *American Journal of Clinical Nutrition* 49: 93–96.

Fallon, A.C. and P. Rozin. 1985. Sex differences in perceptions of desirable body shape. *Journal of Abnormal Psychology* 94:102–105.

Fatis, M., A. Weiner, J.A. Hawkins, and B. Van Dorsten. 1989. Following up on a commercial weight loss program: Do the pounds stay off after your picture has been in the newspaper? *Journal of the American Dietetic Association* 89:547–548.

Forse, A., P.N. Benotti, and G.L. Blackburn. 1989. Morbid obesity: Weighing the treatment options—surgical intervention. *Nutrition Today* 24(Sept/Oct):10–16.

Frisancho, A.R. 1988. Nutritional anthropometry. *Journal of the American Dietetic Association* 88:553–555.

Frisch, R.E. 1987. Nutrition, fatness, puberty, and fertility. *Nutrition and the M.D., Special Report: Obesity and other eating disorders.*

Ganley, R.M. 1989. Emotion and eating in obesity: A review of the literature. *International Journal of Eating Disorders* 8:343–361.

Garn, S.M., T.V. Sullivan, and V. Hawthorne. 1988. Evidence against functional differences between "central" and "peripheral" fat. *American Journal of Clinical Nutrition* 47:836–839.

Gong, E.J., D. Garrel, and D.H. Calloway. 1989. Menstrual cycle and voluntary food intake. *American Journal of Clinical Nutrition* 49:252–258.

Gray, D.S., G.A. Bray, N. Gemayel, and K. Kaplan. 1989. Effect of obesity on bioelectrical impedance. *American Journal of Clinical Nutrition* 50:255–260.

Greenwood, M.R.C., and V. Pittman-Waller. 1988. Weight control: A complex, various, and controversial problem. In *Obesity and weight control*, eds. R.T. Frankle and M-U. Yang. Rockville, MD: Aspen Publishers, Inc.

Grinker, J.A., J. Most, J. Hirsch, L. Borsdorf, and T. Wayler. 1985. Analysis of factors contributing to long-term success among graduates of a residential weight management program for women. *International Journal of Eating Disorders* 4:293–305.

Gwirtsman, H.E., W.H. Kaye, E. Obarzanek, D.T. George, D.C. Jimerson, and M.H. Ebert. 1989. Decreased caloric intake in normal-weight patients with bulimia: comparison with female volunteers. *American Journal of Clinical Nutrition* 49:86–92.

Hammer, R.L., C.A. Barrier, E.S. Roundy, J.M. Bradford, and A.G. Fisher. 1989. Calorie-restricted low-fat diet and exercise in obese women. *American Journal of Clinical Nutrition* 49:77–85.

Herman, C.P. and J. Polivy. 1988. Psychological factors in the control of appetite. In *Control of appetite*, ed. M. Winick. New York: John Wiley & Sons, Inc.

Hill, J.O., P.B. Sparling, T.W. Shields, and P.A. Heller. 1987. Effects of exercise and food restriction on body composition and metabolic rate in obese women. *American Journal of Clinical Nutrition* 46:622–630.

Himms-Hagen, J. 1983. Brown adipose tissue thermogenesis in obese animals. *Nutrition Reviews* 41:261–267.

Hovell, M.F., A. Koch, C.R. Hofstetter, C. Sipan, P. Faucher, A. Dellinger, G. Borok, A. Forsythe, and V.J. Felitti. 1988. Long-term weight loss maintenance: Assessment of a behavioral and supplemented fasting regimen. *American Journal of Public Health* 78(no. 6):663–666.

Hubert, H. 1988. Obesity: A predictor for coronary heart disease. In *Obesity and weight control*, eds. R.T. Frankle and M-U. Yang. Rockville, MD: Aspen Publishers, Inc.

Keesey, R.E. 1988. The body-weight set point. *Postgraduate Medicine* 83(no. 6):114–127.

Kolata, G. 1985. Why do people get fat? *Science* 227:1327–1328.

Kral, J. 1988. Surgery for obesity. In *Obesity and weight control*, eds. R.T. Frankle and M-U. Yang. Rockville, MD: Aspen Publishers, Inc.

Kurtzman, F.D., J. Yager, J. Landsverk, E. Wiesmeier, and D.C. Bodurka. 1989. Eating disorders among selected female student populations at UCLA. *Journal of the American Dietetic Association* 89:45–53.

Lissner, L., J. Stevens, D.A. Levitsky, K.M. Rasmussen, and B.J. Strupp. 1988. Variation in energy intake during the menstrual cycle: Implications for food-intake research. *American Journal of Clinical Nutrition* 48:956–962.

Lohman, T.G. 1981. Skinfolds and body density and their relation to body fatness: A review. *Human Biology* 53:181–225.

Lohman, T.G., M.L. Pollack, M.H. Slaughter, L.J. Brandon, and R.A. Boileau. 1984. Methodological factors and the prediction of body fat in female athletes. *Medicine and Science in Sports and Exercise* 16:92–96.

Mann, G.V. 1981. Menstrual effects of athletic training. In *Medicine and sport*, eds. J. Borms, M. Hebbelinck, and A. Venerado. New York: Karger.

Mayer, J., P. Roy, and K.P. Mitra. 1956. Relation between caloric intake, body weight, and physical work: Studies in an industrial male population in West Bengal. *American Journal of Clinical Nutrition* 4:169–175.

Mayo Clinic Nutrition Letter. 1989. Handling the holidays. *Mayo Clinic Nutrition Letter* 2(no. 12):7.

McArdle, W.D. and M.M. Toner. 1988. In *Obesity and weight control*, eds. R.T. Frankle and M-U. Yang. Rockville, MD: Aspen Publishers, Inc.

Meredith, C.N. 1989. The use of imaging techniques to assess nutritional status. In *Applying new technology to nutrition assessment*. Columbus, Ohio: Ross Laboratories.

Moses, N., M-M Banilivy, and F. Lifshitz. 1989. Fear of obesity among adolescent girls. *Pediatrics* 83:393–398.

Myrvik, Q.N. 1988. Nutrition and immunology. In *Modern nutrition in health and disease*, eds. M.E. Shils and V.R. Young. Philadelphia: Lea & Febiger.

National Center for Health Statistics (NCHS). 1987. Anthropometric reference data and prevalence of overweight, United States 1976–1980. Hyattsville, MD: U.S. Department of Health and Human Services.

National Dairy Council. 1988. Weight control: New findings. *Dairy Council Digest* 59(no. 3):13–18.

National Dairy Council. 1989. Nutrition and a physically active lifestyle. *Dairy Council Digest* 60(no. 4):19–24.

National Institutes of Health (NIH). 1985. *Health implications of obesity.* NIH consensus development conference statement, vol. 5, no. 9. Bethesda, MD: NIH.

National Research Council. 1989. *Diet and health.* Washington, DC: The National Academy Press.

Nauss-Karol, C. and A.C. Sullivan. 1988. Pharmacologic approaches to the treatment of obesity. In *Obesity and weight control,* eds. R.T. Frankle and M-U. Yang. Rockville, MD: Aspen Publishers, Inc.

Perusse, L., A. Tremblay, C. Leblanc, C.R. Cloninger, T. Reich, J. Rice, and C. Bouchard. 1988. Familial resemblance in energy intake: Contribution of genetic and environmental factors. *American Journal of Clinical Nutrition* 47:629–635.

Pi-Sunyer, F.X. 1988a. Obesity. In *Modern nutrition in health and disease,* eds. M.E. Shils and V.R. Young. Philadelphia: Lea & Febiger.

Pi-Sunyer, F.X. 1988b. Exercise in the treatment of obesity. In *Obesity and weight control,* eds. R.T. Frankle and M-U. Yang. Rockville, MD: Aspen Publishers, Inc.

Poehlman, E.T. and E.S. Horton. 1989. The impact of food intake and exercise on energy expenditure. *Nutrition Reviews* 47(no. 5):129–137.

Polivy, J. and C.P. Herman. 1983. *Breaking the diet habit.* New York: Basic Books, Inc., Publishers.

Ravussin, E., S. Lillioja, W.C. Knowler, L. Christin, D. Freymond, W.G. Abbott, V. Boyce, B.V. Howard, and C. Bogardus. 1988. *New England Journal of Medicine* 318:467–472.

Roberts, S.B., J. Savage, W.A. Coward, B. Chew, and A. Lucas. 1988. Energy expenditure and intake in infants born to lean and overweight mothers. *New England Journal of Medicine* 318:461–466.

Rock, C.L. and A.M. Coulston. 1988. Weight-control approaches: A review by the California Dietetic Association. *Journal of the American Dietetic Association* 88:44–48.

Romieu, I., W.C. Willett, M.J. Stampfer, G.A. Colditz, L. Sampson, B. Rosner, C.H. Hennekens, and F.E. Speizer. 1988. Energy intake and other determinants of relative weight. *American Journal of Clinical Nutrition* 47:406–412.

Rosenblatt, E. 1988. Weight-loss programs. *Postgraduate Medicine* 83(no. 6):137–148.

Schiffman, S.S. 1986. Recent findings about taste: Important implications. *Cereal Foods World* 31:300–302.

Sidney, S., G.D. Friedman, and A.B. Siegelaub. 1987. Thinness and mortality. *American Journal of Public Health* 77(no. 3):317–322.

Silverstein, B., B. Peterson, and L. Perdue. 1986. Some correlates of the thin standard of bodily attractiveness for women. *International Journal of Eating Disorders* 5:895–905.

Sims, E.A. 1988. Exercise and energy balance in the control of obesity and hypertension. In *Exercise, nutrition, and energy metabolism,* eds. E.S. Horton and R.L. Terjung. New York: Macmillan.

Sims, E.A., E. Danforth, Jr., E.S. Horton, G.A. Bray, J.A. Glennon, and L.B. Salans. 1973. Endocrine and metabolic effects of experimental obesity in man. *Recent Progress in Hormone Research* 29:457–487.

Steen, S.N., R.A. Oppliger, and K.D. Brownell. 1988. Metabolic effects of repeated weight loss and regain in adolescent wrestlers. *Journal of the American Medical Association* 260:47–50.

Stern, J.S. and P. Lowney. 1986. Obesity: The role of physical activity. In *Handbook of eating disorders,* eds. K.D. Brownell and J.P. Foreyt. New York: Basic Books, Inc.

Stunkard, A.J. 1988. Some perspectives on human obesity: Its causes. *Bulletin of the New York Academy of Medicine* 64(no. 8):902–923.

Stunkard, A.J., T.I. Sorensen, C. Hanis, T.W. Teasdale, R. Chakraborty, W.J. Schull, and F. Schulsinger. 1986. An adoption study of human obesity. *New England Journal of Medicine* 314:193–198.

Sullivan, A.C., C. Nauss-Karol, S. Hogan, and J. Triscari. 1988. Pharmacological modification of appetite. In *Control of appetite*, ed. M. Winick. New York: John Wiley & Sons, Inc.

Surgeon General. 1988. *Surgeon General's report on nutrition and health*. Washington, DC: Department of Health and Human Services.

Taylor, J.L., E.R. Buskirk, J. Brozek, J.R. Anderson, and F. Grande. 1957. Performance capacity and effects of caloric restriction with hard physical work on young men. *Journal of Applied Physiology* 10(no. 3):421–429.

Van Dale, D. and W.H. Saris. 1989. Repetitive weight loss and weight regain: Effects on weight reduction, resting metabolic rate, and lipolytic activity before and after exercise and/or diet treatment. *American Journal of Clinical Nutrition* 49:409–416.

Van Itallie, T.B. and H.R. Kissileff. 1985. Physiology of energy intake: An inventory control model. *American Journal of Clinical Nutrition* 42:914–923.

Vasselli, J.R. and C.A. Maggio. 1988. Mechanisms of appetite and body-weight regulation. In *Obesity and weight control*, eds. R.T. Frankle and M-U. Yang. Rockville, MD: Aspen Publishers, Inc.

Wadden, T.A., T.B. Van Itallie, and G.L. Blackburn. 1990. Responsible and irresponsible use of very-low-calorie diets in the treatment of obesity. *Journal of the American Medical Association* 263:83–85.

Williams, M.H. 1985. *Nutritional aspects of human physical and athletic performance*. Springfield, IL: Charles C. Thomas.

Wurtman, R.J. 1988. Neurotransmitters, control of appetite, and obesity. In *Control of appetite*, ed. M. Winick. New York: John Wiley & Sons, Inc.

Yang, M-U. 1988. Composition and resting metabolic rate in obesity. In *Obesity and weight control*, eds. R.T. Frankle and M-U. Yang. Rockville, MD: Aspen Publishers, Inc.

11

Eating Disorders

In This Chapter

- Eating Disorders Are Difficult to Classify
- Biological, Personal/ Familial, and Societal Factors Have Been Blamed for the Eating Disorders
- There Are Various Treatment Alternatives
- Check for Signs of Disordered Eating

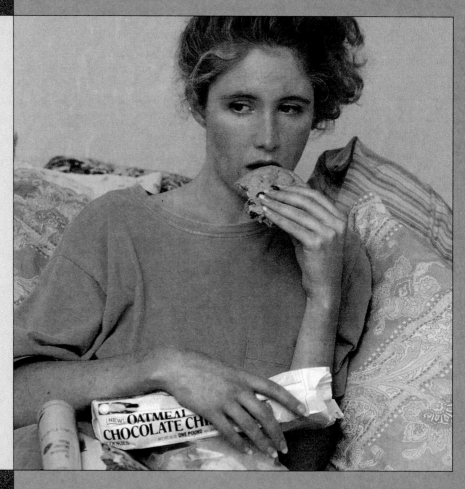

Y ou may already know something about *anorexia nervosa* and *bulimia nervosa* (or simply *bulimia*, as it is often still called in the popular media). These conditions involve abnormal food intake patterns called **eating disorders,** because people who have them misuse the eating function: they may deliberately starve themselves, or they may binge on huge amounts of food and then purge it from their bodies, or they may alternate between these behaviors.

It is not customary to devote much attention to these conditions in an introductory nutrition text, because they are *not primarily nutrition problems.* They are mainly *psychological problems* in which a person has very poor self-esteem and a sense of paralyzing ineffectiveness. Initially, severe dietary restriction provides a sense of self-control and mastery. But since the diet doesn't solve the underlying problems, either the person continues to restrict food intake and lose weight; or the person diets until the urge to eat is overwhelming, then binges, and then repeats the cycle.

In either event, eating disorders often bring about nutritional difficulties and serious health problems. Eating disorders are now well recognized and widespread, affecting some people in almost all of the developed countries. They are most prominent during the adolescent years and the 20s. For these reasons, we believe that eating disorders warrant attention in a college-level nutrition text.

Note that, from time to time, we probably all misuse eating to some degree. For example, if we occasionally eat excessive amounts of food (on Thanksgiving or some other occasion) or eat very little on other days (for instance, on the day after a holiday), this is not indicative of an eating disorder. Eating disorders involve *frequent, extreme eating disturbances that attempt to solve psychological problems*—not occasional, voluntary feasting or fasting. We want to help people understand the difference.

It is important to realize that eating disorders are serious conditions that require treatment: some people die because of them. Many other people find their lives extremely limited by their obsession with food. However, if treated by qualified professionals (who often work as a team), people with eating disorders usually improve. Since the likelihood of recovery is better when the condition is treated early, if you suspect an eating disorder in yourself or somebody else, you should share your concerns with a qualified professional without delay. That person can help decide whether treatment is needed and can direct you or your friend or family member to appropriate help.

Unfortunately, eating disorders often are not recognized early. This stems in part from the fact that our current cultural ideal of a slender appearance, especially for women, reinforces disordered eating behaviors. Therefore, the early signs of eating disorders often invoke an ambivalent response from society (Gordon, 1988), which may interfere with initiating treatment when it could be most helpful.

eating disorder—condition in which a person's food intake deviates markedly from normal intake in an attempt to solve psychological problems

Eating Disorders Are Difficult to Classify

Anorexia nervosa is not a new condition. It was recognized in the late 1800s and may even share some features with the religious fasting of the Middle Ages (Brumberg, 1988). However, intense concern about it and related conditions has developed mainly in the last two decades. Since these disorders have come under scrutiny relatively recently, much remains to be learned about their causes, distinctions, and most effective treatment.

The American Psychiatric Association has taken the lead in trying to standardize terminology and characterize these conditions in the *Diagnostic and Statistical Manual of Mental Disorders, Third Edition–Revised,* usually referred to as the *DSM-III-R* (1987). Tables 11.1 and 11.2 give the diagnostic criteria for **anorexia nervosa** and **bulimia nervosa**.

Because of the many similarities between the two conditions, there is debate among the experts as to whether these are distinct and separate disorders; but, since the typical course of these disorders and the foci of their current treatment are different, it has been practical to regard them as two separate entities (Hsu, 1988a).

anorexia nervosa—an eating disorder in which self-starvation and low body weight are prominent characteristics

bulimia nervosa—an eating disorder in which binging and purging (or other compensatory mechanisms) are prominent characteristics

Table 11.1 Diagnostic Criteria for Anorexia Nervosa

A. Refusal to maintain body weight over a minimal normal weight for age and height, e.g., weight loss leading to maintenance of body weight 15% below that expected; or failure to make expected weight gain during period of growth, leading to body weight 15% below that expected.

B. Intense fear of gaining weight or becoming fat, even though underweight.

C. Disturbance in the way in which one's body weight, size, or shape is experienced, e.g., the person claims to "feel fat" even when emaciated, believes that one area of the body is "too fat" even when obviously underweight.

D. In females, absence of at least three consecutive menstrual cycles when otherwise expected to occur (primary or secondary amenorrhea). (A woman is considered to have amenorrhea if her periods occur only following hormone, e.g., estrogen, administration.)

(From *DSM-III-R,* 1987)

Table 11.2 Diagnostic Criteria for Bulimia Nervosa

A. Recurrent episodes of binge eating (rapid consumption of a large amount of food in a discrete period of time).

B. A feeling of lack of control over eating behavior during the eating binges.

C. The person regularly engages in either self-induced vomiting, use of laxatives or diuretics, strict dieting or fasting, or vigorous exercise in order to prevent weight gain.

D. A minimum average of two binge eating episodes a week for at least three months.

E. Persistent overconcern with body shape and weight.

(From *DSM-III-R,* 1987)

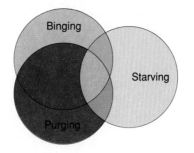

Figure 11.1 Overlap of eating disorders. Binging, purging, and starving are evidence of disordered eating. An affected person may practice just one, two, or all three of these behaviors.

People with both disorders share a phobic fear of fatness and relentless pursuit of thinness; both are done in an attempt to lose weight. Both are characterized by eating behaviors that are clearly outside the norm. Both conditions primarily afflict women, although men are not exempt from either one. In neither disorder is there any physical illness that can account for these attitudes or behaviors.

The most obvious difference between people with these disorders is body weight; people with anorexia nervosa, by definition, have dropped to 85% or less of the average weight for their height, whereas people with bulimia nervosa are more difficult to typify. Many bulimics have experienced large weight swings, and may be below, at, or above recommended weight for their height (Gardner and Fairburn, 1988). There are also some behavioral differences; in anorexia nervosa, more food restriction takes place, and in bulimia nervosa there is more uncontrollable binging. Table 11.3 shows other similarities and differences.

It is apparent, then, that the characteristics of the two groups overlap considerably: almost half of the people diagnosed as having *anorexia nervosa* engage in periodic binging (usually followed by purging), and people who are diagnosed as having *bulimia nervosa* may diet as restrictively as anorexics (starvers) do, at least until the next binge begins. Figure 11.1 represents these overlaps. If it weren't for the differences in body weight, it sometimes would be difficult to distinguish the anorexic with bulimic episodes from the bulimic who periodically starves. Some people cross back and forth over diagnostic lines (Gardner and Fairburn, 1988).

It is inaccurate to think that anorexia nervosa and bulimia nervosa describe the full range of disordered eating behaviors. For example, these two conditions do not account for the person who binges often enough for the eating pattern to be regarded as disordered but who does not exhibit the other characteristics of bulimia nervosa. The *DSM-III-R* has a catch-all category that can accommodate such exceptions: "Eating Disorder Not Otherwise Specified" is simply defined as "disorders of eating that do not meet the criteria for a specific eating disorder." In other words, it is left to the judgment of the mental health worker whether a particular constellation of behaviors might be "disordered."

Some experts suggest that a disorder consisting mainly of frequent binging (without purging or some other compensatory behavior) should be called "bulimia," as distinguished from *bulimia nervosa* (Mitchell and Pyle,

1988). Such a person undoubtedly would become overweight if not obese; but not all cases of obesity should be regarded as eating disorders, since they clearly do not all involve frequent, uncontrollable overeating behaviors of psychological origin.

Because of the confusion that persists in the use of these terms, in this chapter we will describe the most common eating disorders in terms of the behaviors they involve.

Table 11.3 Possible Warning Signals for Anorexia Nervosa or Bulimia Nervosa

Category of Warning Signals	Anorexia Nervosa	Bulimia Nervosa
Eating and related behaviors	Kcaloric intake < 100 kcal/day	Binge eating > twice/week
	Kcalorie counting	Eating used as coping strategy
	Denial of hunger cues	Fasting or restrictive dieting
	Extreme physical activity	Feels lack of control over eating
	Fasting or restrictive dieting	Frequent meal skipping
	Feels controlled by food	Frequent sweets, starches, cravings
	Food avoidances or hoarding	Frequent thoughts about food
	Food seen as good or bad	Guilt after eating/secret eating
	Frequent meal skipping	Purging behavior
	Frequent thoughts about food	Regular alcohol use
		Wide variation in kcaloric intake
Body image and body satisfaction	Body image disturbance	Current or previous overweight
	Fear of weight gain	Fear of weight gain
	Previously overweight	Overconcern with weight/shape
	Thinness as valued goal	Thinness as valued goal
	Weight goal <85% expected weight	Unrealistic weight goal
Health status	Amenorrhea (≥3 months w/no menses)	Bloating/nausea/abdominal pain
	Bloating/nausea	Constipation
	Cold intolerance	Frequent weight fluctuations
	Constipation	Irregular menses (<21 days or >45 days)
	Weight ≤85% expected weight	
Personal functioning	Delayed psychosexual development	Depressed mental state
	Depressed mental state	Negative self-identity
	Individuation difficulties	Perfectionistic
	Negative self-identity	Poor coping with life events
	Perfectionistic	Recent withdrawal from friends
	Poor coping with life events	Substance use/early sexual activity
	Recent withdrawal from friends	
Environmental influences	Enmeshed or overinvolved family	Chaotic or uninvolved family
	Family history of obesity, eating disorder, or weight focus	Family history of obesity, eating disorder, weight or fitness focus
	Few close friends	High achievement expectations
	High achievement expectations	Participation in body-focused activity
	Participation in body-focused activity	

(Adapted from Adams, L.B. and M.B. Shafer. 1988. Early manifestations of eating disorders in adolescents: Defining those at risk. *Journal of Nutrition Education* 20:307–312.)

Bingers and Binger/Purgers

Of all the people who suffer from eating disorders, more of them binge and purge, as opposed to practicing any other type of maladaptive eating behavior.

By **binging,** we mean secretly consuming (or chewing and spitting out) large amounts of food within a couple of hours. The binge usually amounts to many thousands of kcalories and may total as much as 5000 to 20,000 kcalories in a single episode (Mitchell and Pyle, 1988). The food is usually very high in kcalories and easy to eat—the very kinds of foods that are likely to be scrupulously avoided at other times. Binging tends to take place late in the day, and the binger feels he or she can't stop voluntarily—quitting only when pain, sleep, or somebody else interrupts the eating. **Purging** is accomplished through vomiting or the use of laxatives or diuretics. Sometimes instead of purging, the person severely restricts kcalories for a time or exercises excessively. The age of onset of binging and purging is often between 17 and 20 years (Turnbull et al., 1989). In the Slice of Life on p. 364, Lindsey describes what her life was like as a binger/purger.

Many studies have been done to determine the prevalence of binging among high-school and college students, and they have yielded widely varied results. Many of the discrepancies occurred because the behaviors being measured were somewhat different from study to study: standards often varied regarding what constituted a binge or how often the person binged.

A thorough study of an incoming freshman class at an elite private university showed how different the data can be, depending on how the behavior was defined. When asked whether they had practiced binging, 43% of the women and 17% of the men indicated that they had; but when evaluated according to the psychiatric manual's criteria for bulimia nervosa, only 3.8% of the women and 0.2% of the men were found to fit the criteria (Striegel-Moore et al., 1989). There have been similar findings in other studies (Gray and Gray, 1989).

While many people binge periodically, the cases serious enough to be classified as eating disorders are a small proportion of the total. Canadian experts estimate an incidence of bulimia nervosa of 2–3% in females aged 15 to 40, with one male case for every 10 female cases (Woodside and Garfinkel, 1989).

The great majority of binger/purgers are within a normal weight range for their height; usually only about 10% are overweight or obese. Nonetheless, even those of normal weight usually regard themselves as overweight, and many have overfatness in their families. The disorder ordinarily begins during adolescence or early adulthood, usually after a period of dieting.

Physicians and mental health workers who treat binger/purgers note that they often feel inadequate and may feel anxious, angry, and guilty as well. Whatever their weight, they regard themselves as too fat, which is a source of low self-esteem (Mizes, 1988). They frequently alternate between self-restraint and impulsive behavior, and they feel depressed and of particularly low self-worth after a binge. They tend to feel dominated by food and frus-

binging (in the context of eating disorders)—secretly consuming large amounts of high-kcalorie foods in a short time, often stopping only when interrupted by pain, sleep, or another person

purging (in the context of eating disorders)—intentionally clearing food out of the system by vomiting and/or using laxatives and/or diuretics

trated by the control it has over them, generally recognizing that their eating pattern is abnormal.

Besides the emotional chaos experienced by the binger/purger, physical problems can also be created by attempts to compensate for binging. Vomiting, for example, can result in tooth decay from frequent contact with acidic stomach contents. It may also lead to a sore throat and mouth, nasal congestion, electrolyte problems, dehydration, muscle weakness, and menstrual

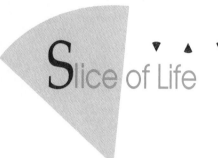

Slice of Life

Life As a Binger/Purger

(From Hall, L. and L. Cohn. 1986. *Bulimia: A guide to recovery.* Santa Barbara: Gurze Books.)

■ Lindsey

. . . I left [for college] in a blatant show of independence and bravery. Once alone in my dorm room, however, I was faced with the isolation and the hateful relationship I had with my Self. I retreated into eating which I knew would numb my anxiety, and I perfected the act of throwing up.

I learned which foods would come back up easily. When I woke in the morning, I often stuffed myself for half an hour and threw up before class. . . . I always thought people noticed when I took huge portions at mealtimes, but I figured they assumed that I was an athlete and burned it off. Sometimes one meal did not satisfy the cravings, and I began to buy food. I always vowed that "this binge will be the last" and that I would magically and with ease metamorphose into a normal human being as soon as I threw up "this last time." I could eat a whole bag of cookies, half a dozen candy bars, and a quart of milk *on top of* a huge meal. Once a binge was under way, I did not stop until my stomach looked pregnant and I felt like I could not swallow one more time.

■ Allison

Allison ignored the instructions on the label of the bottle of laxative and shook the pills out into her hand. Two, four, five . . . that should do it. She popped them into her mouth and swallowed them with a few gulps from a half-finished can of cola.

She felt awful—bloated, fat, and tired—from all she had eaten in the past hour. She hoped that the huge dose of laxative would relieve her of her discomfort before long. Furthermore, she thought the pills would prevent her from "getting fat."

Allison's hopes were largely in vain.

Laxatives hasten emptying of the colon and promote an increased loss of fluid, which results in a temporary feeling of being lighter. But most laxatives do not hurry the passage of food through the small intestine, where digestion and most absorption of energy nutrients take place. As a result, laxatives do not prevent a person from getting most of the kcalories he or she would get from food without the laxative; taking laxatives after overeating does not prevent fat gain from the excess kcalories.

Laxatives, if used repeatedly, can have a very negative consequence: the bowel can actually become dependent on them for functioning. It is unwise to use laxatives routinely, although people in certain circumstances—such as those who are bedridden or quite elderly—may need periodic help from laxatives to relieve constipation. ▲

disturbances. Sometimes people with bulimia nervosa use laxatives in an attempt to prevent their bodies from digesting and absorbing the excesses they consumed. This does not work, as Allison's experience in the Slice of Life on p. 364 explains. Others use diuretics to promote fluid loss and thereby temporarily reduce body weight.

Such pharmacological abuse is dangerous. In addition to problems such as dehydration, electrolyte imbalances, and muscle weakness, the use of diuretics and laxatives can lead to irregular heartbeat, laxative dependence, and rectal bleeding. Because of the electrolyte and water losses that these drugs cause, a binger/purger's weight can easily fluctuate by 10 pounds within a couple of days. At such times, body weight cannot offer a clue as to whether any changes in body fat may have occurred.

Some metabolic studies note a depressed RMR in people with severe binging and purging practices as compared with normal controls; however, these are correlational studies and cannot prove whether one condition caused the other (Bennett et al., 1989; Gwirtsman et al., 1989).

The worst possible outcome of bulimia nervosa is death. Electrolyte imbalances could be the cause, especially if potassium deficiency results in heart failure. Occasionally, death occurs from irreparable rupture of the stomach due to its having been stretched beyond its limit.

Starvers

The typical individual who deliberately self-starves has often been characterized as an upper-middle- or middle-class teenage female; however, in the last 15 years, this social class distribution seems to have disappeared (Woodside and Garfinkel, 1989). It is possible that this reflects an increase in access to treatment by all classes of people (Leichner and Gertler, 1988). The incidence of self-starving is estimated to be approximately 1% among females between the ages of 15 and 40; males in that age range experience the condition only $\frac{1}{20}$ as often (Woodside and Garfinkel, 1989). The age of onset of **starving** behaviors ranges from the early teens through the early 20s and is generally identified sooner than binging and purging (Tufts, 1989).

As young children, most starvers were cooperative, thoughtful, obedient, and eager for praise. Among their peers, starvers tend to be highly competitive, achievement-oriented, and perfectionistic. They are often serious and not very spontaneous (Lucas and Huse, 1988); they tend to be out of touch with their emotions.

In their pursuit of thinness, starvers reduce their food intake drastically, often to just a few hundred kcalories per day. Laura, in the Slice of Life on p. 366, serves as an example.

Starvers misinterpret many messages their bodies try to give them regarding hunger, temperature, pain, and fatigue. For example, when they feel the sensation that a healthy person would recognize as hunger, they do not believe it is caused by *needing* something to eat; rather, they might believe that they have a stomach ache from *having eaten* a few carrot sticks

starving (in the context of eating disorders)—deliberately restricting total food intake to drastically low levels

many hours before. Alternatively, they may experience the physiological sensations of hunger but choose not to respond to the messages; they often derive substitute satisfaction from knowing how much self-control they have exercised.

Eventually, starvers lose so much weight that they experience biochemical and hormonal changes. Their body functions slow down: the gastrointestinal tract works more slowly, resulting in constipation; often there is abdominal pain and a sense of fullness (Lucas and Huse, 1988). BMR goes down, as do blood pressure and pulse, commonly resulting in cold, blue hands and feet; menstruation ceases. A fine body hair (lanugo) often appears, and the complexion becomes sallow. A starver may experience dehydration, decreased kidney function, and dizziness; further, she may develop osteoporosis and abnormalities in heart function.

Most of the physical consequences are reversible if the starver undergoes nutritional rehabilitation (Woodside and Garfinkel, 1989). If there is no intervention and the condition worsens, the most serious possible consequence of prolonged starvation is death.

Slice of Life

A Starver's Diet

(From Stein, P.M. and B.C. Unell. 1986. *Anorexia nervosa: Finding the life line.* Minneapolis: CompCare Publications.)

■ Laura

I ate the same thing every day for six weeks at a time—300 kcalories a day. I'd have tea for breakfast, with artificial sweetener, and lettuce with a few green beans for lunch. I'd wash the beans so there would be no trace of salt on them; I didn't want to retain any liquid. For dinner I'd have two ounces of broiled meat, squeezed until it was like paper to get rid of the grease, and maybe a couple of bites of lettuce.

I couldn't eat in front of people and never ate with the family. I had to have my own food by myself so I could pick at it. If we went out, sometimes I could eat a lettuce salad, but that was all. If I didn't have *my* food, I wouldn't eat.

■ Joe

My parents were divorced when I was ten years old. . . . I was pretty crushed about the divorce, . . . but [after my mother remarried] I grew to feel that my stepbrothers and stepsisters were my actual family. There was a closeness, even though no one in our family shows much emotion. Because we didn't let our emotions show, when I would have a "big" emotion, I hadn't learned what to do with it.

I was twenty years old and a student when my relationship with a girlfriend ended. I was devastated. I became severely depressed and was suicidal during the year after this happened. The breakup happened in the spring, and I was so immobilized that I couldn't go back to school the next fall.

I started eating less and less because I was so depressed. The more weight I lost, the more obsessed I became. I was living with my mother and stepfather and brothers and sisters and would do the meal planning and preparation to help my mom. I was completely preoccupied with food. In looking back, it seems to me I was a typical, textbook anorexic. ▲

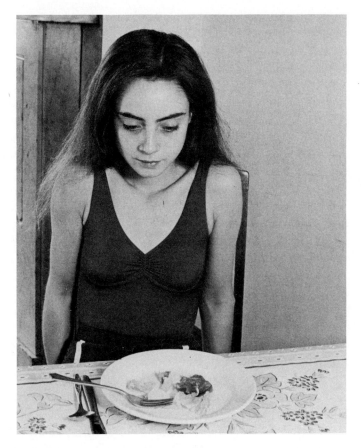

A starver. A person with a starving eating disorder limits her energy intake to very low levels, although she often pushes herself to do physically demanding solitary athletic activities. Thoughts about eating and not eating occupy a large part of her time. Approximately half of the people who are starvers also alternately binge and purge.

While all of this is happening, the starver denies that anything is wrong; in fact, she often maintains that she is still overfat and ought to lose more weight. She takes great satisfaction in her incredible self-control:

> I had started other projects in the past and then dropped them when I couldn't do them perfectly. I was so proud of myself and on a "high" because I had finally found something I could do better than anyone else. Everyone I knew complained of failing to lose weight on diets. My doctor later said he didn't know how I had mustered the energy to take care of the house, the kids, and my husband on so little nutrition.
>
> I was oversensitive to touch, cold, noise. I lost lots of hair and my periods stopped. But this was "my thing," and I didn't notice the destruction because I was totally wrapped up in it. I had no friends at all. Losing weight was the focus of my entire world. (From Stein, P.M. and B.C. Unell. 1986. *Anorexia nervosa: Finding the life line.* Minneapolis: CompCare Publications.)

If she is a student, she may study harder than ever but get less done (Sibley and Blinder, 1988). At least in the earlier stages of the disorder, she is likely to drive herself to perform demanding physical activities despite her low energy intake. Eventually, the starver experiences a substantial decrease in aerobic capacity (Einerson et al., 1988), which limits physical endurance.

Even with the excessive physical activity, sleep disorders are common (Lucas and Huse, 1988). She avoids eating most foods, even though she is frantically preoccupied with food and eating, and she often deliberately puts herself in proximity to food by cooking for other people (Sibley and Blinder, 1988). Gradually, she becomes more socially isolated.

Because starving occurs so much more often in females than in males, we have frequently referred to "she" or "her" in describing the starver above. Some men do experience the disorder, however, as Joe testifies in the Slice of Life on p. 366. Experts hypothesize that the lower incidence of eating disorders in males may occur because they received less social pressure to be thin; therefore, males who develop eating disorders may have stronger *internal* incentives for doing so (Andersen, 1988).

Because starvers sometimes join athletic teams to support their determination to exercise hard and regularly, it is important for coaches and trainers to educate themselves about this disorder (Smith and Worthington-Roberts, 1989). The classic activities to which people with starving tendencies are drawn are gymnastics, distance running, swimming, ballet and other types of dancing, rowing, and bicycling, but starvers may be attracted to many other activities as well. A perceptive coach or trainer should recognize a person who is vehement about weight loss and overzealous about exercise and see that he or she undergoes evaluation for an eating disorder.

Not every instance of excessive weight loss among athletes is indicative of a true eating disorder having a psychiatric component; an athlete's weight loss might be a temporary reaction to the extreme pressure athletes undergo to maintain a certain competitive weight. Nonetheless, the athlete should be evaluated and, if there is no eating disorder, should receive nutrition counseling and follow-up monitoring for appropriate food intake. It is a good idea to have someone other than the coach responsible for supervising the weight control of athletes (Smith, 1980).

Although not athletic in nature, another activity that is associated with an unusually high incidence of self-starving is modeling. Unfortunately, some people who train and manage female models reinforce such eating behaviors by encouraging weight loss or maintenance of unnaturally low body weight.

Models reflect the attitudes of society about what amount of body fatness is thought to be beautiful. As was discussed in Chapter 10, current societal standards for women in the U.S. seem too low to be consistent with good health.

Combined Starver/Binger/Purger

> Every morning at 6:30 without fail, I would lie in bed planning exactly what I would and would not eat that day, and every night I would lie there and count up the calories of that meagre supply. In short, I was obsessed with food.
>
> During the week I purged myself, starving myself, dreading the weekend ahead when I knew very well I was likely to go on a binge, eating all in sight, shoveling it in, to make up for what I had deprived myself of in the week. The guilt that followed these binges was unbearable. It made me lose any confidence I

might have had in myself and in my strict self-discipline which seemed all important. . . .

My periods had been non-existent for a good two years; my hair was falling
out; I had constant indigestion; I looked like a bag of bones and desperately
needed help. (From Crisp, A. H. 1980. *Anorexia nervosa: Let me be.* London: Academic Press.)

As we mentioned earlier, approximately half of the people diagnosed as
having anorexia nervosa practice some binging and purging, and many people diagnosed as having bulimia nervosa periodically self-starve. These two
groups resemble each other quite closely, except for body weight. Here, we
consider them together as one group.

People who self-starve, binge, and purge tend to be somewhat more able
to acknowledge and express their emotions than starvers, although they still
have considerable difficulty in this regard. They seek out more involvement
with others than starvers do but remain somewhat socially isolated. Mental
health workers note that they tend to be more impulsive and are more likely
to engage in socially unacceptable behaviors such as stealing. They are also
more prone to use alcohol and other drugs than starvers are. As you would
suspect, the physical problems that starver/binger/purgers develop can include the consequences of both sets of behaviors, as discussed earlier.

We must also acknowledge that the change from one set of disordered
behaviors to another can also take place within a much longer time frame
than the week mentioned above. A person who has been primarily a starver
for months or years might at some later time practice binging and purging as
her dominant pattern (or vice versa), thereby crossing diagnostic boundaries
(Chaitin, 1988). With such behavior changes, the affected person might experience weight changes of 50 pounds or more.

Because eating (or not eating) is prompted by strong *psychological* factors,
her *physiological* cues regarding hunger and satiety are largely denied; she
has become very practiced in overriding them. Similarly, as she moves
through various weight ranges, she has little residual sense of what a "normal" or "good functional weight" is for herself.

I used to believe that if I were thin, a man would like me and take me away
from all the chaos in my life. But that theory didn't work because I got too thin;
men don't like you too thin, either. The funny thing is: I can't remember being
in-between. I lost weight and then I gained weight. I can't remember ever thinking that whatever I weighed was the "right" weight. I never felt I was "there."
(From Stein, P.M. and B.C. Unell. 1986. *Anorexia nervosa: Finding the life line.* Minneapolis: CompCare Publications.)

Biological, Personal/Familial, and Societal Factors Have Been Blamed for the Eating Disorders

Nobody really knows why eating disorders develop, but there is no shortage
of theories. The factors thought to prompt them can be biological determi-

nants, personal development and family interactions, and societal pressures. Specific initiating incidents may also provoke disordered eating behaviors. While it is possible that one of these factors alone may be the cause, it is equally possible that complex chains of events interact to finally precipitate the illness (Hsu, 1988b).

Biological Determinants

The likelihood of developing an eating disorder may be increased by genetic factors. Studies of twins with eating disorders and chromosome studies suggest the possibility that a predisposition to eating disorders may exist (Scott, 1986). However, more research is needed on this subject.

Some experts propose that biochemical abnormalities may be responsible for eating disorders. There is no doubt that people with severe eating disorders (especially self-starving) exhibit abnormal levels of certain hormones and some neurotransmitters; but this may be an *effect rather than a cause* of inappropriate intakes (Newman and Halmi, 1988). Most of these abnormalities are relieved and finally disappear as the starver returns to normal weight (Woodside and Garfinkel, 1989).

An observation that appears to support the possibility of a biochemical cause, though, is that many female starvers stop menstruating (a hormonally controlled function) well before they have lost enough weight for malnutrition to be the sole cause. Since emotional disturbances of various types can cause hormonal changes, however, this also may be an *effect* of the eating disorder (Hsu, 1988b). Still, researchers have not ruled out the possibility that there may be a pre-existing central disturbance that is "unmasked" by abnormal eating.

Some scientists have suggested that there may be a parallel between substance addiction and the eating disorders. A psychiatrist points out that both substance abuse and eating disorders show elements of "dyscontrol" or "ill-control" of drives (Edelstein, 1989). Both may somehow stimulate the pleasure centers of the brain (Rusting, 1988). Some people with eating disorders have been treated successfully with medications used for treatment of substance abuse, but this does not prove that the conditions are of similar origin. Further, even if a connection is found, this does not prove a biochemical cause for the eating disorders; it is still debated whether substance abuse is due to genetic or environmental causes or to a combination of factors.

Personal Development and Family Interactions

Researchers have tried to characterize people with eating disorders and the families they are part of. Such studies do not all agree, but certain trends emerge, as this section will describe. Keep in mind that such studies simply show a correlation between eating disorders and certain personal and family characteristics; they do not prove that the characteristics *cause* the eating disorders.

Personal Development Hilde Bruch, a psychiatrist who was an early leader in the study and treatment of eating disorders, typified the eating-disordered person as feeling "a paralyzing sense of ineffectiveness." As children, they may have felt that they were the "property" of their parents and were treated as something to complement the parents' needs (Hsu, 1988b). When the stresses of the adolescent years and the prospect of separation from family (such as going away to college) confront such a teenager, she may perceive her body as the one domain over which she can exercise control and through which she can achieve a sense of self. This may be behind the relentless pursuit of thinness and may initiate the weight-loss dieting that commonly precedes an eating disorder.

Another interpretation of why the person wants to become thin is to maintain the look (and position in the family) of a preadolescent. By retreating into a child-like body, she can avoid the responsibilities associated with maturing (Crisp, 1988) or delay the challenge of coping with a world that seems to operate differently than her family (Tuft's University, 1989). Research has shown eating disturbances to be more common in college undergraduate women who have been less successful at separating emotionally from their parents, especially their mothers (Zakin, 1989).

Family Characteristics Many researchers and clinicians note that the families of people with eating disorders often have interpersonal problems—especially difficulties in the parents' marital relationship—that interfere with healthy family functioning. Some experts theorize that the person with the eating disorder recognizes that these problems exist and is worried that the family might break apart. The eating disorder provides a common concern for the parents and serves to unite them. Because of this perceived usefulness, the child works to maintain the disorder. Despite their problems, eating-disordered families avoid discussing feelings and conflicts between parents and children (Kog and Vandereycken, 1989). There also is more depression and other psychiatric illness in families with a member who has an eating disorder. The incidence of such illnesses is approximately three times as high in these families as it is among non-eating-disordered families (Strober and Katz, 1988).

Some factors distinguish the families of people with one type of eating disorder from those with another. The family of the starver appears to be a model unit at first glance, but there are usually problems beneath the surface. Open conflict is avoided, and the families tend to be so "enmeshed" that it is difficult for each member to develop an individual identity and feel in charge of his or her own behavior. (Interestingly, enmeshment has also been noted in families of obese adolescents [Brone and Fisher,1988].)

The parents in such families tend to be overprotective, overinvolved, and rigid. Parents tend to communicate a double message of nurturant affection combined with neglect of their daughter's need to express her feelings (Humphrey, 1989).

> During my childhood, everything was really rigid and planned. We had piano lessons Thursday, other lessons Sunday, and, of course, school. Instead of going out to play, we would work with our dad on math problems—not schoolwork, just exercises he had us do.
>
> The atmosphere at home was really strict, so there wasn't any real encouragement to socialize. My parents and my brothers were so close. I guess I felt ignored and wasn't sure if my parents loved me. I felt very intimidated by my father. (From Stein, P.M. and B.C. Unell. 1986. *Anorexia nervosa: Finding the life line.* Minneapolis: CompCare Publications.)

The family of the binger/purger, on the other hand, is more chaotic. Even though there is more conflict within the household, discussion of feelings is suppressed. The family is less cohesive than that of the starver; the parents can hardly be accused of being overinvolved or overprotective (Stern et al., 1989). Family members feel that their needs for emotional involvement and support go unmet, and they generally do not have good ways of dealing with tension. Furthermore, other family members often have emotional disorders (Chaitin, 1988); these are seen in the families of approximately half of binger/purgers (Turnbull et al., 1989). Family members may also practice antisocial behaviors such as substance abuse and sexual abuse (Wooley and Wooley, 1986).

It is interesting that the type of eating disorder a person develops seems in keeping with the personality of the family from which she came: the person from the family that restrains feelings and maintains external orderliness is the person that restrains her eating; the person from the family where chaos and acting-out behaviors are more common acts out in an extreme way in regard to her eating.

Many experts caution against making too much of the matter of family interactions; they doubt that these conditions *alone* could precipitate eating disorders, even if some causal connection is established (Sibley and Blinder, 1988; Stern et al., 1989). Also, the characterizations above are not true for all cases; there are many exceptions. A final important point is that research on families has invariably been done *after* the eating disorders have been diagnosed; therefore, the families have been living with these exasperating conditions for some time before being studied. It is possible that some of the abnormal behaviors seen in the families may be stress reactions to the presence of the eating disorders (Hsu, 1988b).

Societal Pressures

Society also plays a role in promoting eating disorders.

Contemporary American culture has idealized the *thin* female form. Chapter 10 discussed the fact that societal ideals for female body weight are below the natural weights many girls and women would maintain if they ate in response to physiological hunger and satiety signals. This pressure— intensified by their own desire to weigh less—prompts many females to diet

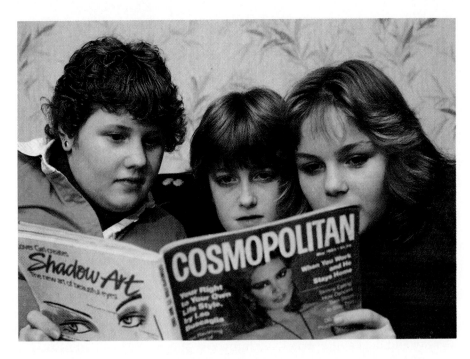

Social pressure and eating disorders. Some experts suggest that the current lean ideal, particularly for women, causes many people to continually attempt to restrict their energy intake even if their weight is acceptable from a health perspective. Such ongoing food denial may precede an eating disorder.

excessively. Because very severe dieting usually leads to overeating and weight regain, a person may attempt a more radical or prolonged regimen in the future. In some people, this may lead to an eating disorder.

Not only does society regard the thin female form as most attractive, but it has also given it connotations of strength, independence, and achievement. This attitude parallels changes taking place in our society, in which adolescent women are now being told that they must prepare for responsible careers, land important jobs, be self-reliant, maintain a love relationship, be a parent, manage a household, and stay in fashion. The pressure to be outstanding in so many diverse roles can be tremendous. One expert notes, "It is quite obvious that the conflict between so many irreconcilable demands on her time . . . exposes the modern woman to a terrible social ordeal" (Palazzoli, 1978).

Not only does the modern young woman feel conflict in regard to time use; she also feels conflict in defining her gender. The current societal expectation to be highly successful in a challenging career may seem to be a "masculine" ideal, which may be difficult to integrate into a feminine self-image (Hsu, 1988b). This role diffusion presumably increases her insecurity; this may heighten her striving for self-control and may encourage her attempt to severely restrict her eating.

Initiating Incidents

Clinicians who treat people with eating disorders find that their patients often connect specific kinds of incidents with the triggering of their bizarre food habits. Sometimes it is unkind remarks about their bodies—whether or not they are accurate—that the person remembers as provoking the disordered eating behaviors.

One person remembers it: "I remember the day I started my diet, the diet that led me down the anorexia road. I asked my husband, 'Don't you think I'm too heavy?' He replied, 'Yeah, you *are* getting big in the rear end.' I can tell you the exact day and the year. I was bound and determined to get that weight off" (Stein and Unell, 1986). Such experiences, played against a backdrop of developmental difficulties, unhealthy family relationships, and societal demands, may together set the stage for an eating disorder.

There Are Various Treatment Alternatives

Experts have developed several approaches to treatment, based on research and their experience in dealing with eating disorders. The objectives of such programs are to help people with eating disorders learn to eat appropriately in response to hunger and satiety signals and to take proper steps toward doing what they want to accomplish in life. They also need to learn how to identify and deal appropriately with their emotions in a way that is socially acceptable and physically and psychologically healthy.

Often, treatment can be accomplished on an outpatient basis. A multidisciplinary team consisting of professionals who have specialized in treating people with eating disorders appears to provide the most effective treatment (American Dietetic Association, 1988). The team is likely to be made up of several of the following: a physician, a dietitian, a mental health worker, and/or a nurse-practitioner or nurse.

The treatment varies, depending on the nature of the eating behaviors. Typical current therapies are described below.

Treatment for Disorders That Include Starving

Some clinics treat only the starver; others believe the whole family should be involved, especially when the person with the disorder is quite young and will be living in the household for some time to come. Many treatment teams use both approaches together. A helpful focus of family therapy is developing a balance between the need for autonomy and the need for supportive relationships (Sargent and Liebman, 1988).

Treatment for starvers involves nutritional rehabilitation, resolution of the disturbed pattern of family interaction, and individual psychotherapeutic help. It is important that the starvation state be corrected early in treatment because a starving person is often not receptive to psychotherapy and may not be able to think clearly (Garner, 1985). At the same time that it works toward restoration of physical status, nutritional rehabilitation benefits the psychological state, thereby improving chances for recovery of other aspects of mental health.

Note that it is not enough that the person achieve a normal body weight; without adequate psychotherapy, the disorder will resume as soon as treatment is discontinued. Similarly, psychotherapy alone is not an effective treatment. Drugs may be prescribed, although they are thought to have a limited role (Tolstoi, 1989).

How successful is treatment? We'll give you the worst news first: studies show that approximately 6% of patients who practiced self-starving were so resistant to treatment that they died of their disorder. On a more positive note, approximately three-fourths of the patients had more acceptable body weights at follow-up than when they entered treatment. Between half and three-fourths resumed menstruation, although menstrual irregularity was common. Many patients continued to have eating problems and/or psychiatric difficulties to some degree, but approximately 90% were able to maintain full-time employment (Lucas and Huse, 1988).

The long-term health effects are not clear. Some researchers believe that former starvers, even though recovered, may be more prone to developing osteoporosis because their poor food intakes and low estrogen (female hormone) levels resulted in less-than-normal bone mass (Chapter 13 discusses osteoporosis more fully). Researchers will monitor whether people with new cases of osteoporosis (especially younger women) have a history of eating disorders. A former patient reflects on what her treatment did for her:

> After fourteen weeks' hospitalization on a strict regimen, bed rest, and family therapy, I am now 28 pounds heavier, happy most of the time, and most important of all I understand myself far better than I ever have done. I can't say I know

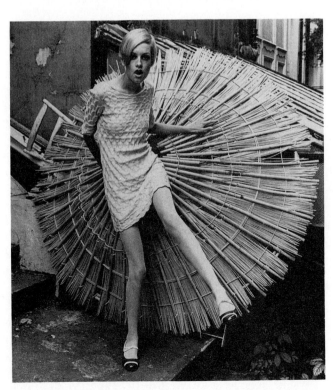

Coming soon . . . the long-term health effects of eating disorders. In the 1960s, adolescent girls tried to get as thin as Twiggy, the most recognized model of the decade. In their quest, some developed eating disorders. Even though they were subsequently "cured," we do not know whether there are lingering ill effects. We will find out as the teenage girls of the 1960s become middle-aged women in the 1990s.

myself perfectly yet, but being able to answer for my actions and emotions is a much more positive way of going through life than denying my mind and my body.

At last, as well as others valuing my own worth, I do too. I intend to respect both my body and my mind from now on. (From Crisp, A. H. 1980. *Anorexia nervosa: Let me be.* London: Academic Press.)

Treatment for Disorders That Include Binging/Purging

There are also varying approaches to treatment for binging/purging. Except in the most severe cases, this disorder is generally treated on an outpatient basis. Group therapy is sometimes used with good result; because binger/ purgers are generally more spontaneous, outgoing, and socially adept, they are more likely to form functional groups than are starvers (Dixon, 1988).

Treatment may include various medications; antidepressants are often prescribed. Generally speaking, pharmacological agents have been found to be more helpful for binger/purgers than for starvers (Walsh, 1988). Psycho-therapy and behavior modification may also be used. A few patients re-spond to a minimal intervention such as several educational group sessions, consultation with a dietitian or nutritionist, and support to cope with any weight change that may occur (Woodside and Garfinkel, 1989).

There are not yet enough data available on the outcome of treatment of binging/purging for us to give them here. It is apparent for all types of eating disorders, however, that the sooner a person seeks treatment, the better the chances are for a more complete recovery.

Check for Signs of Disordered Eating

How can a person know whether she or he has an eating disorder? This section offers some guidance. But note: *we do not intend that you should diagnose eating disorders in yourself or others.* Only experienced clinicians should assume that responsibility.

In order to know whether to seek evaluation, it is important to have some kind of self-screening technique. These questions may be helpful:

- Is your usual daily kcaloric intake roughly equivalent to your energy output? If there is a difference of more than 1000 kcalories between what you eat and the energy you expend in a typical day, the answer is "no."
- Do you fear that once you start to eat foods that you enjoy, you will not be able to stop eating?
- Do you hoard or hide food?
- Does it take you more than half an hour to eat a meal or snack when you are eating alone and are not involved in another activity at the same time?
- Do you have any health problems that can be linked to your eating practices, such as absence of menstruation or low body weight?
- Does eating or the anticipation of eating create strong negative feelings in you, such as dread or disgust? Does the sight of others eating a normal meal create feelings of disgust?

If you answered "no" to the first question or "yes" to any of the others, it may be reasonable to consider professional evaluation. Remember, *these questions are not diagnostic criteria for eating disorders;* they are simply designed to help you make a preliminary distinction between normal and abnormal eating behaviors. Surely, a "wrong answer" to one of the above questions does not mean that a person has a disorder, but a few such answers would make the matter worth checking.

This chapter's Nutrition for Living section suggests sources of help if you think you may have an eating disorder.

Sometimes friends of people with eating disorders suspect the problem, recognize that it is a serious matter, and want to help. The best help friends can give is to urge the affected person to get treatment: confront her or him with your concern.

Be forewarned that if she or he is a starver, your friend may deny the problem. Quite likely, she will be proud of her behavior and might even think that you are jealous of her. On the other hand, people who binge and purge know that their behavior is abnormal, but they are likely to deny their disorder or get angry because they are acutely embarrassed about it. An alternative is to contact a residence hall staff member, the student health service, or the dean of students' office about your friend. On many college campuses, these people are prepared to intervene, evaluate the situation, and help people get into treatment if necessary.

Whether it is you or a friend that is involved, remember that early treatment brings the greatest likelihood of success.

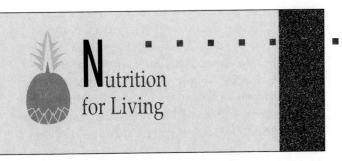

Nutrition for Living

Getting Help When You Need It

If you think you have an eating disorder, *get specialized treatment now.* We cannot help you here, nor are most doctors trained to deal with such conditions.

If you don't know of a local expert or treatment facility, ask for a referral from your general physician or a staff member of your university health center. An alternative is to contact one of the organizations that maintains lists of people and places offering specialized treatment; they can tell you what is available in your area. One organization we have found to be responsive to inquiries is:

■ American Anorexia/Bulimia Association, Inc. (AABA)
418 East 76th Street
New York, NY 10021

If you need help, get it. Don't delay.

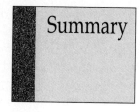

Summary

▶ **Eating disorders** that involve **starving, binging,** and/or **purging** are not primarily *nutrition* problems but *psychological* ones. It is important to understand that everyone occasionally under- or overeats but that people who have eating disorders do so *frequently* and *drastically*. These disorders are serious conditions and require professional treatment.

▶ Two of the more common eating disorders are **anorexia nervosa** (in which starving and low body weight are prominent characteristics) and **bulimia nervosa** (in which binging and purging dominate). However, there is much overlap between their characteristics. Some people alternately starve and binge and purge.

▶ The various types of eating disorders have potential negative physical consequences including tooth decay; dehydration; menstrual disturbance; electrolyte imbalance; inability to correctly interpret the body's messages about hunger, pain, and fatigue; and—in the most extreme cases—death.

▶ Biological determinants, personal development and family interactions, and societal pressures have all been blamed for the eating disorders, but no one really knows why they develop. Some clinicians have found that their patients connect specific incidents with the triggering of their abnormal eating habits. It seems likely that the cause of these disorders is multifactorial.

▶ True eating disorders need specialized professional treatment. You should not attempt to diagnose an eating disorder in yourself or anyone else, but if you suspect abnormal eating behavior, seek professional evaluation immediately; earlier treatment is more likely to be successful. Most people who are treated for eating disorders do improve.

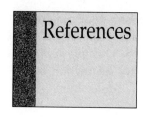

References

American Dietetic Association. 1988. Position of the American Dietetic Association: Nutrition intervention in the treatment of anorexia nervosa and bulimia nervosa. *Journal of the American Dietetic Association* 88:68–71.

American Psychiatric Association. 1987. *Diagnostic and statistical manual of mental disorders. Third edition–revised (DSM-III-R).* Washington, DC: The American Psychiatric Association.

Anderson, A.E. 1988. Anorexia nervosa and bulimia nervosa in males. In *Diagnostic issues in anorexia nervosa and bulimia nervosa,* eds. D.M. Garner and P.E. Garfinkel. New York: Brunner/Mazel, Publishers.

Bennett, S.M., D.A. Williamson, and S.K. Powers. 1989. Bulimia nervosa and resting metabolic rate. *International Journal of Eating Disorders* 8:417–424.

Brone, R.J. and C.B. Fisher. 1988. Determinants of adolescent obesity: A comparison with anorexia nervosa. *Adolescence* 23:155–169.

Brumberg, J.J. 1988. *Fasting girls: The emergence of anorexia nervosa as a modern disease.* Cambridge: Harvard University Press.

Chaitin, B.F. 1988. The relationship of the eating and affective disorders. In *The eating disorders,* eds. B.J. Blinder, B.F. Chaitin, and R.S. Goldstein. New York: PMA Publishing Corp.

Crisp, A.H. 1988. Some possible approaches to prevention of eating and body weight/shape disorders, with particular reference to anorexia nervosa. *International Journal of Eating Disorders* 7:1–17.

Dixon, K.N. 1988. Group psychotherapy for anorexia nervosa and bulimia. 1988. In *The eating disorders,* eds. B.J. Blinder, B.F. Chaitin, and R.S. Goldstein. New York: PMA Publishing Corp.

Edelstein, E.L. 1989. *Anorexia nervosa and other dyscontrol syndromes.* London: Springer-Verlag.

Einerson, J., A. Ward, and P. Hanson. 1988. Exercise responses in females with anorexia nervosa. *International Journal of Eating Disorders* 7:253–260.

Garner, D.M. 1985. Iatrogenesis in anorexia nervosa and bulimia nervosa. *International Journal of Eating Disorders* 4:701–726.

Garner D.M. and C.G. Fairburn. 1988. Relationship between anorexia nervosa and bulimia nervosa: Diagnostic implications. In *Diagnostic issues in anorexia nervosa and bulimia nervosa*, eds. D.M. Garner and P.E. Garfinkel. New York: Brunner/Mazel, Publishers.

Gordon, R.A. 1988. Sociocultural interpretation of the current epidemic of eating disorders. In *The eating disorders: Medical and psychological bases of diagnosis and treatment*, eds. B.J. Blinder, B.F. Chaitin, and R.S. Goldstein. New York: PMA Publishing Corp.

Gray, G.E. and L.K. Gray. 1989. Nutritional aspects of psychiatric disorders. *Journal of the American Dietetic Association* 89:1492–1498.

Gwirtsman, H.E., W.H. Kaye, E. Obarzanek, D.T. George, D.C. Jimerson, and M.H. Ebert. 1989. Decreased caloric intake in normal-weight patients with bulimia: comparison with female volunteers. *American Journal of Clinical Nutrition* 49:86–92.

Hall, L. and L. Cohn. 1986. Bulimia: A guide to recovery. Santa Barbara, CA: Gurze Books.

Hsu, L.K. 1988a. Classification and diagnosis of the eating disorders. In *The eating disorders*, eds. B.J. Blinder, B.F. Chaitin, and R.S. Goldstein. New York: PMA Publishing Corp.

Hsu, L.K. 1988b. The etiology of anorexia nervosa. In *The eating disorders*, eds. B.J. Blinder, B.F. Chaitin, and R.S. Goldstein. New York: PMA Publishing Corp.

Humphrey, L.L. 1989. Observed family interactions among subtypes of eating disorders using structural analysis of social behavior. *Journal of Consulting and Clinical Psychology* 57:206–214.

Kog, E. and W. Vandereycken. 1989. Family interaction in eating disorder patients and normal controls. *International Journal of Eating Disorders* 8:11–23.

Leichner, P. and A. Gertler. 1988. Prevalence and incidence studies of anorexia nervosa. In *The eating disorders: Medical and psychological bases of diagnosis and treatment*, eds. B.J. Blinder, B.F. Chaitin, and R.S. Goldstein. New York: PMA Publishing Corp.

Lucas, A.R. and D.M. Huse. 1988. Behavioral disorders affecting food intake: Anorexia nervosa and bulimia. In *Modern nutrition in health and disease*, eds. M.E. Shils and V.R. Young. Philadelphia: Lea and Febiger.

Mitchell, J.E. and R.L. Pyle. 1988. The diagnosis and clinical characteristics of bulimia. In *The eating disorders*, eds. B.J. Blinder, B.F. Chaitin, and R.S. Goldstein. New York: PMA Publishing Corp.

Mizes, J.S. 1988. Personality characteristics of bulimic and non-eating-disordered female controls: A cognitive behavioral perspective. *International Journal of Eating Disorders* 7:541–550.

Newman, M.M. and K.A. Halmi. 1988. The endocrinology of anorexia nervosa and bulimia nervosa. *Endocrinology and Metabolism Clinics of North America* 17:195–212.

Palazzoli, M.S. 1978. *Self-starvation*. New York: Jason Aronson.

Rusting, R. 1988. Starvaholics? *Scientific American* 11:36.

Sargent, J. and R. Liebman. 1988. Family therapy for eating disorders. In *The eating disorders*, eds. B.J. Blinder, B.F. Chaitin, and R.S. Goldstein. New York: PMA Publishing Corp.

Scott, D.W. 1986. Anorexia nervosa: A review of possible genetic factors. *International Journal of Eating Disorders* 5:1–20.

Sibley, D.C. and B.J. Blinder. 1988. Anorexia nervosa. In *The eating disorders*, eds. B.J. Blinder, B.F. Chaitin, and R.S. Goldstein. New York: PMA Publishing Corp.

Smith, N.J. 1980. Excessive weight loss and food aversion in athletes simulating anorexia nervosa. *Pediatrics* 66:139–142.

Smith, N.J. and B. Worthington-Roberts. 1989. *Food for sport*. Palo Alto, CA: The Bull Publishing Company.

Stein, P.M. and B.C. Unell. 1986. *Anorexia nervosa*. Minneapolis: CompCare Publications.

Stern, S.L., K.N. Dixon, D. Jones, M. Lake, E. Nemzer, and R. Sansone. 1989. Family environment in anorexia nervosa and bulimia. *International Journal of Eating Disorders* 8:25–31.

Striegel-Moore, R.H., L.R. Silberstein, P. Frensch, and J. Rodin. 1989. A prospective study of disordered eating among college students. *International Journal of Eating Disorders* 8:499–509.

Strober, M. and J.L. Katz. 1988. Depression in the eating disorders: A review and analysis of descriptive, family, and biological findings. In *Diagnostic issues in anorexia nervosa and bulimia nervosa,* eds. D.M. Garner and P.E. Garfinkel. New York: Brunner/Mazel, Publishers.

Tolstoi, L.G. 1989. The role of pharmacotherapy in anorexia nervosa and bulimia. *Journal of the American Dietetic Association* 89:1640–1646.

Tuft's University. 1989. Is an eating disorder developing in your family? *Tuft's University Diet and Nutrition Letter* 7 (no. 3):3–6.

Turnbull, J., C.P. Freeman, F. Barry, and A. Henderson. 1989. The clinical characteristics of bulimic women. *International Journal of Eating Disorders* 8:399–409.

Walsh, B.T. 1988. Pharmacotherapy of eating disorders. In *The eating disorders,* eds. B.J. Blinder, B.F. Chaitin, and R.S. Goldstein. New York: PMA Publishing Corp.

Woodside, D.B. and P.E. Garfinkel. 1989. An overview of the eating disorders anorexia nervosa and bulimia nervosa. *Nutrition Today* 24:27–29.

Wooley, S. and O. Wayne Wooley. 1986. Thinness mania. *American Health* October, 1986:68–74.

Zakin, D.F. 1989. Eating disturbance, emotional separation, and body image. *International Journal of Eating Disorders* 8:411–416.

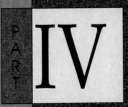
MICRONUTRIENTS:
REGULATORS AND RAW
MATERIAL

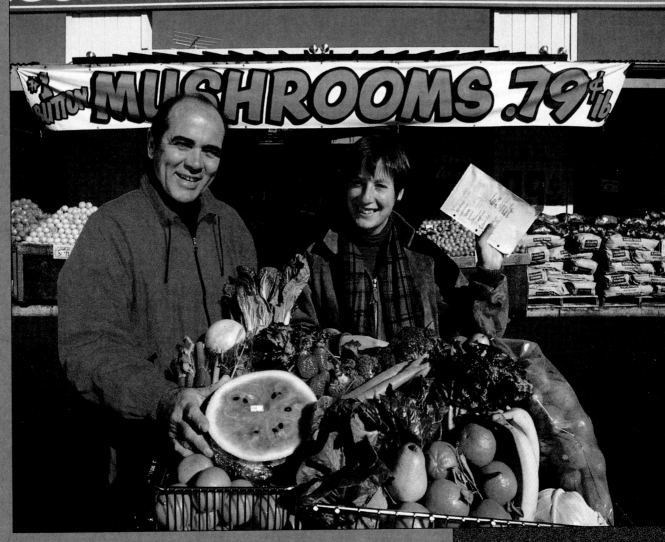

12

Vitamins

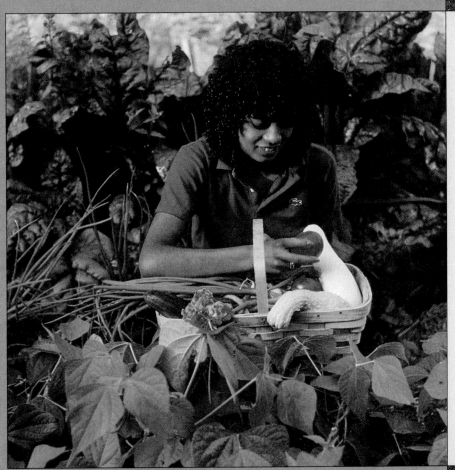

In This Chapter

- Vitamins Have Similarities but Differ in Several General Ways
- Key Concepts About Vitamins Are As Important As Individual Facts
- Additional Important Concepts Warrant Emphasis

ew people need to be convinced that vitamins are important. An FDA study shows that 36% of the U.S. population takes vitamin and mineral supplements regularly (Moss et al., 1989), and it is estimated that $2 billion is spent each year on these products.

Although the common assumption that this class of nutrients provides energy is not accurate, it is true that vitamins are essential for the body's functioning. In this chapter, we will describe what vitamins do. Further, we emphasize that a *well-chosen diet can supply all the vitamins that most people need.*

Nonetheless, we will also deal with the matter of vitamin supplements, since they are so commonly used. Although supplements can be helpful in some circumstances, many nutritionists believe that the pendulum has swung too far in the direction of their use. This concern is based on the fact that large excesses of some vitamins can cause serious damage; some people take dangerously large doses because of inaccurate claims about the benefits supplemental vitamins can provide.

Many newspapers and magazines contain articles that are excessive in their claims of what vitamins can accomplish and what doses should be taken: *"Miracle vitamin beats tiredness"* one headline claims, and then the article goes on to recommend levels that are hundreds of times the RDA for certain vitamins. Another article suggests large multivitamin supplements for athletes, the formulation varying with the sport. To many people, such materials convey the impression that the larger the doses you take, the better off you are.

In this chapter, we want to help you find the middle ground: the point at which you take in enough vitamins to carry out the functions that vitamins are needed to perform, but not so much that they cause damage. We'll start by describing the nature of vitamins—how these substances are alike, and how they differ.

Vitamins Have Similarities but Differ in Several General Ways

vitamins—organic compounds present in small amounts in foods, and needed in small amounts by the body as regulators of metabolic functions

The thirteen known **vitamins** are organic substances that occur in small amounts in foods; they are needed by the human body in minute amounts as regulators of metabolic functions. Vitamins generally do not require digestion but are absorbed intact through the small intestine.

We need relatively small amounts of these substances because vitamins are not used up in one biochemical reaction: one molecule is used repeatedly. Only gradually are vitamins degraded (broken apart) and in need of replacement. Consider vitamin B-12, the vitamin needed in the smallest amount. Just 1 gram of vitamin B-12 can fulfill the RDA of one-half million people for one day. Even the vitamin we need in the largest amount, vitamin C, has a recommended intake of only 60 mg/day. A gram of it can supply 17 people for one day.

Various Solubilities, Absorption Efficiencies, and Storage Capacities

Traditionally, the vitamins are subdivided according to whether they are soluble in fat or in water. The fat-soluble vitamins are A, D, E, and K; the water-soluble vitamins are thiamin, riboflavin, niacin, vitamin B-6, folic acid, vitamin B-12, pantothenic acid, biotin, and vitamin C.

The maximum amount of a vitamin that body tissues can maintain is called the **saturation level.** The saturation levels of various vitamins differ. In general, fat-soluble vitamins can be stored in larger quantities than water-soluble vitamins.

saturation level—the maximum amount of a substance a tissue can maintain

Whether a vitamin is fat-soluble or water-soluble also influences how well it is absorbed, which depends in part on what is in the gut. For example, the presence of fat in the chyme facilitates the absorption of fat-soluble vitamins.

Various Structures, Forms, and Potencies

Aside from the fact that they are all organic, vitamins are otherwise structurally unrelated: there is no characteristic organization of the carbon, hydrogen, and oxygen in a vitamin molecule. Furthermore, some vitamins also contain nitrogen, sulfur, or cobalt in their structures. You can see how dissimilar vitamin structures are by looking at Appendix I.

Some of the vitamins have several different but closely related chemical forms that can function as that vitamin. These different forms can even occur in the same food at the same time. For example, nicotinamide and nicotinic acid, two forms of niacin, can be simultaneously present in one food. (These compounds are not the same as nicotine in tobacco.)

Sometimes a compound that is rather unlike a nutrient can be converted into one by the body. Such early versions of nutrients are called *precursors;* vitamin precursors are called **provitamins.** For example, there are about 50 carotenoids that are provitamins for vitamin A, one of which is beta-carotene (β-carotene); and the amino acid tryptophan can be considered a provitamin of niacin.

provitamins—vitamin precursors that the body can convert into the active form of a vitamin

Because vitamins and provitamins occur in different forms, a single vitamin can be known by a multitude of chemical names. You might encounter these names on the labels of food products to which vitamins have been added or on the labels of vitamin supplements. Such names are alternatives to the letter names, or letter/number names, that many vitamins were given when they were first discovered. Often, when vitamins are shown on an ingredient list, the letter/number names accompany the chemical names (Figure 12.1). We will give you the various common names and forms as we discuss each vitamin.

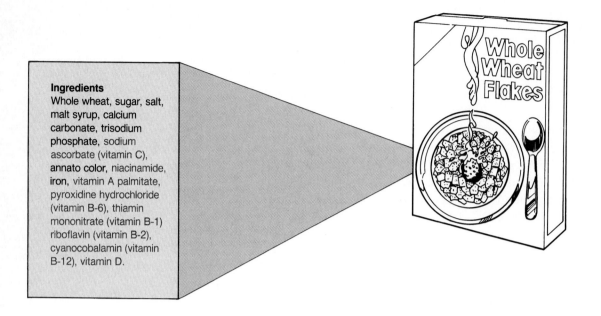

Ingredients
Whole wheat, sugar, salt, malt syrup, calcium carbonate, trisodium phosphate, sodium ascorbate (vitamin C), annato color, niacinamide, iron, vitamin A palmitate, pyroxidine hydrochloride (vitamin B-6), thiamin mononitrate (vitamin B-1) riboflavin (vitamin B-2), cyanocobalamin (vitamin B-12), vitamin D.

Figure 12.1 How added vitamins are shown on ingredient lists. Labels of foods with added vitamins usually give both the common name and the name of the specific chemical compound used.

The form in which a vitamin occurs can influence its potency. For example, the potency of different forms of vitamin A varies considerably. There are several reasons. With vitamin A, a much smaller proportion of the provitamin carotene is absorbed than is retinol, another form of vitamin A. The efficiency of the conversion of different carotenoids to vitamin A in the body also varies.

While discussing forms of vitamins, it is appropriate to comment on "natural" versus synthetic vitamins, since some people assume that there are substantial differences between the two. The fact is that "natural" and synthetic vitamins, if they are in the same form, are identical: although they have different origins, they are not chemically different.

However vitamins, whether in foods or in supplements, are not alone: other substances are present with them. For example, many vegetables with carotenoids also contain vitamin C, fiber, and a variety of carbohydrates; and carotenoid supplements, whether they are made from "natural" or synthetic carotene, contain fillers in addition to the carotenoids. All things considered, "natural" carotene supplements may be less pure and/or concentrated than synthetic carotene. But either type of supplement probably has more of the carotenoids and fewer of the other substances than are found in good food sources of carotenoids.

The effect of these other substances is unpredictable, because (depending on what they are and how much is present) they can either enhance, detract from, or have no effect at all on the vitamin's activity in the body. Therefore, it is impossible to generalize whether vitamins from "natural" supplements, from synthetic supplements, or from food will be more effective in the body.

Finally, the Slice of Life on page 387 points out the difficulty in defining "natural" vitamins. Consumers can be misled into thinking they're getting something they're not when they reach for the package with "natural" on the label.

Various Toxicity Levels

The level of intake at which a vitamin becomes toxic (able to harm the body) varies with several factors. Because the body can store more of a fat-soluble vitamin, it has a greater potential to reach excessive levels and become toxic than a water-soluble vitamin. In the past, it was generally assumed that an excess of water-soluble vitamins would simply be excreted in the urine; however, we now know that, like fat-soluble vitamins, they can also become toxic at high doses.

The chemical potency of the form of the vitamin is another factor related to its toxicity; the more potent the form, the smaller the amount required to achieve toxicity. The time in which the vitamin is ingested also matters. One unusually large dose of a vitamin every six months might not be harmful, but repeated intakes of that same amount every day may be toxic.

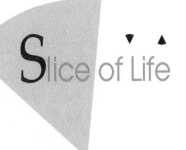

Slice of Life

How Natural Are "Natural" Vitamins? Will the Answers Change?

The article from which this was excerpted was written by a pharmacist with the Consumers Cooperative of Berkeley, Inc.

> Spurred by our growing sales . . . I visited two manufacturers of "natural" vitamins in Southern California. These companies make capsules, tablets, and other dosage forms sold under some of the most famous brand names found in "health food" stores. . . .
>
> During the visits, it became clear that many vitamin products labeled "natural" or "organic" are not really what I had imagined those terms to mean.
>
> For example, their "Rose Hips Vitamin C Tablets" are made from natural rose hips combined with chemical ascorbic acid, the same vitamin C used in standard pharmaceutical tablets. Natural rose hips contain only about 2% vitamin C, and we were told that if no vitamin C were added the tablet "would have to be as big as a golf ball." (Kamil, 1974)

Would you have guessed that the amount of vitamin C coming from rose hips was just a tiny fraction of the amount added as a synthetic chemical?

For many years, the terms *natural* and *organic* had no legal definitions; the practice described above was legal, although it was misleading. Several individual states, including Wisconsin, have worked toward giving meaning to these terms for use within their own borders. Federally, the FDA is still attempting to create a definition for nationwide use, but as of July, 1990, no definition had been accepted.

It is easier to define these terms when related to *foods* than to *supplements*. In order for a food to be labeled as an "organic food," it must have met the conditions under which such foods must be grown as defined by the state. Such conditions are likely to include the avoidance of synthetic fertilizers and pesticides. It is possible to test for the presence of synthetic pesticides, so to this extent at least, the appropriate use of the term can be verified.

On the other hand, *"natural" vitamin supplements or foods to which "natural" vitamins are added* pose a particularly difficult problem. The difficulty is not as much with making the regulation as with enforcing it; there would be no way to test whether the vitamins were of natural or of laboratory origin, because both types have the same chemical structure (see text). Enforcing the regulation fairly would be impossible. ▼

Various Stabilities

Some vitamins are less stable than other nutrients. They can be degraded by oxygen, light, various pH conditions, heat, and/or the passage of time. Because people are greatly concerned with how vitamin losses occur in foods and how to prevent them, we talk more extensively about this topic in Chapter 14 (on processing).

Various Units of Measurement

Most vitamins are quantified by their mass in milligrams and micrograms. Another unit related to mass that has been used in the past for some vitamins (vitamins A and D) is the International Unit (IU).

equivalents—unit now coming into use as an indicator of vitamin activity in the body

Now that scientists are aware that different forms of some vitamins and their precursors have varying potencies, they use units called **equivalents** to reflect as accurately as possible the amount of vitamin activity the various forms provide. The 1989 RDA recommends intakes of vitamins A, E, and niacin in equivalents (see inside back cover). However, many food composition tables still express levels of these vitamins in IUs, and until food composition tables can be completely revised to match the newer equivalent values, comparing such values will be like comparing apples to oranges. We will discuss how to deal with these temporary discrepancies at appropriate points in this chapter.

Key Concepts About Vitamins Are As Important As Individual Facts

The classic way to teach about vitamins is to deal with them one by one and discuss their functions, typical intakes, and dietary sources and the effects of their deficiency and excess. At the very time nutritionists do this, they know that in a sense the approach is misleading because it insinuates that a particular vitamin has very limited functions in only certain tissues. In this approach, vitamin A is often cited as the vitamin that keeps skin from getting rough, for example. Although certain types of cells may exhibit obvious symptoms more quickly than others when a particular vitamin deficiency occurs, *almost all vitamins function in almost all body cells; every vitamin has widespread effects on the body.*

Another problem with teaching about vitamins one by one is that this approach insinuates that vitamins function in isolation. In reality, *vitamins interact with many other nutrients,* including other vitamins. For example, carotenoid and vitamin A absorption and utilization are enhanced by dietary fat and vitamin E. This means that if a person drastically changes his or her intake of one vitamin, the utilization and even functions of many other nutrients are likely to be affected as well. The interaction of nutrients is a relatively new and important area of research; you can expect to hear much more about it in the future.

Despite the flaws inherent in presenting vitamins one by one, it still makes sense to organize material in this way. But as you read, keep in mind the two concepts discussed above. Other important concepts are discussed in a section following the material about the individual vitamins. All these themes are at least as important as the details about specific vitamins.

There is much to say about the 13 vitamins. Table 12.1 gives an overview of some of the facts about them. We will begin by discussing the fat-soluble vitamins.

Vitamin A

When we talk about vitamin A in food, we may be referring to any of several different chemical forms of vitamin A: both preformed (already formed) versions and provitamins of vitamin A are found in food. The most common preformed version present in food is *retinol*; others are *retinal, retinaldehyde,* and *retinoic acid.* The last of these, retinoic acid, cannot be converted by the body into retinol, so it cannot perform all the functions retinol can.

There are hundreds of compounds called *carotenoids* that occur, for the most part, in plant materials and have some structural similarity to vitamin A. About 50 of them can be converted into retinol by the body, so only these are provitamins of vitamin A and, if converted to retinol, perform the functions of vitamin A. The most important of these provitamin A compounds is *beta-carotene* (β-carotene).

Functions and Effects of Deficiency   Vitamin A plays a well-defined role in the eye; it is a component of rhodopsin and iodopsin, which are colored, light-sensitive substances in the retina. When light falls on these compounds, they undergo changes that are translated into messages about what was seen. Then they are converted back to their original form. If vitamin A has been deficient in the diet, these conversions occur more slowly than normal, and there is a time lag before the eye can see again. Since this occurs particularly when the eye is trying to adapt from bright light to darkness, the condition is called **night blindness.** Night blindness is reversible. Only retinol or carotenoids that can be converted to retinol, not retinoic acid, can prevent night blindness.

night blindness—condition in which eyes cannot adapt quickly from bright light to darkness, and temporary blindness occurs; caused by vitamin A deficiency

Vitamin A, although it was the first vitamin discovered, still puzzles scientists who are trying to explain how it functions within body cells. It appears that vitamin A acts directly on the nucleus of cells and affects *gene expression;* that is, it affects DNA and ultimately the type and/or amount of protein synthesized by the cell. This affects the growth and health of cartilage, bone, and body coverings and linings (epithelial tissues). Epithelial tissues include the corneas of the eyes; the mucous membranes, including the linings of nasal passages, gastrointestinal tract, and genitourinary tract; and the skin. This maintenance of epithelial tissue is one of several ways in which vitamin A maintains immune function.

Table 12.1 Key Information About the Vitamins

Vitamin	RDA for Healthy Adults Ages 19–50	Major Dietary Sources	Major Functions	Signs of Severe, Prolonged Deficiency	Signs of Extreme Excess
Fat-Soluble					
A	Females: 800 RE[a] Males: 1000 RE[a]	Fat-containing and fortified dairy products; liver; provitamin carotene in orange and deep green fruits and vegetables	Vitamin A is a component of rhodopsin; carotenoids can serve as antioxidants; still under intense study	Night blindness; keratinization of epithelial tissues including the cornea of the eye (xerophthalmia) causing permanent blindness; dry, scaling skin; increased susceptibility to infection	*Preformed vitamin A:* damage to liver, bone; headache, irritability, vomiting, hair loss, blurred vision; *13-cis retinoic acid:* some fetal defects; *Carotenoids:* yellowed skin
D	<25 years: 10 μg >25 years: 5 μg	Fortified and full-fat dairy products, egg yolk (diet often not as important as sunlight exposure)	Promotes absorption and use of calcium and phosphorus	Rickets (bone deformities) in children; osteomalacia (bone softening) in adults	Calcium deposition in tissues leading to cerebral, CV, and kidney damage
E	Females: 8 α-tocopherol equivalents Males: 10 α-tocopherol equivalents	Vegetable oils and their products; nuts, seeds; present at low levels in other foods	Antioxidant to prevent cell membrane damage; still under intense study	Possible anemia and neurological effects	Generally nontoxic, but at least one type of intravenous infusion led to some fatalities in premature infants; may worsen clotting defect in vitamin K deficiency
K	Females: <25: 60 μg >25: 65 μg Males: <25: 70 μg >25: 80 μg	Green vegetables; tea	Aids in formation of certain proteins, especially those for blood clotting	Defective blood coagulation causing severe bleeding on injury	Liver damage and anemia from high doses of the synthetic form menadione
Water-Soluble					
Thiamin (B-1)	Females: 1.1 mg Males: 1.5 mg	Pork, legumes, peanuts, enriched or whole-grain products	Coenzyme used in energy metabolism	Nerve changes, sometimes edema, heart failure; beriberi	Generally nontoxic, but repeated injections may cause shock reaction
Riboflavin (B-2)	Females: 1.3 mg Males: 1.7 mg	Dairy products, meats, eggs, enriched grain products, green leafy vegetables	Coenzyme used in energy metabolism	Skin lesions	Generally nontoxic

Vitamin	RDA for Healthy Adults Ages 19–50	Major Dietary Sources	Major Functions	Signs of Severe, Prolonged Deficiency	Signs of Extreme Excess
Niacin	Females: 15 niacin equivalents Males: 19 niacin equivalents	Nuts, meats; provitamin tryptophan in most proteins	Coenzyme used in energy metabolism	Pellagra (multiple vitamin deficiencies including niacin)	Flushing of face, neck, hands; potential liver damage
B-6	Females: 1.6 mg Males: 2.0 mg	High-protein foods in general	Coenzyme used in amino acid metabolism	Nervous, skin, and muscular disorders; anemia	Unstable gait, numb feet, poor coordination
Folic acid	Females: 180 μg Males: 200 μg	Green vegetables, orange juice, nuts, legumes, grain products	Coenzyme used in DNA and RNA metabolism; single carbon utilization	Megaloblastic anemia (large, immature red blood cells); GI disturbances	Masks vitamin B-12 deficiency; interferes with drugs to control epilepsy
B-12	2 μg	Animal products	Coenzyme used in DNA and RNA metabolism; single carbon utilization	Megaloblastic anemia; pernicious anemia when due to inadequate intrinsic factor; nervous system damage	Thought to be nontoxic
Pantothenic acid	4–7 mg[b]	Animal products and whole grains; widely distributed in foods	Coenzyme used in energy metabolism	Fatigue, numbness, and tingling of hands and feet	Generally nontoxic; occasionally causes diarrhea
Biotin	30–100 μg[b]	Widely distributed in foods	Coenzyme used in energy metabolism	Scaly dermatitis	Thought to be nontoxic
C (ascorbic acid)	60 mg	Fruits and vegetables, especially broccoli, cabbage, cantaloupe, cauliflower, citrus fruits, green pepper, kiwi fruit, strawberries	Functions in synthesis of collagen; is an antioxidant; aids in detoxification; improves iron absorption; still under intense study	Scurvy; petechiae (minute hemorrhages around hair follicles); weakness; delayed wound healing; impaired immune response	GI upsets, confounds certain lab tests

[a] RE = retinol equivalents (Because many food composition tables still list the vitamin A activity of foods as IU, it may be helpful to recognize that previous RDAs for vitamin A were 5000 IU [men] and 4000 IU [women].)

[b] Estimated Safe and Adequate Daily Dietary Intake in 1989 RDAs

References: 1) RDA Subcommittee, 1989. *Recommended Dietary Allowances.* Washington, DC: National Academy Press. 2) Shils, M.E. and V.R. Young. 1988. *Modern Nutrition in Health and Disease.* Philadelphia: Lea & Febiger.

xerophthalmia—condition in which cornea of the eye becomes keratinized, which can result in permanent blindness if untreated; caused by severe, prolonged vitamin A deficiency

antioxidant—substance that prevents oxygen from combining with other substances to which it might cause damage

Figure 12.2 Changes in the cornea due to vitamin A deficiency. Here you see one of the stages of eye damage from vitamin A deficiency. The cornea is dull and opaque, and the membrane covering the white of the eye has become wrinkled. If not treated, the membranes will tear and cause blindness. (From *Nutrition Today*, March/April, 1988, p. 36.)

If vitamin A is deficient in the body, *keratinization* occurs—that is, epithelial tissue becomes abnormally rough. The skin becomes dry and rough and mucous membranes may crack and hemorrhage. The most devastating example of this effect occurs in the cornea of the eye (the clear covering over the front of the eyeball); in severe and prolonged cases of vitamin A deficiency, keratinization can cause blindness. The term used to refer to severe vitamin A deficiency symptoms in the eye is **xerophthalmia.** Figure 12.2 shows one stage in the development of blindness from vitamin A deficiency. Although this disease is not often seen in the developed countries, it causes blindness in an estimated one-half million children annually (Bauerfeind, 1988). Figure 12.3 shows in which parts of the world blindness due to vitamin A deficiency is common.

Inadequate intake of *carotenoids* may put people at greater risk of another health problem—cancer. Several investigators have noted that the intake of more carotenoids was associated with a lower risk of cancer, particularly of the lung (Public Health Service, 1988). The mechanism is unclear but probably involves the ability of carotenoids to serve as **antioxidants** without being converted to retinol (Bendich and Olson, 1989). Remember, though, that this statistical correlation does not *prove* that carotene reduces the risk of cancer: other factors in foods that contain carotenoids (such as fiber and undefined chemicals) may also affect the incidence of cancer.

Recommended and Typical Intakes   Currently the RDAs for vitamin A for women and men are 800 and 1000 retinol equivalents (RE), respectively. According to survey data, the average adult male in the United States consumes more than 1400 RE of vitamin A daily (HNIS, 1986). Averages are sometimes misleading: another large survey found that although the average individual from 1 to 74 years of age consumed more than the RDA for vitamin A, 42% consumed less than one-half the RDA for males on the day surveyed (National Center for Health Statistics, 1979). This is not necessarily a problem because a large intake one day is saved for use on another day—your body stores vitamin A in the liver. This situation also demonstrates the

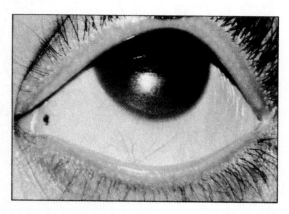

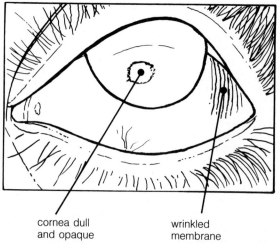

cornea dull
and opaque

wrinkled
membrane

difficulty of trying to predict the adequacy of your diet on the basis of one day's intake.

Dietary Sources As you can see in Table 12.2, the fruit and vegetable group contains a number of foods that are outstanding sources of vitamin A. The fruits and vegetables that generally have the highest amount of vitamin A are the carotene-containing deep orange and dark green varieties. The best among them are apricots, broccoli, cantaloupe (muskmelon), carrots, pumpkin, winter squash, sweet potatoes, and spinach and other dark, leafy greens. Another food that provides a large amount of vitamin A in one serving is liver; here, the major form of vitamin A is retinol. Dairy products and eggs provide significant amounts of both retinol and carotenoids.

As was discussed in the beginning of the chapter, your body cannot use all forms of vitamin A equally well. Retinol (found mainly in animal sources) is much better utilized than carotenoids (found mainly in plant sources). Even though we generally consume more carotenoids, USDA scientists have estimated that carotenoids contribute less than one-third of the total vitamin A *activity* in the diets of Americans.

Although experts now express vitamin A requirements as retinol equivalents (RE), many food composition tables still list the vitamin A content of foods the old way—in international units (IU). The RE values are based on new understandings about the usefulness of various forms of vitamin A and

Figure 12.3 Geographical distribution of vitamin A and xerophthalmia. (From *Nutrition Today*, March/April, 1988, p. 35.)

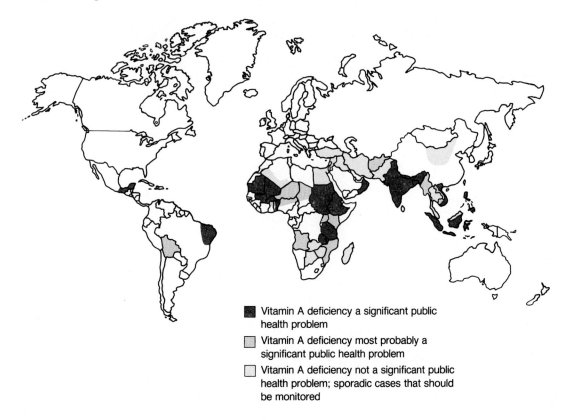

Vitamin A deficiency a significant public health problem

Vitamin A deficiency most probably a significant public health problem

Vitamin A deficiency not a significant public health problem; sporadic cases that should be monitored

Table 12.2 Vitamin A in Some Foods

The RDA for men is 1000 RE/day; for women, 800 RE/day.

Food	Household Measure	IU	RE	RE of Vitamin A (0 200 400 600 800 1000)
Fruits and vegetables				
Apple	1 medium	74	7	
Apricots, canned juice pack	½ cup	2098	210	
Broccoli, frozen, cooked	½ cup	1740	174	
Cantaloupe	½ cup	2579	258	
Carrot, raw	7½ inches long	20,253	2025	2025
Corn, canned	½ cup	128	13	
Green beans, frozen, cooked	½ cup	359	36	
Lettuce, iceberg	1 cup	185	20	
Orange juice, frozen, reconstituted	½ cup	97	10	
Peach, fresh	1 medium	465	47	
Spinach, frozen, cooked	½ cup	8779	878	
Grain products				
Bread, white, enriched	1 slice	tr	tr	
Cornflakes	1 cup	1000	303	
Total® fortified cereal	1 cup	5893	1786	1786
Pasta, cooked	½ cup	0	0	
Milk and milk products				
Buttermilk from skim milk, not fortified	1 cup	81	20	
Skim milk, vitamin A fortified	1 cup	500	140	
Milk, whole, not fortified	1 cup	307	76	
Cheese, cheddar	1⅓ ounces	400	115	
Meats and meat alternates				
Beef, ground, broiled	2 ounces	0	0	
Chicken, fried	2 ounces	39	12	
Eggs	2 large	520	156	
Kidney beans, canned	1 cup	0	0	
Liver, beef, fried	2 ounces	20,562	6110	6110
Combination foods				
Bean burrito (2)	7¾ ounces	332	33	
Beef chunky soup, canned	1 cup	2611	261	
Cheese pizza	⅛ of 15-inch pie	727	140	
Cream of mushroom soup made with milk	1 cup	154	38	
Nachos with cheese	6–8	559	92	
Limited extras				
Butter	1 teaspoon	153	38	
Carbonated beverages	12 ounces	0	0	
Sugar, honey	1 tablespoon	0	0	

Data Sources: (1) HNIS. Agricultural handbook 8 series on composition of foods. Washington, D.C.: U.S. Department of Agriculture. (2) Appendix E, this textbook.

394

are therefore more valid. In Table 12.2, where the vitamin A contents of some foods are given in both RE and IU, note that no single mathematical conversion factor was used across the board (Bendich and Langseth, 1989). However, if you are using a food composition table that defines vitamin A only in IU (as is true of Appendices E and F) and you want to compare those values with the RDA that is expressed in RE, divide the IU values by 10 for foods of plant origin and by 5 for foods of animal origin to get a *rough* estimate of RE values.

Consequences of High Intake   It is possible to consume high levels of vitamin A as carotene in vegetables and fruits. The skin of individuals (especially children) who consume excess amounts of deep yellow and green vegetables with every meal may turn yellow; excess carotene has no other known detrimental consequences. This effect can be reversed by eating less of the carotene-rich foods. On the other hand, routine overconsumption of vitamin A as retinol (more than 50,000 IUs daily) may result in toxicity (Bendich and Langseth, 1989). Symptoms may include skin lesions, hair loss, and—eventually—liver and bone damage. A few patients who unwittingly overdosed themselves with vitamin A supplements developed such elevated pressure in fluids around the brain that physicians suspected brain tumors before they recognized the real problem (Evans and Lacey, 1986). A similar condition has been seen in patients who ate liver several times per week, which caused a symptom the *Journal of the American Medical Association* dubbed "liver lover's headache" (Selhorst et al., 1984).

A caution must also be given against taking a particular synthetic form of vitamin A called *13-cis-retinoic acid* during pregnancy. The brand name of this drug is Accutane, and it is sometimes prescribed for treatment of severe cystic acne. Because it is known to cause malformation in animal fetuses, it is never prescribed for a woman who is pregnant or intends to become pregnant during the course of drug use, but there have been cases in which women taking the drug have become pregnant. A study of 59 such pregnancies resulted in 12 spontaneous abortions, 21 malformed infants, and only 26 infants without major malformations (Lammer et al., 1985). A chemical with this potential for harm must be totally avoided by women intending to become pregnant during the course of drug treatment and must be prescribed very cautiously even under circumstances in which its use seems indicated.

Synthetic vitamin A compounds have also been used in certain skin creams to treat acne and/or wrinkling caused by sun damage. Its effectiveness for treating acne is better established than for sun damage (Roberts, 1988). There is no evidence that such *topical* application for either purpose is a risk during pregnancy.

Vitamin D

Vitamin D is a unique vitamin because it can be produced by the body. This occurs when ultraviolet light from the sun changes a compound in the skin called 7-dehydrocholesterol into vitamin D.

In food, vitamin D occurs as various forms of *cholecalciferol* (vitamin D of animal origin) and *ergocalciferol* (vitamin D of plant origin).

Functions and Effects of Deficiency   After vitamin D is modified slightly in the liver and kidneys, it serves as a hormone in the body. The primary roles of vitamin D are to enhance the intestinal absorption of calcium and phosphorus, to promote retention of calcium that might otherwise be lost in the urine, and to mobilize calcium from bone if necessary. All these activities work together to maintain the levels of calcium and phosphorus in the blood that are necessary for normal nerve and muscle activity. In addition, enhancement of calcium absorption and retention helps to promote calcium deposition in bone when circulating levels of calcium are maintained (DeLuca, 1988).

If the level of vitamin D is inadequate in the body over a period of time, bones will fail to mineralize or will progressively demineralize in order to keep serum calcium levels within normal levels. The problem is that this results in bone softening. When this occurs in children, the condition is called **rickets.** It is characterized by abnormal bone development that may result in bowed legs and other deformities. When vitamin D deficiency occurs in adults, the condition is called **osteomalacia.**

rickets, osteomalacia— progressive demineralization of bone in children and adults, respectively; caused by vitamin D deficiency

Recommended Intakes   Because vitamin D is linked closely to bone growth and maintenance, the RDA for this nutrient is highest for those who still have the potential to grow. For children and young adults through age 24, the recommended intake is 10 μg. At age 25 it drops to 5 μg. During pregnancy and lactation, an intake of 10 μg is recommended.

It is debatable whether an RDA for vitamin D for adults is necessary. That is, many adults produce in their bodies as much vitamin D as they need, provided they get enough sun. But since the amount of internally produced vitamin D can be variable, the adult RDA fills in the gaps if insufficient vitamin D is produced in the body.

The amount of vitamin D produced in a person's skin depends on many factors: the surface area exposed to sunlight, the amount of pigment in the skin (dark skin increases the amount of sunlight needed to initiate vitamin D production), the time of day, the season, the latitude, whether a sunscreen has been applied (sunscreens with a skin-protection factor of 8 or higher block vitamin D production), and even a person's age (production diminishes with age). Because of all these variables, statements regarding how much sun is required to produce sufficient vitamin D have to be full of qualifications. For example, one expert recommends that elderly white people living in Boston in the summertime should expose hands, arms, and face to doses of sun that are less than would cause reddening—usually 10–15 minutes, depending on the person's skin pigmentation, two or three times a week (Holick, 1987).

Dietary Sources   There are no naturally excellent sources of vitamin D among the foods people normally eat. However, there is a good fortified source—milk fortified with vitamin D. Table 12.3 reveals that two servings will provide the adult RDA. Other significant sources are egg yolks and products made with fortified milk.

Cod-liver oil is a very potent source of vitamin D. Because of the toxicity of vitamin D, if cod-liver is ingested for any reason, the amount taken should be carefully controlled to avoid toxicity.

Consequences of High Intake   Vitamin D is regarded as the most toxic of all the vitamins. Excess intakes of vitamin D lead to high blood calcium levels and deposition of calcium in soft tissue, resulting in irreversible renal (kidney) and cardiovascular damage (RDA Subcommittee, 1989). Note this statement from the 1989 RDA: "Since the toxic level of vitamin D may in some

Table 12.3 Vitamin D in Some Foods

The RDA for men and women through age 24 is 10 μg/day; after that, 5 μg/day.

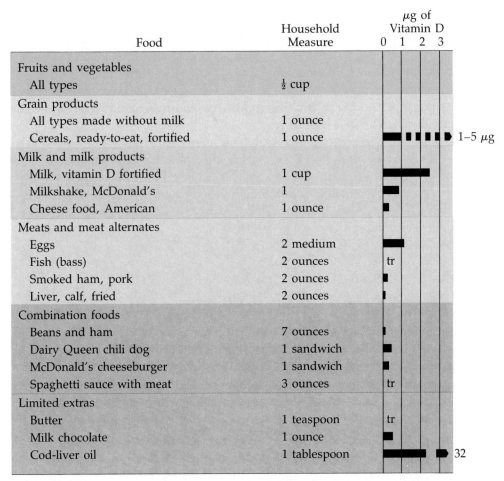

Data adapted from 1) Pennington, J.A. 1989. *Food values of portions commonly used.* New York: Harper & Row and 2) Pennington, J.A. and H.N. Church. 1985. *Food values of portions commonly used.* Philadelphia: J.B. Lippincott.

cases be only 5 times the RDA . . . , dietary supplements may be detrimental for the normal child or adult who drinks at least two glasses of vitamin D fortified milk per day."

There is no need to worry that excess sunlight will result in internal production of toxic levels of vitamin D. It has been found that following the initial period of sun exposure, the skin produces progressively less provitamin for vitamin D (Holick, 1987). (Of course, prolonged exposure to sun exacts a different, unrelated penalty—increased risk of skin cancer.)

Vitamin E

Vitamin E occurs in food as compounds called *tocopherols* and *tocotrienols*. The most active form of vitamin E is *alpha-tocopherol (α-tocopherol)*; other forms, such as *beta-tocopherol* or *gamma-tocopherol*, are only 1–50% as active.

Functions and Effects of Deficiency   Many researchers believe that vitamin E performs primarily as an antioxidant; it prevents oxygen from combining with other substances and damaging them. For example, the presence of vitamin E is thought to protect vitamin A from being oxidized. Vitamin E also protects polyunsaturated fatty acids (PUFAs) from oxidation. This occurs not only in foods, but also in the body, where PUFAs are part of cell membranes. It has been suggested that vitamin E may help protect against certain types of cancer, but this requires much further study (Surgeon General, 1988). The data are sketchy.

Vitamin E deficiency is so rare that for many years this vitamin was said to be "in search of a disease." This fact seemed to invite nutrition hucksters to make unfounded claims about what diseases it could cure or prevent. (Have you seen ads for vitamin E that suggest it can protect you from heart disease or cyclical fibrocystic breast disease, or cure you of muscular dystrophy, or improve your sexual or athletic performance? These are examples of unsupported claims.) Although vitamin E deficiency is almost impossible to induce in healthy subjects, it can occur in premature infants (Gutcher, Ranor, and Farrell, 1984), and it might occur in somebody who is unable over a period of years to absorb fat and fat-soluble vitamins.

Recommended and Typical Intakes   Because there is such great variation in the activity of the various forms of vitamin E, recommended intakes of vitamin E are designated in equivalents. An equivalent has the vitamin E activity equal to that of 1 mg of α-tocopherol. The RDA recommends 10 α-tocopherol equivalents for adult males and 8 α-tocopherol equivalents for adult females.

The body's actual need for vitamin E varies with the degree of unsaturation of fats in the diet. The RDA for vitamin E is based on typical intakes by Americans. Since vitamin E protects the unsaturated bonds from oxidation, anyone who drastically increases his or her intake of polyunsaturated fatty acids needs more vitamin E.

Scientists at USDA estimate that in the United States, the average consumption of α-tocopherol by men and women is 9.8 and 7.1 α-tocopherol equivalents daily, respectively (HNIS, 1986). Both amounts are slightly less than the RDA. Data on the presence in food of other forms of vitamin E besides α-tocopherol are very limited; therefore these estimates of vitamin E intake may be somewhat low.

Dietary Sources   Among ordinary foods, plant oils (including those in grains, nuts, and seeds) provide the highest levels of vitamin E. Notice in Table 12.4 that the best sources of the most active form of vitamin E (α-tocopherol) are products that include plant oils. This means that mayonnaise and other salad dressings, many margarines, and many oils used as ingredients are good contributors of vitamin E.

A few points should be made about these outstanding vitamin E sources. First of all, many of these foods belong to the limited extras group, which makes them exceptions to the general rule that limited extras are low in micronutrients. Second, since plant foods that contain high levels of polyunsaturated fats usually also contain high levels of vitamin E, the higher need for the vitamin may be automatically satisfied when the fat is eaten. However, there is variation in the type and quantity of vitamin E compounds present in foods high in PUFAs. Third, Table 12.4 lists only the α-tocopherol content of foods. The total vitamin E activity of some foods would be higher, perhaps by 20%. Finally, you may sometimes see tocopherol listed as an ingredient in bacon. It has not been put there to improve your vitamin E status; it has been approved for use as an additive in bacon to inhibit the formation of nitrosamine, a carcinogen. (More about nitrosamine in Chapter 15.) This shows that substances we value for one attribute may have other useful characteristics as well.

Toxicity   Because of the many claims made for vitamin E, many people have consumed vitamin E supplements. Few side effects have been noted (Bendich and Machlin, 1988). However, excess intake of vitamin E may worsen a coagulation defect produced by vitamin K deficiency. An increased death rate was noted among low-birth-weight infants given an intravenous preparation of vitamin E; the cause was not identified, but the product was removed from the market (Anon, 1987).

Vitamin K

The forms of vitamin K that are synthesized by green plants are called *phylloquinones,* and those synthesized by bacteria are called *menaquinones.* A type of menaquinone is produced by humans when given a synthetic form of vitamin K called *menadione.*

Functions and Effects of Deficiency   Vitamin K is essential for the formation of several proteins necessary for blood clotting as well as for the synthesis of a variety of other proteins whose functions are still undefined. When people are very deficient in vitamin K, it takes longer than normal for their blood to clot when bleeding occurs. (Vitamin K is unrelated to the disease *hemophilia;* in that condition, other factors needed for blood clotting are deficient.)

Table 12.4 Vitamin E in Some Foods

The RDAs for men and women are 10 and 8 α-tocopherol equivalents/day, respectively.

Food	Household Measure	mg of α-Tocopherol[a]
Fruits and vegetables		
Apple	1 medium	
Corn, canned	4 ounces	
Peas, frozen	4 ounces	
Potato, boiled	1 medium	
Strawberries, raw	$\frac{1}{2}$ cup	
Grain products		
Bread, white	1 slice	
Pasta, cooked	$\frac{1}{2}$ cup	
Wheat flakes	1 ounce	
Milk and milk products		
Cheese, cheddar	$1\frac{1}{3}$ ounces	
Milk, whole	1 cup	
Meats and meat alternates		
Beef steak, broiled	2 ounces	
Chicken, frozen, fried	2 ounces	
Eggs, cooked	2 large	
Haddock, broiled	2 ounces	
Peanuts, dry roasted	2 ounces	
Combination foods		
Beef stew, canned	8 ounces	
Cheeseburger	1 sandwich	
Ravioli, chicken, canned	8 ounces	
Limited extras		
Butter	1 teaspoon	
Margarines made with soybean oil	1 teaspoon	
Mayonnaise made with soybean oil	1 tablespoon	
Milk-chocolate candy	1 ounce	

(Chart scale: 0 1.0 2.0 3.0 4.0 5.0)

[a] The bars on this chart represent the amount of the most active form of vitamin E (α-tocopherol) found in the specified servings of food. Since many other, less active forms of vitamin E are present at the same time, the total vitamin E activity of these foods is likely to be somewhat higher than these figures suggest.

Data adapted from 1) Pennington, J.A. 1989. *Food values of portions commonly used.* New York: Harper & Row and 2) Pennington, J.A. and H.N. Church. 1985. *Food values of portions commonly used.* Philadelphia: J.B. Lippincott.

Recommended Intakes In 1989, for the first time, RDAs were established for vitamin K; they are 80 μg per day for men and 65 μg per day for women. Little is known about typical intakes of vitamin K, but they have been assumed to be adequate because most individuals have normal blood clotting times. In one recent survey, diets of college-aged males were analyzed and found to contain on average 77 μg of vitamin K daily (Suttie et al., 1988). This suggests that some people may consume less than adequate amounts.

At birth, infants have very low levels of vitamin K in their bodies. If they become injured in some way—either internally or externally—their blood does not clot as quickly as an adult's blood, and excessive bleeding is likely. As a safeguard, it is recommended (and widely practiced) that infants be given an injection of vitamin K soon after birth or daily oral supplements for a short period (RDA Subcommittee, 1989).

Dietary Sources Green vegetables and tea are the leading dietary sources of vitamin K; this suggests one reason why it is important to consume green vegetables regularly. Lesser amounts are available from eggs and dairy fats. Part (but probably not all) of the body's need for vitamin K may be met by menaquinone synthesized by bacteria in the gut (RDA Subcommittee, 1989). (Individuals regularly taking large doses of antibiotics [which kill useful intestinal bacteria as well as pathogenic organisms] may require more dietary vitamin K because of reduced synthesis in the gut.) More information on dietary sources and better means of assessing the requirements for vitamin K are needed.

Thiamin, Riboflavin, and Niacin

It is logical to discuss thiamin, riboflavin, and niacin together because these water-soluble vitamins are often found in the same foods and they have related functions.

There are alternate names for these vitamins. Thiamin is also known as *vitamin B-1*, and riboflavin is referred to as *vitamin B-2*. The numbering scheme came about when early vitamin researchers named an important water-soluble factor in food *vitamin B;* when they later realized that this factor consisted of several different compounds, they attached the numbers to distinguish them from each other.

The term *niacin* refers to several compounds: *nicotinamide*, which is the active form of the vitamin, and *nicotinic acid,* which the body readily converts to the active form. (Neither of these compounds is the same as nicotine in tobacco.) In addition, the essential amino acid *tryptophan* can be converted into niacin by the body.

Functions and Effects of Deficiency Thiamin, riboflavin, and niacin all serve as **coenzymes;** that is, they unite with specific protein precursors called *apoenzymes* to create *active enzymes*. Figure 12.4 shows this relation-

coenzymes—vitamin-containing substances that unite with enzyme precursors to create active enzymes

Figure 12.4 Vitamins, coenzymes, and enzymes. Coenzymes containing vitamins are essential components of many enzymes. If the vitamin is deficient, the enzyme is inactive. However, an excess of the vitamin cannot create enzyme activity above a predetermined level.

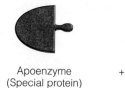

Apoenzyme
(Special protein)

+

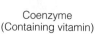

Coenzyme
(Containing vitamin)

=

Active enzyme

ship. Once an apoenzyme is fitted with coenzyme (vitamin), an additional amount of the vitamin can't increase the activity of the enzyme any further. The extra vitamin is a waste; it must be excreted or it can become toxic.

The enzymes activated by thiamin, riboflavin, and niacin have roles in energy-producing biochemical reactions involving carbohydrates, fats, proteins or amino acids, and alcohol. Figure 12.5 gives an indication of how these vitamins (and others you will read about later) enter into energy metabolism.

Since these vitamins often occur in the same foods, if intake of one of these vitamins is very poor, intakes of the other two are also likely to be low. This is especially frequent in developing parts of the world.

beriberi—disease resulting from thiamin deficiency

Severe and prolonged thiamin deficiency results in the disease **beriberi** (literally, "I cannot"). It is characterized by neuromuscular changes that may result in paralysis of the legs or heart failure; sometimes edema occurs. In developed countries, the only people apt to develop thiamin deficiency are alcoholics (more on this in Chapter 18). Riboflavin deficiency results in skin lesions that are indistinguishable from the lesions caused by several other deficiencies. **Pellagra,** the symptoms of which were historically described as diarrhea, dermatitis, dementia (mental illness), and death, is often ascribed to niacin deficiency.

pellagra—disease resulting from niacin deficiency (or possibly a combination of vitamin deficiencies)

Of these three, pellagra has probably affected the greatest number of people as an isolated disease. The disease (but not its cause) has been known for centuries. During an outbreak in the United States between 1905 and 1910, a scientist noted that the diets of people with pellagra were lacking in meat, milk, and eggs and that when dietary intake of these foods increased, the patients improved.

This finding suggested that pellagra was a nutritional deficiency rather than a disease caused by a microorganism. The theory was later confirmed when another researcher administered body substances including waste products from those affected with pellagra to healthy volunteers; the healthy people did not get the disease. (Such a research proposal would probably not be approved today by a committee concerned with the ethical use of human subjects.) Although pellagra was believed to be caused by niacin deficiency alone, this is probably an oversimplification (Carpenter and Lewin, 1985).

Recommended and Typical Intakes   In keeping with their primary roles in energy metabolism, these vitamins should be consumed (according to RDA committee recommendations) in amounts directly proportional to energy intake: the more kcalories a person's diet contains, the higher the intake of these vitamins should be. This is accomplished fairly effortlessly since foods that provide a lot of energy are also likely to contain these vitamins (provided they are not low-nutrient-density foods). The RDAs established for men and women reflect appropriate vitamin intakes for people in the United States with average energy usage. For thiamin and riboflavin, the adult RDAs are between 1 and 2 mg/day; for niacin, they are between 13 and 19 niacin equivalents. The average American consumes more than 100% of the RDA for these vitamins (HNIS, 1985).

Niacin is one of the vitamins whose requirements are expressed in equivalents (NE). This approach makes it possible to take into account niacin that can be converted from the amino acid tryptophan (60 mg tryptophan = 1 NE) as well as the preformed versions.

Dietary Sources   A national survey showed grain products, fruits, and vegetables to be the origin of approximately 40–60% of the thiamin, riboflavin, and niacin Americans consume. Whole grains make a significant contribution, as do enriched and fortified grain products. (More will be said about enrichment and fortification in Chapter 14.) Milk and milk products and meats and meat alternatives can also be excellent sources, as shown in Table 12.5.

Consequences of High Intake   Niacin is the only one of these three vitamins for which many instances of toxic effects have been reported (McCormick, 1989). High doses of nicotinic acid, a form of niacin, can cause transient flushing (particularly of the face and neck), widespread itching, and nausea; but these symptoms often decrease with time. Occasionally, chronic use of high doses of nicotinic acid is associated with high blood sugar and uric acid and with liver damage.

The vitamin supplement industry has promoted the idea that high intakes of thiamin, riboflavin, niacin, and assorted other vitamins will help relieve psychological stress. But one pharmaceutical company that produces a so-called stress vitamin supplement was taken to court and fined for making false and misleading claims to this effect (Nutrition Forum, 1986). There have also been claims that megavitamin therapy was helpful in the treatment of schizophrenia; but when these treatments were tested in well-designed studies, they were not found to be effective (Ban, 1981). It is important to remember that although a prolonged deficiency of niacin can cause mental symptoms, very high doses of niacin cannot cure mental illness of other causes in an adequately nourished person.

Similarly pharmaceutical companies sometimes imply that B vitamins are

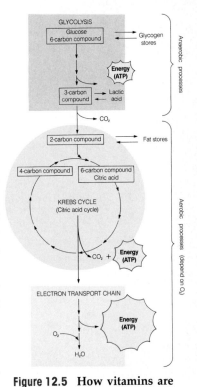

Figure 12.5 How vitamins are involved in metabolism.
Many of the water-soluble vitamins are involved in the biochemical pathways that produce energy from foods. Thiamin, riboflavin, niacin, biotin, and pantothenic acid are part of coenzymes for various reactions in glycolysis. Those same five vitamins—plus vitamin B-6, folic acid, and vitamin B-12—are part of coenzymes needed for conversion of protein, fat, and glycogen into compounds that ultimately can be used in the citric acid cycle and the electron transport chain.

sources of energy. This is not true. They are not a source of kcalories (energy).

Large doses of vitamins have sometimes been used in an attempt to achieve legitimate therapeutic benefits; in such cases, the vitamin is functioning as a drug rather than as a nutrient. For example, large doses of niacin (3–12 g/day) are sometimes used to lower blood cholesterol levels in patients whose high cholesterol levels do not respond adequately to modifications of their diets (Anon., 1989). This therapy is promising, but the toxic side effects of niacin are sometimes problematic; therefore, this drug therapy should *be used only by patients under a physician's close supervision.*

Table 12.5 Thiamin, Riboflavin, and Niacin in Some Foods

The RDA for thiamin for women aged 19–50 is 1.1 mg; for men it is 1.5 mg.

The RDA for riboflavin for women aged 19–50 is 1.3 mg; for men it is 1.7 mg.

The RDA for niacin for women aged 19–50 is 15 niacin equivalents (NE); for men it is 19 NE. The niacin values on this table do not account for the presence of the niacin precursor tryptophan. Foods with significant levels of protein (which contains the amino acid tryptophan) have greater niacin activity than these values show.

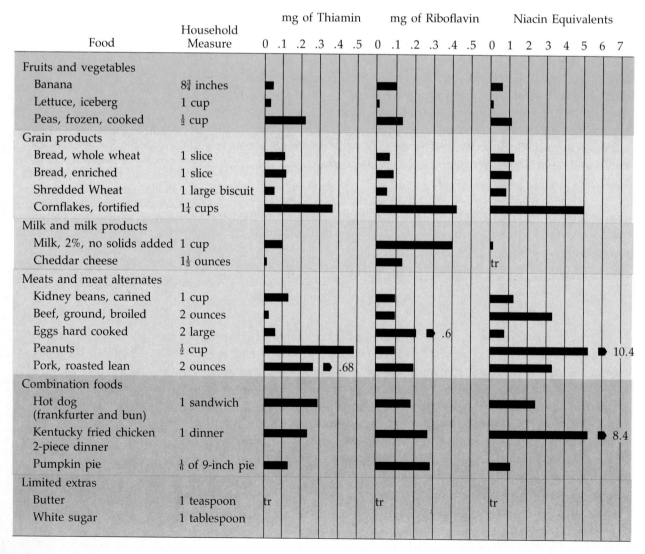

Vitamin B-6

Vitamin B-6 occurs in food in three forms: *pyridoxine, pyridoxamine,* and *pyridoxal.* They are closely related structurally and have equivalent vitamin activity.

Functions and Effects of Deficiency Like other B vitamins, vitamin B-6 serves as a coenzyme. Many reactions involved in protein metabolism, such as the conversion of essential amino acids to nonessential amino acids, require vitamin B-6. Vitamin B-6 also participates in the production and transformation of tryptophan to niacin as well as other important body reactions. Symptoms seen in association with vitamin B-6 deficiency most often involve nervous system problems such as depression, confusion, and convulsions; dermatitis; and anemia.

Recommended and Typical Intakes Because of the importance of vitamin B-6 in protein metabolism, this vitamin is thought to be needed in direct proportion to the amount of protein in the diet. The adult RDAs for vitamin B-6 of 2.0 mg/day for men and 1.6 mg/day for women are based on average American protein intakes.

In 1985, the average vitamin B-6 intake of adult men in the United States was slightly below the RDA, but that of women was less than 75% of the RDA. It seems that American women don't do as good a job of getting this vitamin as they do most others. However, this does not necessarily mean that all American women are deficient in vitamin B-6; deficiency can be determined only by biochemical testing.

Dietary Sources Meats and meat alternates are generally good sources of vitamin B-6. Fruits and vegetables are less consistent sources. Grain and milk products provide lesser amounts, as shown in Table 12.6. Suggestions for increasing the intake of this vitamin are to include larger servings of nuts, flesh proteins, and/or the better fruit and vegetable sources. However, your body does not generally utilize vitamin B-6 from plant sources as well as those from animal sources. This decrease in bioavailability (biological utilization) of vitamin B-6 only further emphasizes the potential for inadequate intakes by some. (The concept of bioavailability will be more thoroughly discussed in Chapter 13 [on minerals].)

Consequences of High Intake Excess vitamin B-6 is excreted in the urine. In the past, this led people to believe that it was harmless—until reports of toxicity started to appear in the medical literature. Individuals who took anywhere from 200 to 6000 mg of vitamin B-6 per day, which is 100 times to 3000 times the RDA, developed sensory neuropathies (nerve disorders) (Schaumberg et al., 1983; Parry and Bredesen, 1985). Symptoms appeared one month to three years after starting vitamin B-6 supplementation.

Why had people been taking these huge amounts of vitamin B-6? They took them because they thought the supplements would give them relief

premenstrual syndrome (PMS)— physical and/or emotional symptoms experienced by some women before menstruation that decrease or disappear during or after menstruation

from **premenstrual syndrome** (especially water retention), provide a general sense of well-being, and offer improvement of a psychiatric condition. However, in a well-designed clinical study, no benefits from therapy with vitamin B-6 could be shown (Mira et al., 1988).

The next Slice of Life (on page 407) describes one person's experience with vitamin B-6 supplementation.

Table 12.6 Vitamin B-6 in Some Foods

The RDA for vitamin B-6 for women is 1.6 mg; for men it is 2.0 mg.

Food	Household Measure	mg of Vitamin B-6
Fruits and vegetables		
Apple	1 medium	
Banana	8¾ inches	
Cantaloupe	½ cup	
Green beans, frozen, cooked	½ cup	
Potato, baked	1 large	
Prunes, cooked	½ cup	
Spinach, chopped, raw	½ cup	
Grain products		
Bread, whole wheat	1 slice	
Cookies, chocolate chip	2 average	
Crackers, Saltines	4 squares	
Tortilla, corn	1 average	
Popcorn, popped, oil	3 cups	
Milk and milk products		
Cheese, cheddar	1⅓ ounces	
Milk, skim or whole	1 cup	
Meats and meat alternates		
Beef, lean, cooked	2 ounces	
Chicken, light meat, no skin, cooked	2 ounces	
Cod, baked	2 ounces	
Eggs	2 large	
Lima beans, canned	1 cup	
Peanut butter	¼ cup	
Tuna, canned in water	2 ounces	
Combination foods		
Chicken à la king, frozen	1 cup	
Macaroni and cheese, homemade	1 cup	
Split-pea soup with ham, canned	1 cup	
Limited extras		
Butter	1 teaspoon	tr
Carbonated beverages	12 ounces	
Coffee	6 ounces	

Folic Acid and Vitamin B-12

Folic acid and vitamin B-12 are discussed together because each is a part of coenzymes involved in DNA and RNA metabolism.

Each of these vitamins includes a number of compounds. The terms *folate* and *folacin* are used to describe compounds that have nutritional properties of folic acid (also known as *pteroylglutamic acid*). Vitamin B-12 includes a group of cobalt-containing compounds known as *cobalamins*.

Slice of Life

Harm from a Vitamin Rather Than Help

Six months ago, Samantha had started taking supplements of vitamin B-6 in the hope that it would make her problems with premenstrual syndrome go away. She had read in a magazine that vitamin B-6 supplements could provide relief, and that was a wonderful prospect.

Samantha hated the week before her menstrual period—she always felt bloated, tired, irritable, and depressed. She craved certain foods. Sometimes she had headaches and backaches, and it was hard for her to concentrate. Her boyfriend had once asked her, "What's making you so grouchy these days, Sam? It's just not like you."

Maybe these supplements would be the solution. The article said to take 1000 mg per day. She had done that for the first month without results, so in the second month she increased her intake to 2000 mg per day. That month, she wasn't sure it was helping; to hurry things along, she started taking 3000 mg.

Then some strange things began to happen. When she bent her head down, a tingling sensation ran down her neck and back, into her legs and to the soles of her feet. At other times, her feet felt numb, her coordination was off, and she had to

steady herself. Then the numbness went to her hands as well, and she became clumsy when handling things. At this point, she knew something was seriously wrong, but she didn't suspect the supplements.

A neurologist made the connection. In addition to her muscular problems, he found that her sensations of touch, temperature, pinpricks, vibration, and joint position were severely impaired in both arms and legs. Biochemical tests confirmed his suspicion that Samantha was experiencing vitamin B-6 toxicity.

Fortunately, the damage to her nervous system was not permanent. A year after discontinuing the supplements, she felt fairly normal and could function as before.

Of course, she still was contending with premenstrual syndrome, but after this experience, she was convinced not to use large doses of any nutritional supplements even though she still occasionally saw that advice in magazines and newspapers. Instead, she sought the help of a gynecologist who recommended more moderate measures: a balanced diet, an exercise program, and medication for the most troublesome symptoms. The physician pointed out that much remains to be learned about the cause and treatment of PMS; one of the unexpected findings along the way has been the discovery that large doses of vitamin B-6 can be a potentially dangerous treatment (Schaumburg et al., 1983). ▲

Functions and Effects of Deficiency Since DNA and RNA are the substances that direct cell division, these vitamins are especially important during periods of growth. In addition, folic acid and vitamin B-12 are important in the metabolism of certain amino acids (see Figure 12.5) and the transfer of single carbon units between various biochemical compounds in the body.

Deficiencies of either of these vitamins produce a form of anemia characterized by large, immature red blood cells, a condition called **megaloblastic anemia.** In cases where anemia has been produced by an inadequacy of vitamin B-12, treatment with large amounts of folic acid will normalize the red blood cells. However, folic acid cannot substitute for B-12 in other ways; for example, it cannot prevent the nerve damage that vitamin B-12 deficiency also produces. It is dangerous to take folic acid if it is possible that B-12 deficiency is the problem; the folic acid will mask the B-12 deficiency, and the nerve damage will progress insidiously. For this reason, it is critical that the cause of the megaloblastic anemia be accurately determined so that the appropriate vitamin can be given to treat the deficiency.

At least one large survey has indicated that the infants of women who had consumed multivitamin supplements containing folic acid during the first six weeks of pregnancy had a reduced risk of neural tube defects (birth defects affecting the central nervous system) compared with women who did not take the supplements (Milunsky et al., 1989). The data are speculative and *at most* warrant use of a standard one-a-day multivitamin during pregnancy.

Recommended and Typical Intakes

The RDA for folic acid for men is 200 μg; for women it is 180 μg. The 1989 RDA advises pregnant women to get 400 μg per day through careful selection of food; this recommendation contrasts with previous ones that encouraged physicians to prescribe folate supplements for their pregnant patients. Except during pregnancy, Americans appear generally to take in enough folic acid.

For vitamin B-12, the RDA is 2 μg for both men and women. Most people's intake of vitamin B-12 comfortably exceeds the RDA. Vegans are at risk for B-12 deficiency because, as you will see in the next section, vitamin B-12 is not produced by plants. Vegans need a supplement of vitamin B-12 or to consume foods fortified with vitamin B-12. If a pregnant or lactating woman does not consume vitamin B-12, the baby may experience a deficiency (Specker et al., 1988).

The presence of vitamin B-12 in the diet does not guarantee that it will be absorbed. Absorption of this vitamin depends on the presence of a substance called **intrinsic factor,** which is produced by the lining of the stomach. If intrinsic factor is absent, only about 1% of dietary B-12 is absorbed; when intrinsic factor is present, amounts up to the RDA may be absorbed from one meal (Herbert and Colman, 1988). The production of intrinsic factor sometimes decreases in the elderly, so older people may become defi-

megaloblastic anemia—form of anemia characterized by large, immature red blood cells

intrinsic factor—substance produced by the stomach lining; enhances vitamin B-12 absorption

cient in the vitamin even if their diets contain RDA levels of it. This deficiency disease is called **pernicious anemia;** people who have it are usually given periodic injections of vitamin B-12.

pernicious anemia—anemia resulting from the inadequate production of intrinsic factor, which leads to the inadequate absorption of vitamin B-12 despite its presence in the diet

Dietary Sources Several foods in each of the food groups contain significant amounts of folic acid. The only type of basic food notably low in this vitamin is flesh protein (Table 12.7). Contributors of relatively large amounts of folic acid are fruits, vegetables, legumes, and some grain products. (The terms related to *folic acid* come from the same root word as *foliage*.)

The food sources of vitamin B-12 are considerably different from those of folacin. Foods of animal origin are the only reliable sources of vitamin B-12 (Table 12.7). Since vegans avoid these foods, they need to consume a vitamin B-12 supplement or a food fortified with the vitamin to achieve the recommended level of intake.

Pantothenic Acid and Biotin

The vitamins pantothenic acid (or *pantothenate*) and biotin are both components of enzymes involved in energy metabolism. Pantothenic acid is also involved in the synthesis of other vital body substances.

The Greek word from which *pantothenic* was derived means "from all sides," and the reference is appropriate because of the widespread distribution and usefulness of this nutrient. Pantothenic acid is so generally available among common foods that scientists have been unable to induce a deficiency experimentally.

A deficiency of biotin can produce diverse problems such as dermatitis and neuromuscular disorders. Healthy individuals who eat a reasonably balanced diet are unlikely to experience a biotin deficiency, but deficiencies of biotin occur in patients with genetic defects (McCormick, 1988). A deficiency could be caused by consumption of large amounts of a compound that could bind the vitamin in the intestine and make it unavailable for absorption. (Raw egg whites contain such a compound, called *avidin*. You would have to consume most of your diet as raw egg white to induce such a deficiency.)

Vitamin C

Vitamin C has a couple of aliases—*ascorbic acid* and *ascorbate*. This vitamin is probably the most familiar to the general public; it is also the most popular vitamin supplement (Nutrition Reviews, 1990). Even though this vitamin–like all vitamins–is essential, whether it deserves this elevated public status is debatable.

Functions and Effects of Deficiency The disease resulting from a deficiency of vitamin C is **scurvy.** It was first recognized by the Egyptians before

scurvy—disease resulting from vitamin C deficiency

1500 BC. It was the scourge of Greek and Roman armies and navies because typical military rations were devoid of good sources of vitamin C. Scurvy also plagued the crewmen who came to America with explorer Jacques Cartier in the 1500s. Fortunately, the Indians knew the cure: they steeped a tea from the needles of a certain type of evergreen tree and gave it to the sick

Table 12.7 Folic Acid and Vitamin B-12 in Some Foods

The RDAs for folic acid for women and men are 180 and 200 μg, respectively. The RDA for vitamin B-12 for both women and men is 2 μg.

Food	Household Measure	μg of Folic Acid (0 100 200)	μg of Vitamin B-12 (0 1.0 2.0 3.0)
Fruits and vegetables			
Banana	$8\frac{3}{4}$ inches		
Broccoli, fresh, cooked	$\frac{1}{2}$ cup		
Green beans, cooked	$\frac{1}{2}$ cup		
Lettuce, iceberg	1 cup		
Lettuce, romaine	1 cup		
Orange juice	$\frac{1}{2}$ cup		
Potatoes, mashed	$\frac{1}{2}$ cup		
Grain products			
Bread, whole wheat	1 slice		
Cake, chocolate with icing	1 wedge		
Cornflakes, fortified	$1\frac{1}{4}$ cups		
Rice, brown, cooked	$\frac{1}{2}$ cup		
Milk and milk products			
Milk, whole	1 cup		
Cheese, cheddar	$1\frac{1}{3}$ ounces		
Yogurt	1 cup		
Meats and meat alternates			
Beef, lean, cooked	2 ounces		
Chicken, dark, cooked	2 ounces		
Codfish, baked	2 ounces		
Salmon, canned	2 ounces		
Eggs, hard cooked	2 large		
Peanuts	$\frac{1}{2}$ cup		
Pinto beans	1 cup		
Walnuts, English	$\frac{1}{2}$ cup		
Combination foods			
Beef, macaroni, and tomato-sauce casserole	1 cup		
Chicken curry, homemade	1 cup		
Enchilada, cheese	4 ounces		
Limited extras			
Butter	1 teaspoon	tr	tr
Mayonnaise	1 tablespoon	tr	

men. The needles, we now know, contained small amounts of vitamin C. Because of the lifesaving brew, the tree was named *arborvitae,* meaning "tree of life." Later, in the 1700s, British sailors cured or prevented scurvy by eating citrus fruit and so earned themselves the nickname limeys.

Although a great deal of research has been done on vitamin C over the years, we do not yet understand exactly what vitamin C does at the cellular level (Hornig et al., 1988). It is needed for the formation of collagen, the protein that serves so many connective functions in the body. Among the body's collagen-containing materials and structures are the framework of bone; the gingivae (gums); and the binding materials in skin, muscle, and scar tissue. Vitamin C is also necessary for the production of certain hormones and neurotransmitters, and it is needed for the metabolism of some amino acids and vitamins.

In addition, it aids blood cells in fighting infection, the liver in detoxifying dangerous substances, and the gut in absorbing iron from foods. With such wide-ranging functions, it is not surprising that the symptoms of vitamin C deficiency are diverse: generalized feelings of weakness, bleeding gums and loosened teeth, easy bruising and small hemorrhages in the skin, and impaired immune function.

Recommended and Typical Intakes The adult RDA for vitamin C is 60 mg/day. Generally, Americans do not find it difficult to achieve this intake: the average consumption exceeds 135% of the RDA (HNIS, 1985). However, the 1989 RDA Subcommittee recommends that regular cigarette smokers consume at least 100 mg of vitamin C daily, since it is metabolized more rapidly in smokers. This suggests that smokers should be deliberate about including *two* servings of a good source of vitamin C in their diets every day.

Dietary Sources Many common fruits and vegetables have such a high content of vitamin C that they furnish half or more of the RDA in one serving. The citrus fruits have a well-deserved reputation in this regard, but they are not alone: broccoli, cabbage, cantaloupe (muskmelon), cauliflower, green peppers, and strawberries are also excellent sources. Many other fruits and vegetables make smaller though still significant contributions, but nature has provided very little vitamin C in other types of foods (Table 12.8).

Vitamin C is *added* to many products, however. Many kinds of beverages are supplemented with vitamin C: fruit juices, fruit-flavored drinks, and some carbonated beverages are fortified with it; even some cereals are. Some people also take concentrated vitamin C in pill form. Considering all these sources, both natural and supplemental, it is no wonder that Americans generally get more than the RDA for vitamin C.

Consequences of High Intake Many people experience diarrhea when they consume too much vitamin C. Large doses of vitamin C also interfere with several laboratory tests; for example, the standard test for colon cancer may yield a false-negative result in those who have taken large amounts of vitamin C (Hornig et al., 1988).

Large excesses of vitamin C have been accused of causing other negative effects, but such effects have not been proved in controlled studies (Hornig et al., 1988). For example, several scientists still think that some people may require more vitamin C to prevent scurvy after their bodies have become used to very large doses (Omaye et al., 1988), but this is debatable.

Table 12.8 Vitamin C in Some Foods

The RDA for vitamin C for both women and men is 60 mg.

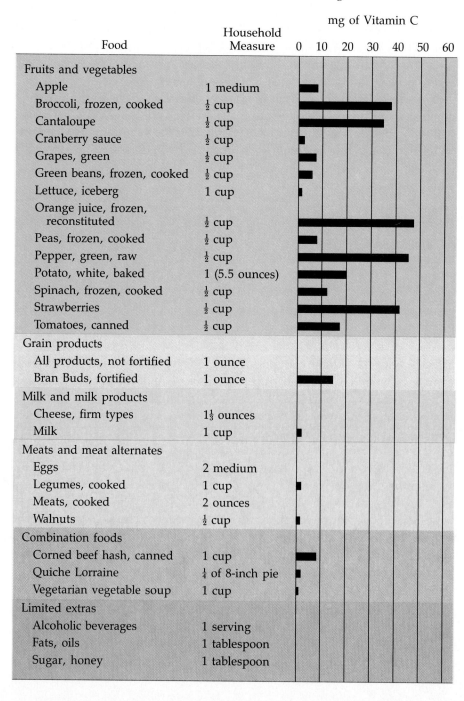

Food	Household Measure	mg of Vitamin C
Fruits and vegetables		
Apple	1 medium	
Broccoli, frozen, cooked	½ cup	
Cantaloupe	½ cup	
Cranberry sauce	½ cup	
Grapes, green	½ cup	
Green beans, frozen, cooked	½ cup	
Lettuce, iceberg	1 cup	
Orange juice, frozen, reconstituted	½ cup	
Peas, frozen, cooked	½ cup	
Pepper, green, raw	½ cup	
Potato, white, baked	1 (5.5 ounces)	
Spinach, frozen, cooked	½ cup	
Strawberries	½ cup	
Tomatoes, canned	½ cup	
Grain products		
All products, not fortified	1 ounce	
Bran Buds, fortified	1 ounce	
Milk and milk products		
Cheese, firm types	1⅓ ounces	
Milk	1 cup	
Meats and meat alternates		
Eggs	2 medium	
Legumes, cooked	1 cup	
Meats, cooked	2 ounces	
Walnuts	½ cup	
Combination foods		
Corned beef hash, canned	1 cup	
Quiche Lorraine	¼ of 8-inch pie	
Vegetarian vegetable soup	1 cup	
Limited extras		
Alcoholic beverages	1 serving	
Fats, oils	1 tablespoon	
Sugar, honey	1 tablespoon	

Pharmaceutic Uses of Vitamin C   Vitamin C has been actively promoted for preventing and curing colds and cancer. We need to examine these claims.

We can attribute the idea that massive doses of vitamin C prevents colds to Linus Pauling, who won a Nobel Prize in physical chemistry in the mid-1950s. He formed the hypothesis that humans, because their bodies do not produce ascorbic acid as do those of many other animals, need megadoses of it to achieve the levels produced (and therefore assumed to be needed) by these other animals.

Based on observations of animals whose bodies function quite differently from those of humans, he recommended taking as much as several grams of vitamin C every day. (The RDA is 60 mg.) He claimed there would be many benefits, including fewer colds. Many people, influenced by his excellent reputation and the simplicity of his recommendation, began taking the doses he recommended. Subsequently, various double-blind studies involving hundreds of subjects were conducted to test the effect of supplemental vitamin C on the incidence and treatment of colds. This chapter's Critical Thinking discusses this research and helps you consider options for your own use.

The other issue is cancer: can supplements of vitamin C be used to prevent cancer or extend the life of a person who has it? The evidence argues against a treatment role. Although Linus Pauling and colleagues claim that large doses of vitamin C can extend the life of people with cancer and help them feel better, a study done at the Mayo Clinic demonstrated no benefit from the vitamin C therapy (Nutrition Reviews, 1986).

Scientists do not agree on whether vitamin C can help prevent cancer. Like vitamin E, it is an antioxidant. Furthermore, vitamin C may have a protective effect among smokers and people who frequently consume nitrosamine, a compound that causes stomach cancer (Surgeon General, 1988). (Nitrosamines will be discussed further in Chapter 15 [on toxicants].)

The Surgeon General's Report on Nutrition and Health sums up the controversy this way: "Despite limitations in data, the American Cancer Society guidelines recommend foods rich in vitamins A and C and the National Cancer Institute suggests eating a variety of fruits and vegetables, thus ensuring an adequate supply of vitamin C. There is no adequate evidence that larger amounts of vitamin C provide any additional benefits."

Nonvitamins

Some substances that are not essential for humans have been touted recently. Although several of these are involved in metabolic reactions, they are produced in adequate amounts within the healthy body, so they cannot be categorized as vitamins. Among these substances are rutin, inositol, carnitine, para-aminobenzoic acid (PABA), bioflavinoids (dubbed "vitamin P" by some), and lipoic acid.

Choline is another nonvitamin of particular interest. It is a component of the neurotransmitter acetylcholine, which is present in lower-than-normal levels in people who have certain nervous disorders. For this reason, it is being tested as part of the treatment for those conditions. There is no evidence, however, that normally healthy people would benefit in any way from taking supplemental choline. Choline is usually found in foods as a component of the phospholipid lecithin (Chapter 7).

Although these substances are not vitamins, they are nonetheless marketed by some dietary supplement manufacturers, who welcome having another product to sell. For normally healthy people who consume them, the only possible benefit is from the placebo effect—that is, if consumers believe that the substance will make them feel better, there may be some perceived improvement.

Other nonvitamins are more worrisome to scientists because they may actually be harmful in some instances. "Vitamin B-17," or laetrile, is one

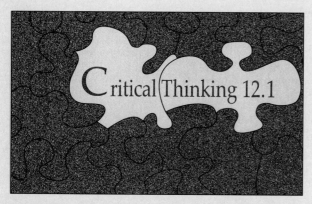

Do Vitamin C Supplements Prevent Colds?

The situation

The person you share an apartment with has just come down with a cold. She feels miserable—not only because of the cold, but also because she does not feel well enough to continue studying for a particularly important exam she has tomorrow.

You are at the beginning of a very demanding couple of weeks yourself, and catching a cold would certainly interfere with accomplishing everything you need to. You think about what you might do to avoid the cold. One thing that crosses your mind is vitamin C; you have heard that taking vitamin C supplements can prevent a cold or cure it faster if you do get one. You wonder how much you would need to take.

Is the information accurate and relevant?

■ It is true that vitamin C is important to the functioning of the immune system; if a person's average intake of vitamin C is substantially below the RDA for a long period of time, the function of the immune system is impaired. This would make a person less able to combat all types of contagions effectively, not just colds.

■ Other nutrients are also needed for the immune system to function effectively. If the intake of almost any of the vitamins is deficient for a long period of time, immune functions are compromised; the same is true if there is long-standing protein deficiency.

■ Studies have been done regarding the effectiveness of vitamin C supplements in preventing and treating colds, with mixed results (next section).

What else needs to be considered?

A number of studies have been done to determine whether vitamin C supplements prevent colds, and the results do not agree. One scientist claims to have clinical evidence that such supplements are effective, but the research has not yet been published (Dick, 1989). In most large epidemiologic studies, however, there was no *statistically sig-*

such substance. Laetrile contains the poison cyanide, making consumption of large amounts dangerous. Although laetrile has sometimes been used as a cancer treatment, scientific tests find it ineffective for this purpose; the primary concern is that its use may delay or substitute for treatments that *could* slow down or arrest the disease (more on laetrile in Chapter 15).

Additional Important Concepts Warrant Emphasis

Now that we have dealt with various details about vitamins, it is appropriate to stand back and identify some other concepts about them.

nificant difference in the incidence of colds between groups that received supplemental vitamin C and those that did not.

Some studies showed a *very small* decrease in the number of colds among people taking vitamin C (Anderson, 1978). Another study (Baird et al., 1979) demonstrated that 80 mg of vitamin C had a *slight effect similar to that of the larger doses* of purified vitamin C used in several earlier studies. If vitamin C does slightly reduce a person's likelihood of getting colds, this study indicates that the same benefit can be had from drinking an extra cup of orange juice per day; the large supplements of vitamin C appear to yield no better results.

Another point of interest is that large epidemiologic studies of vitamin C supplements and colds often did not include an assessment of the amount of vitamin C in the diets of the subjects. It is possible that people who appeared to benefit from the supplements had been consuming inadequate levels in their diets, and the supplements made up for the dietary deficiencies.

As far as the *treatment* of colds is concerned, the evidence is somewhat more positive; vitamin C supplements taken during a cold reduced the severity of the symptoms in some people during the first few days of the cold (Anderson, 1978). Also, some people taking supplements spent less time at home with the cold—an average of half a day less. This may be due to the antihistaminic effect that vitamin C sometimes has (Clemetson, 1980).

Nonetheless, the total number of days that people's colds lasted did not differ from one group to the other (Anderson, 1978).

The authors of the 1989 RDA noted: "Several reviewers have concluded that any benefits of large doses of ascorbic acid for these conditions are too small to justify recommending routine intake of large amounts . . . ."

What do you think?

- Option 1   You decide to follow the Basic Food Guide for selecting your daily food, making sure you get *one* good source of vitamin C every day.
- Option 2   You decide to follow the Basic Food Guide for selecting your daily food and make sure you get *two* good sources of vitamin C every day.
- Option 3   You decide to take a supplement of 60 mg of vitamin C every day (the adult RDA).
- Option 4   You decide to take a daily multivitamin supplement that does not exceed 100% of the U.S. RDA for any of the nutrients.

Do you see any other safe and effective nutrition-related options? Which makes the most sense to you? What additional strategies could you use to reduce your risk of catching the cold?

Vitamin Deficiencies

Generally, vitamin deficiencies occur when:

1. The diet is limited to only a few types of foods.
2. The diet is limited in overall quantity.
3. The individual cannot absorb or utilize vitamin(s) to a normal extent owing to inborn problems, disease conditions, or alcohol or other drug use.
4. The requirements for vitamins are unusually high when there is rapid growth or disease.

Most of the people who experience vitamin deficiencies are those who simply do not get enough to eat; most of them live in the developing countries. They are more likely to have multiple deficiencies than a single, independent vitamin deficiency. The notable exception is vitamin A; in areas of the world where good sources of vitamin A are not commonly consumed, this deficiency does often occur by itself.

Each vitamin affects the whole body; a person who has a vitamin deficiency often feels weak, fails to grow or reproduce, and is more susceptible to illnesses. Marginal deficiencies are apt to be related to impaired immune function (Beisel, 1982). In addition, some vitamin deficiencies have obvious effects on specific body tissues. Certain signs and symptoms are associated with particular deficiency diseases, but such clues by themselves are not adequate for diagnosing vitamin deficiencies. Biochemical tests should be used to identify both serious and less severe vitamin deficiencies.

The amount of time it takes to develop a vitamin deficiency varies greatly according to the vitamin, the severity of the deficiency, and other dietary factors. Scurvy probably develops the fastest—in about two months. Deficiencies of vitamin A or B-12 take a great deal longer to develop. Age is also a factor; deficiencies tend to develop more rapidly in children than in adults, and individual variability has an effect independent of age.

Vitamin Toxicities

People who ingest very large amounts of vitamins also put themselves at risk for developing health problems. Vitamin toxicities are more apt to occur when:

1. Individuals regularly consume nutrient supplements, especially those containing large amounts of one nutrient, for several weeks or months.
2. Body size is small; for example, children and women are more prone to toxicity because the dose per body mass is greater.
3. Development is still occurring; that's why fetuses and young infants are more apt to suffer permanent effects.

Therefore, although it is *possible* to incur vitamin toxicity by eating too much food with a very high vitamin density (such as liver), the most common cause of vitamin toxicity is the ingestion of vitamin supplements in excessive quantities for a long period of time. Most people who incur vitamin toxicities have been overdosing at ten or more times the RDA (often referred to as *megadosing*) for anywhere from a few months to a few years before they seek help for their vitamin-caused problems. But you can't count on it taking that long: sometimes toxicities occur more quickly and with less excessive intakes, especially in the case of vitamin D.

Every year, approximately 4000 people receive treatment for vitamin supplement poisoning (Dubick and Rucker, 1983). Many are unaware that substances that are essential at one level can be harmful at higher doses. This is an important concept to understand, since approximately 36% of the American public takes vitamin supplements regularly (Moss et al., 1989). One distinguished nutritional scientist has noted that "some food faddists are performing self-experimentation studies with combinations and doses of single nutrients never previously envisioned [by scientists]" (Beisel, 1982).

Toxicity can affect all the body's tissues and systems, just as deficiencies can. Just as there are classic symptoms of vitamin deficiency, typical indicators of vitamin excesses are increasingly being recognized.

The Advisability of Vitamin Supplementation

The preceding sections suggest that there are benefits and risks to vitamin supplementation. How can you know who will be helped and who will be harmed? Who needs vitamin supplements and who doesn't?

In 1987, the American Medical Association's Council on Scientific Affairs offered guidance in a report called "Vitamin Preparations as Dietary Supplements and as Therapeutic Agents." It emphasized that most healthy adult men and women eating a typical, varied diet do not need vitamin supplements but that there are various categories of people who *do* benefit from supplements.

The types of people the report focused on were those who have medically diagnosed vitamin deficiencies, those who have certain pathological conditions or diseases, and those who routinely take medications that increase the need for vitamins (more on this in Chapter 18). Vitamin supplements should be prescribed as a part of treatment for people in these categories according to each patient's individual needs.

The AMA's report also describes several groups of generally healthy people who benefit from supplemental vitamins. *Vegans* need to get vitamin B-12 from supplements because it is not generally available in their diets; *vegan children* may also need supplemental riboflavin and vitamin D. *Pregnant and lactating women* may benefit from a multivitamin supplement, since their needs are somewhat higher at these times. (However, not all experts agree with the need for vitamin supplements during pregnancy [see footnote, Table 12.9].) A good general rule is not to take supplements that pro-

Vitamin supplementation.
Approximately 36% of Americans take vitamin supplements routinely. In some instances, modest supplements of up to 100% of the U.S. RDA are useful; however, at high intakes there is a danger of overdose.

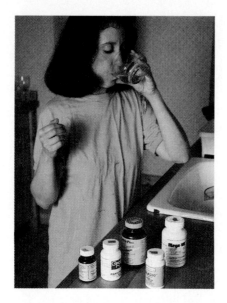

vide more than 100% of the U.S. RDA for any nutrient (National Research Council, 1989).

All *newborns* need to receive vitamin K, and *infants under one year of age* may need various vitamin supplements, depending on what kind of milk they are fed (more on this in Chapter 16). The *elderly*, too, may benefit from supplements, especially if their food intake diminishes. In fact, *anyone whose energy intake decreases dramatically for any reason*—and this includes weight-reduction dieting—would probably benefit from a modest vitamin supplement.

These points are summarized in Table 12.9.

Table 12.9 Healthy People for Whom Vitamin Supplements Are Recommended

Advisability of Supplementation	Who Needs Supplement	Vitamin(s) to Be Supplemented
Recommended in all cases	Newborns	Vitamin K
	Vegans	Vitamin B-12; possibly riboflavin and vitamin D, especially for vegan children
Often recommended	Pregnant[a] and lactating women	Multivitamin
	Infants up to 1 year of age	Depends on what milk is used; pediatrician should advise
	Older adults	Multivitamin
	People with low energy intake, including those on weight-reduction diets	Multivitamin

[a] Moderate vitamin supplementation during pregnancy has been a longstanding medical practice. However, the Committee on Nutritional Status During Pregnancy and Lactation, of the National Academy of Sciences, stated in their 1990 report *Nutrition During Pregnancy* that the increased needs for vitamins during pregnancy could be met with a well-selected diet alone (Committee on Nutritional Status, 1990).

Note that taking a vitamin supplement does not ensure that all a person's nutritional needs will be met. Since there are approximately 50 essential nutrients, getting an adequate intake of only the 13 vitamins does not constitute good nutrition. This chapter's Nutrition for Living offers guidelines for achieving adequate vitamin intake.

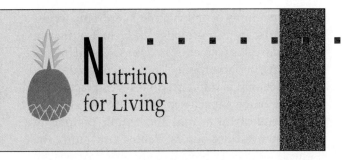

Nutrition for Living

Most people have heard that they can get the vitamins they need from food, but the marketplace sends the conflicting message to use vitamin supplements and eat foods that have had nutrients added to them. Some straightforward guidelines may help resolve the inevitable confusion.

The purpose of this section is to suggest how all three sources of vitamins—foods as nature produced them, foods fortified with vitamins during processing, and concentrated vitamin supplements—can be sensibly used to achieve the levels of vitamins you need and to avoid risk of toxicity.

■ If you consume the types of food in at least the minimal amounts recommended by the Basic Food Guide, you will get adequate intakes of most vitamins on most days. Remember: that means consciously choosing one source of a significant amount of vitamin C and one source of vitamin A each day. If you need to eat more than is suggested by the minimal number of servings (many people do), select most of your additional food from the basic food groups.

■ Foods that are fortified with vitamins during processing can make valuable contributions to your nutrient intake, especially if the fortification replaces vitamins lost during processing. However, be aware that fortification does not usually replace all lost nutrients (see Chapter 14).

■ Some foods are so heavily fortified that they contain 100% of a day's vitamin needs per serving. This is not necessary and usually represents overkill. Some say such foods are vitamin pills masquerading as foods. In some cases, fortified foods represent silly applications of a basically useful process. For example, adding a few vitamins to chewing gum or candy does not do much to improve overall nutrition, and it may delude people into thinking that those foods are more nutritious than they are.

■ If you choose to take a vitamin supplement, take a multivitamin that provides no more than 100% of the U.S. RDA. This should not be construed as a general recommendation to take supplements. Rather, since we acknowledge that it is a common practice among healthy people, it is reasonable for us to suggest how to do it safely.

Summary

▶ Few people need to be convinced that vitamins are important, but not everyone realizes that a well-chosen diet can supply all the vitamins that most people need, or that vitamin supplements taken in very high doses can be dangerous.

▶ **Vitamins** are regulators of metabolic functions; they are needed only in minute amounts. Vitamins A, D, E, and K are fat-soluble; thiamin, riboflavin, niacin, B-6, folic acid, B-12, pantothenic acid, biotin, and vitamin C are water-soluble. In general, the body can accumulate more of the fat-soluble vitamins; therefore, they have more potential to cause harm. However, toxicities due to overingestion of water-soluble vitamins can occur.

▶ The vitamins are structurally unrelated to each other. A number of vitamins exist as several slightly different chemical forms that all function in the body as that vitamin. The body can also convert vitamin precursors called **provitamins** into active forms. The form in which a vitamin occurs can affect its potency, but whether the vitamin was produced ''naturally'' or synthetically makes no difference.

▶ Several units of measurement are used to quantify vitamins. Now that scientists are aware of the varying potencies of different forms of some vitamins and their precursors, a unit called **equivalents** is coming into common use to reflect as accurately as possible the amount of vitamin *activity* the various forms provide.

▶ Almost all vitamins are at work in almost all body cells, so every vitamin has a widespread effect on the body, and body functions (such as energy production, growth, reproduction, and immune function) are influenced by many vitamins simultaneously. Tables 12.2–12.8 list common food sources of vitamins, and Table 12.1 summarizes their major functions and signs of deficiency and excess.

▶ Some substances that have recently been touted as vitamins are in fact produced in adequate amounts by healthy people; thus, they technically are not vitamins and certainly need not be supplemented in the diet. Other nonvitamins are toxic and can cause harm to people who consume them.

▶ Extreme vitamin deficiencies are rare in the developed countries but still occur in many parts of the world. Such deficiencies usually arise when food is limited in type and/or quantity, when the individual cannot absorb or utilize vitamins to a normal extent, and in individuals whose need for vitamins is high owing to rapid growth or disease. Worldwide, most people who have vitamin deficiencies simply do not get enough to eat and are likely to have multiple deficiencies rather than a shortage of a single vitamin. There is considerable variation in both the signs and symptoms of deficiencies and the time it takes for a particular deficiency to develop.

▶ Large excesses of vitamins are dangerous, though it is rare for an individual to consume harmful amounts of any vitamin in ordinary foods. Vitamin toxicity is more often the result of ingesting vitamin supplements in excessive quantities over a long period of time. The level of toxicity for a given vitamin is influenced by several factors including storage capacity in the body, level of intake, chemical form, and the length of time in which the overdose occurs. People who suffer the ill effects of toxicity have usually been taking vitamin megadoses for anywhere from a few months to a few years.

▶ Most healthy people do not need to take vitamin supplements at all. Vegetarians who do not eat any animal products do need supplemental vitamin B-12, and supplements can be helpful during pregnancy and lactation, periods of rapid growth, and for the elderly. Vitamin supplements may also have limited use for individuals who are taking certain kinds of drugs or whose energy intake has decreased dramatically.

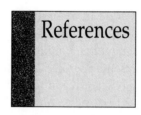

References

Anderson, T.W. 1978. Vitamin C and the common cold. *Contemporary Nutrition* 3 (no.10).

Anon. 1987. Mystery of the E-ferrol syndrome. *Nutrition Reviews* 45:76–78.

Anon. 1989. Secondary prevention of coronary disease with lipid-lowering drugs. *Lancet* (March 4, 1989): 473–474.

Bailey, L.B. 1988. Factors affecting folate bioavailability. *Food Technology* 42:206–212, 238.

Baird, I.M., R.E. Hughes, H.K. Wilson, J.E. Davies, and A.N. Howard. 1979. The effects of ascorbic acid and flavonoids on the occurrence of symptoms normally associated with the common cold. *American Journal of Clinical Nutrition* 32:1686–1690.

Ban, T.A. 1981. Megavitamin therapy in schizophrenia. In *Nutrition and Behavior*, ed. S.A. Miller. Philadelphia: The Franklin Institute Press.

Bauerfeind, J.C. 1988. Vitamin A deficiency: A staggering problem of health and sight. *Nutrition Today* 23:34–36.

Beisel, W.R. 1982. Single nutrients and immunity. *American Journal of Clinical Nutrition* 35:417–468.

Bendich, A. and L. Langseth. 1989. Safety of vitamin A. *American Journal of Clinical Nutrition* 49:358–371.

Bendich, A. and L.J. Machlin. 1988. Safety of oral intake of vitamin E. *American Journal of Clinical Nutrition* 48:612–619.

Bendich, A. and J.A. Olson. 1989. Biological action of carotenoids. *FASEB Journal* 3:1927–1932.

Carpenter, K.J. and W.J. Lewin. 1985. A reexamination of the composition of diets associated with pellagra. *Journal of Nutrition* 115:543–552.

Clemetson, C.A. 1980. Histamine and ascorbic acid in human blood. *Journal of Nutrition* 110:662–668.

Committee on Nutritional Status During Pregnancy and Lactation. 1990. *Nutrition During Pregnancy*. Washington, DC: National Academy Press.

Council on Scientific Affairs, American Medical Association. 1987. Vitamin preparations as dietary supplements and as therapeutic agents. *Journal of the American Medical Association* 257:1929–1936.

DeLuca, H.F. 1988. Vitamin D and its metabolites. In *Modern nutrition in health and disease*, eds. M.E. Shils and V.R. Young. Philadelphia: Lea & Febiger.

Dick, E.C. 1989. Personal communication. University of Wisconsin Department of Preventive Medicine, Madison, WI 53706.

Dubick, M.A. and R.B. Rucker. 1983. Dietary supplements and health aids—a critical evaluation. Part 1—Vitamins and minerals. *Journal of Nutrition Education* 15(no.2):47–53.

Erdman, J.W., C.L. Poor, and J.M. Dietz. 1988. Factors affecting the bioavailability of vitamin A, carotenoids, and vitamin E. *Food Technology* 42:214–216.

Evans, C.D. and J. H. Lacey. 1986. Toxicity of vitamins: Complications of a health movement. *British Medical Journal* 292:509–510.

Gutcher, G.R., W.J. Raynor, and P.M. Farrell. 1984. An evaluation of vitamin E status in premature infants. *The American Journal of Clinical Nutrition* 40:1078–1089.

Herbert, V. and N. Colman. 1988. Folic acid and vitamin B-12. In *Modern nutrition in health and disease*, eds. M.E. Shils and V.R. Young. Philadelphia: Lea & Febiger.

HNIS (Human Nutrition Information Service). 1985. Nationwide food consumption survey: Continuing survey of food intakes by individuals. NFCS CSFII Report No. 85-1. Hyattsville, MD: U.S. Department of Agriculture.

———. 1986. Nationwide food consumption survey: Continuing survey of food intakes by individuals: Men 19–50 years, 1 day, 1985. Report No. 85-3. Hyattsville, MD: United States Department of Agriculture.

Holick, M.F. 1987. Photosynthesis of vitamin D in the skin: Effect of environmental and life-style variables. *Federation Proceedings* 46:1876–1882.

Hornig, D.H., U. Moser, and B.E. Glatthaar. 1988. Ascorbic acid. In *Modern nutrition in health and disease*, eds. M.E. Shils and V.R. Young. Philadelphia: Lea & Febiger.

Kamil, A. 1974. How natural are those "natural" vitamins? *Nutrition Reviews* (Supplement 1) 32:34.

Lammer, E.J., D.T. Chen, R.M. Hoar, N.D. Agnish, P.J. Benke, J.T. Braun, C.J. Curry, P.M. Fernhoff, A.W. Grix, I.T. Lott, J.M. Richard, and S.C. Sun. 1985. Retinoic acid embryopathy. *New England Journal of Medicine* 313:837–841.

Leklem, J.E. 1988. Vitamin B-6 bioavailability and its application to human nutrition. *Food Technology* 42:194–196.

McCormick, D.B. 1988. (4 chapters) Thiamin. Riboflavin. Niacin. Biotin. In *Modern nutrition in health and disease*, eds. M.E. Shils and V.R. Young. Philadelphia: Lea & Febiger.

Mira, M., P.M. Stewart, and S.F. Abraham. 1988. Vitamin and trace element status in premenstrual syndrome. *American Journal of Clinical Nutrition* 47:636–641.

Moss, A.J., A.S. Levy, I. Kim, Y.K. Park. 1989. Use of vitamin and mineral supplements in the United States: Current users, types of products, and nutrients. *Advance Data* 174:1–20.

National Center for Health Statistics. 1979. *Dietary intake source data, United States, 1971–1974.* U.S. Department of Health, Education, and Welfare (DHEW) Publication No. (PHS)79–1221. Hyattsville, MD: DHEW.

National Research Council. 1989. *Diet and health.* Washington, DC: National Academy Press.

Nutrition Forum. 1986. "Stress vitamin" manufacturer agrees to stop false and misleading claims. *Nutrition Forum* 3:28.

Nutrition Reviews. 1986. A proposition: Megadoses of vitamin C are valuable in the treatment of cancer. *Nutrition Reviews* 44:28–32.

Nutrition Reviews. 1990. Use of vitamin and mineral supplements in the United States. *Nutrition Reviews* 48: 161–162.

Omaye, S.T., J.H. Skala, and R.A. Jacob. 1988. Rebound effect with ascorbic acid in adult males. *American Journal of Clinical Nutrition* 48:379–381.

Parry, G.J. and D.E. Bredesen. 1985. Sensory neuropathy with low-dose pyridoxine. *Neurology* 35:1466–1468.

Public Health Service. 1988. *The Surgeon General's report on nutrition and health.* Washington, DC: U.S. Department of Health and Human Services.

RDA Subcommittee. 1989. *Recommended dietary allowances.* Washington DC: National Academy Press.

Roberts, L. 1988. Question raised about antiwrinkle cream. *Science* 240:564.

Schaumberg, H., J. Kaplan, A. Windebank, N. Vick, S. Rasmus, D. Pleasure, and M.J. Brown. 1983. Sensory neuropathy from pyridoxine abuse: A new megavitamin syndrome. *New England Journal of Medicine* 309:445–448.

Selhorst, J.B., E.A. Waybright, S. Jennings, and J.J. Corbett. 1984. Liver lover's headache: Pseudotumor cerebri and vitamin A intoxication. *Journal of the American Medical Association* 252:3365.

Specker, B.L., D. Miller, E.J. Norman, H. Greene, K.C. Hayes. 1988. Increased urinary methylmalonic acid excretion in breast-fed infants of vegetarian mothers and identification of an acceptable dietary source of vitamin B-12. *American Journal of Clinical Nutrition* 47:89–92.

Suttie, J.W., L.L. Mummah-Schendel, D.V. Shah, B.J. Lyle, and J.L. Greger. 1988. Vitamin K deficiency from dietary vitamin K restriction in humans. *American Journal of Clinical Nutrition* 47:475–480.

13

Minerals

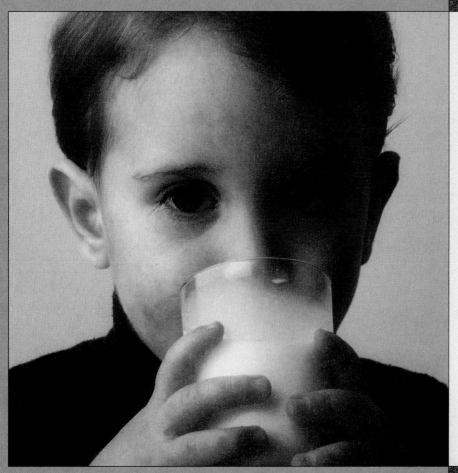

In This Chapter

- Minerals Are Elements
- Varying Bioavailability
  Makes Mineral Needs
  Difficult to Establish
- The Necessary Levels of
  Essential Minerals Are
  Available from Foods
- Mineral Intake Should Be
  Neither Too Low Nor Too
  High
- There Are Several Ways to
  Evaluate Your Mineral Intake

any consumers think of minerals as almost indistinguishable from vitamins. Frequent references are made to *vitamins and minerals* together, as though they were one large nutrient group.

It is true that there are similarities between these two groups: they are both micronutrients whose importance to humans has been appreciated mainly in this century. Like vitamins, minerals are widespread in basic foods but are nonetheless aggressively marketed by the supplement industry. Professional nutritionists are concerned that some misleading—or even false—advertising claims about the benefits of mineral supplements encourage people to consume them at toxic levels.

There are also major differences between the two groups. One distinction is that vitamins are organic (carbon-containing) compounds, whereas minerals are inorganic.

Minerals Are Elements

minerals—chemical elements other than carbon, hydrogen, oxygen, and nitrogen that make up the body

Minerals are the chemical elements other than carbon, hydrogen, oxygen, and nitrogen that make up the body. Carbon, hydrogen, oxygen, and nitrogen account for 96% of body weight; minerals constitute only about 4%. Minerals in the body make up in number what they lack in gross weight: at least 20 are commonly found in humans, and as many as 60 have been identified in living organisms.

Categories

Minerals are usually divided into two categories. Those present in the human body in amounts greater than 0.01% of body weight (or needed in the diet in amounts of 100 mg or more per day) are called **macrominerals** or **major minerals.** Calcium, phosphorus, sulfur, potassium, sodium, chloride, and magnesium are macrominerals.

macrominerals (major minerals)—those minerals present in the body in amounts greater than 0.01% of body weight

The macrominerals present in your body in the largest amounts are calcium (approximately 2 pounds) and phosphorus (approximately 1½ pounds). Figure 13.1 shows the amounts typically present in an adult male.

The minerals that are present in your body in quantities smaller than 0.01% of body weight are called **trace minerals** or **trace elements.** They include iron, iodine, fluoride, zinc, selenium, copper, chromium, manganese, molybdenum, cobalt, silicon, arsenic, nickel, and vanadium.

trace minerals (trace elements)—those minerals present in the body in amounts less than 0.01% of body weight

Iron and zinc are the most prevalent trace elements in your body, which probably contains 2 to 4 grams of each of them. Most of the other trace minerals are present in much smaller quantities—perhaps just one-thousandth as much.

To help you visualize how small the amounts of trace elements in your body are, imagine that your normal body weight is one ton (2000 pounds).

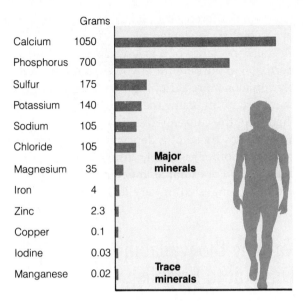

Grams

Calcium	1050
Phosphorus	700
Sulfur	175
Potassium	140
Sodium	105
Chloride	105
Magnesium	35
Iron	4
Zinc	2.3
Copper	0.1
Iodine	0.03
Manganese	0.02

Major minerals

Trace minerals

Figure 13.1 Some of the minerals in a 70-kg man.
Amounts of the major minerals and a few of the essential trace minerals are shown. Other trace minerals occur in the body in even smaller amounts than those listed.

Assuming normal trace mineral composition, you would contain only 1.8 ounces of iron, 1.1 ounces of zinc, 0.05 ounce of copper, 0.01 ounce of iodine, 0.003 ounce of chromium, 0.001 ounce of cobalt, and 0.0004 ounce of vanadium.

Relative Importance

At this time scientists do not think that the body requires all the chemical elements it contains: only some of the minerals found in the human body have been found to be essential for growth, reproduction, and health. Although you might expect that the distinction between essential and nonessential minerals should be easy for scientists to make, they do not unanimously agree on the status of some of the minerals.

A major reason for the disagreement is that the tests to determine essentiality are difficult to conduct and interpret. A traditional test is to show that serious negative consequences result when animals' diets contain very low levels of the test nutrient for a certain period of time. Keeping all vestiges of trace elements out of test diets and the environment of test animals is extremely difficult, however, so designing a study in which the effects of a specific trace mineral deficiency can be demonstrated is a major obstacle.

Disagreements among scientists about the essentiality of particular minerals also reflect differences in judgment. For example, some scientists regard fluoride as essential; others do not. These differing judgments arise from two facts: the presence of fluoride in the diet significantly discourages tooth decay, but poor growth and death do not result from lack of fluoride. Table 13.1 identifies the minerals thought by some experts to be essential for animals; it is likely that humans need them as well. The fact that this table does not agree completely with the RDA listing of essential minerals underscores the differences in judgment and the limited amount of data available for several trace elements.

The importance of a given mineral to your health is not necessarily proportional to the amount in your body. For example, the human body probably contains more aluminum, which is not believed to be essential to health, than chromium, manganese, and certain other essential trace minerals. Furthermore, the consequences of essential *trace* mineral deficiency can be just as severe as those of a deficiency of a *major* essential mineral.

As with other essential nutrients, mineral intakes in excess of need can be dangerous. For example, the minerals zinc and iron are essential for life, but if they are ingested in very large quantities, they are toxic.

Varying Bioavailability Makes Mineral Needs Difficult to Establish

bioavailability—degree to which the body is able to use a substance in the form or amount present

A key concept regarding minerals is that the **bioavailability** (usefulness to the body) of a given ingested mineral varies a great deal depending on the

Table 13.1 Minerals—Essential and Nonessential

Minerals Believed Essential for Animals

Calcium	Arsenic	Manganese
Phosphorus	Chromium	Molybdenum
Sulfur	Cobalt	Nickel
Potassium	Copper	Selenium
Sodium	Fluoride[a]	Silicon
Chloride	Iodine	Vanadium
Magnesium	Iron	Zinc

Minerals Not Proven to Be Required for Animals

Aluminum	Germanium	Strontium
Antimony	Gold	Thallium
Barium	Lanthanum	Titanium
Beryllium	Lead	Uranium
Bismuth	Mercury	Zirconium
Bromine	Niobium	Boron[b]
Cadmium	Radium	Lithium[b]
Cesium	Rubidium	Tin[b]
Gallium	Ruthenium	
	Silver	

[a]Scientists have not demonstrated that fluoride is essential for life itself, but it is well documented that its presence in the diet has a beneficial effect on dental health.

[b]Scientists have shown these elements to be essential in isolated studies. These data need to be confirmed by other investigators before these minerals are classified as essential.

Reference: Nielsen, F.H. 1988. Ultra trace minerals. In *Modern nutrition in health and disease,* eds. M.E. Shils and V.R. Young. Philadelphia: Lea & Febiger.

circumstances. Many factors influence mineral bioavailability—some decrease it and others increase it. As mentioned in Chapter 12, we are beginning to learn that bioavailability is also an issue for certain vitamins such as vitamin B-6 and folic acid. Bioavailability of minerals, on the other hand, has been studied much more intensively for many years.

In general, healthy people absorb more than 90% of the protein, carbohydrate, and fat in their diets, but they do not absorb minerals as efficiently. In fact, in controlled studies adults have been found to absorb an average of only about 5% of the manganese, 5–10% of the iron, 10–20% of the zinc, and 15–40% of the magnesium and calcium in their diets.

Differences in food composition can cause large variations in the bioavailability of minerals. For example, healthy adults have been found to absorb anywhere from 1% to over 35% of their dietary iron intake, depending on the composition of the diets (Monsen, 1988). Studies have also shown the absorption of calcium to range from less than 5% to more than 60% of what was ingested. Bioavailability of minerals can be influenced by other factors as well, such as an individual's health and the use of medications. These factors usually influence mineral bioavailability by altering absorption, excretion, storage, or transport of minerals.

Dietary Factors That Improve Mineral Bioavailability

Few dietary factors actually improve the body's use of minerals. Much of this discussion centers on iron because more is known about the bioavailability of this mineral than about that of others.

The iron in your diet can be classified into two categories: heme iron and nonheme iron. **Heme iron,** as the name implies, is found in the hemoglobin of blood and in the myoglobin of animal flesh; it accounts for about 40–50% of the iron in meat, fish, and poultry. **Nonheme iron** accounts for the remaining iron in these foods. All the iron in eggs, milk, and plant foods is considered nonheme iron. These classifications are important because scientists have found that people usually absorb 15–35% of the heme iron in their diets but only 1–20% of the nonheme iron.

heme iron—a form of iron that is part of hemoglobin or myoglobin in meat, fish, and poultry

nonheme iron—iron present in the diet other than heme iron (includes iron in milk, eggs, and plant products)

What does this mean in practical terms? Let's assume that you consumed equal amounts of iron in two meals. In one meal the iron was provided by meat, and in the other meal it was provided by cereal. You would absorb more iron from the meal containing the meat.

There are at least two ways to improve the absorption of nonheme iron; they are discussed in the upcoming sections. Vegetarians are often particularly interested in this matter, although it warrants general concern: in a national survey, nonheme iron accounted for more than 90% of the iron in the diets of most adults (Raper et al., 1984).

Ascorbic Acid for Iron One way to improve the absorption of nonheme iron is to increase the amount of vitamin C (ascorbic acid) in the diet. Scientists have found that adding 75 mg of ascorbic acid to a meal can increase more than twofold the absorption of nonheme iron from that meal. This means that adding 6 ounces of orange juice to a breakfast of toast and eggs can double the bioavailability of the iron in the toast and eggs. Similarly, adding canned tomatoes to a rice casserole can improve the bioavailability of the iron in the rice. (Unfortunately, ascorbic acid has not been found to improve the absorption of other minerals in humans.)

Unidentified Meat Factor for Iron   A second dietary factor that can increase the absorption of nonheme iron is known as the **unidentified meat factor.**

Although scientists do not know exactly what substance in meat is responsible for this effect, they do know that adding 3 ounces of meat, fish, or poultry to a meal can increase more than twofold the absorption of the nonheme iron in the meal. In other words, adding ham or tuna to a macaroni and cheese casserole increases the bioavailability of the iron in the macaroni and cheese. At the same time, the heme iron in the meat or fish is absorbed with characteristic efficiency.

It is important to be aware of one other fact when you use these principles: ascorbic acid and/or unidentified meat factor must be consumed *at the same meal as the nonheme iron* in order to increase its bioavailability. The orange juice or sausage you consume at breakfast will not influence the absorption of the nonheme iron eaten at supper. Rather, moderate amounts of vitamin C–rich foods or meat added to each meal will probably improve your utilization of iron more than eating a large amount of these foods at just one meal during the day.

Iron in Breast Milk for Infants   Nutritionists have found that infants absorb the iron and zinc in breast milk more efficiently than the iron and zinc in cow's milk or infant formulas. Reasons for this phenomenon have been advanced but not proved (Lönnerdal, 1987). In general, the balance of levels of various minerals (including calcium, iron, and zinc) and the presence of proteins, peptides, and other factors that bind with zinc and iron appear together to optimize absorption of zinc and iron from human milk by infants. (See Chapter 16 on the nutrition of mothers and infants.)

Dietary Factors and Other Minerals   Although less research has been done regarding the bioavailability of other minerals, it is known that an adequate supply of vitamin D, either in the diet or synthesized in response to sunlight, is needed for optimal absorption of calcium and phosphorus. Also, the presence of lactose in foods may facilitate calcium and magnesium absorption, but this effect may not occur consistently. Additional dietary protein may increase zinc absorption (Greger, 1989a).

Unfortunately, scientists do not yet know as much as they should about the mineral forms or dietary factors that improve the absorption of minerals, but research is in progress.

unidentified meat factor— substance present in meat that can increase the bioavailability of nonheme iron consumed at the same meal

Factors That Depress Mineral Bioavailability

A number of substances people consume inhibit absorption of minerals. The practical importance of each is based not only on their ability to decrease absorption of minerals but also on the amount of these compounds in the diet.

Dietary Fiber and Related Substances Dietary fiber and some organic compounds found in foods with fiber decrease the absorption of minerals. Probably the most important of these substances is **phytate,** an organic compound that contains phosphorus. Fiber and phytate are commonly found in whole grains, bran, and soy products, as shown in Figure 13.2.

Human and animal studies have shown that adding phytate either alone or with fiber to a meal can decrease the absorption of zinc, calcium, magnesium, and sometimes iron. The phosphorus that is included in the phytate structure is not usually well absorbed either.

Because phytate and fiber decrease the absorption of calcium, it might seem logical to supplement diets containing lots of phytate with calcium, but the addition of calcium to a high phytate diet causes a further decrease in zinc absorption. Phytate–zinc complexes are fairly insoluble in the gut, but phytate–calcium–zinc complexes are even less soluble.

Yeast contains an enzyme that breaks down phytate. For this reason, the minerals in a whole-grain, yeast-leavened bread may have a higher bioavailability than those in a whole-grain unleavened bread or cereal.

Most North Americans probably do not consume enough fiber and phytate to decrease their absorption of minerals significantly. However, poor individuals in developing countries and vegetarians in the developed coun-

phytate—phosphorus-containing organic compound found in some plant materials; decreases mineral absorption

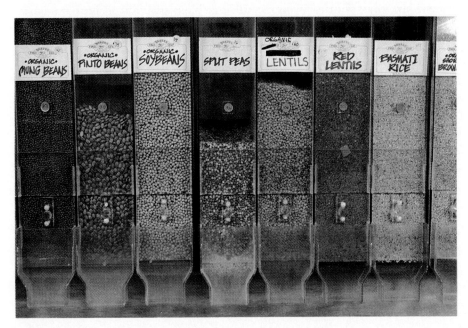

Figure 13.2 Various compounds in foods can decrease mineral bioavailability. Although whole grains and legumes contain fairly large amounts of minerals, they also include fiber and phytate, which reduce mineral bioavailability.

tries may consume considerable amounts of fiber and phytate; this is of particular concern if their intake of some minerals, especially calcium and zinc, is low to begin with. Individuals who regularly supplement their diets with generous portions of bran may also decrease their absorption of minerals. Over a long period, this could lead to mineral deficiencies, particularly if the dietary intake is inadequate or marginal.

Other Organic Dietary Components   Studies in the developing countries have shown that the consumption of large amounts of tea by infants (Merhav et al., 1988) and coffee by pregnant women (Muñoz et al., 1985) has been associated with an increased incidence of anemia. It is likely that **tannins,** more correctly called **polyphenols** (organic compounds that have an astringent quality), were the component in the tea that caused the poorer utilization of iron. Some grain, particularly sorghum, can also contain very high levels of tannins.

tannins (polyphenols) and oxalates—naturally occurring compounds that can depress utilization of some minerals in some situations

Oxalates, which are organic acids found in spinach, rhubarb, and chocolate, may also depress the absorption of calcium (Weaver et al., 1987). Large amounts of ascorbic acid can decrease copper utilization (Johnson and Murphy, 1988). The importance of these factors needs further evaluation.

High levels of dietary protein can also negatively affect calcium bioavailability, but the effect is at the excretion stage rather than at absorption. Large intakes of protein tend to increase the urinary excretion of calcium, resulting in a net loss of that mineral. Dietary phosphorus affects both absorption and excretion of calcium: high intake of phosphorus sometimes can decrease calcium absorption, but will simultaneously decrease urinary calcium excretion, usually to a greater extent. The result is that if the high-protein foods a person eats are also high in phosphorus (as is true of meats and milk), calcium may be protected (Greger, 1989a). You can see that the effect of protein and phosphorus levels on calcium bioavailability in humans is an important but often controversial topic.

Other Minerals   Minerals can also compete with each other for absorption. Scientists have found that when diets are supplemented with calcium, absorption of magnesium, zinc, and iron can be depressed, especially if dietary phosphorus levels are high. This effect is apt to be significant when the amount of calcium consumed from supplements is very high (Greger et al., 1987).

Similarly, it has been found that the supplementation of human diets with zinc can depress the absorption of copper (Solomons, 1988). Other interactions of this sort exist between minerals, such as between zinc and iron, and between manganese and iron. Consumers must be aware that supplementation of diets with minerals "just to be sure" can sometimes create problems instead of solving them.

Although we have emphasized the negative aspect of minerals in preventing absorption, this phenomenon can be beneficial at times. Researchers have shown that calcium and iron can depress the bioavailability of lead;

therefore, children absorb less lead (which is toxic) from paint chips or other sources when they have consumed adequate amounts of calcium and iron. Similarly, mercury in fish is less toxic when adequate dietary selenium has been consumed.

Pica Some people eat substances that most individuals in our society would not consider to be food for example, clay, laundry starch, fireplace ashes, newspaper, and paint chips. (Some people claim that paint chips taste sweet.) This custom is called **pica,** and it is practiced most often by women and children. It seems to be taught within certain cultures.

pica—the ingestion of non-food substances such as clay, laundry starch, or chalk

Pica can have two effects on the mineral nutriture of people who practice it. First, toxic substances may be present in the items consumed, as is true of lead-based paints. Repeated ingestion of chips of such paints is likely to result in lead toxicity; this type of pica is seen primarily among young children. Second, the items eaten may contain substances that inhibit mineral absorption. The types of clay that are consumed by some women in the southern part of the United States and in the Middle East often contain compounds that interfere with iron and zinc absorption. The effect is accentuated if mineral intake is low.

Medications The interactions between medications and nutrients are many and complex. Consumers should be aware that medications, even over-the-counter drugs, can affect the utilization of and requirements for dietary minerals, just as they can for vitamins. For example, aluminum-containing antacids can decrease the absorption of dietary phosphorus and fluoride. These antacids are commonly available; some people consume them as freely as candy without realizing their possible negative nutritional effects.

The opposite is also true; not only can drugs influence the utilization of minerals, but minerals can influence the utilization of drugs. If you take the antibiotic tetracycline with a glass of milk, the calcium in the milk will bind to the tetracycline; neither will be absorbed.

Physiological Factors That Affect Bioavailability

Your physiological status also plays a role in how well your body absorbs the minerals you consume. For example, scientists know that people who have low body reserves of iron absorb both heme and nonheme iron more efficiently than individuals who have larger body stores. In other words, the individuals who have greater need for the iron absorb a higher proportion of it. Similar observations have been made for calcium, phosphorus, magnesium, and zinc.

Fortunately, the bodies of healthy individuals can make adjustments to different diets and to the total environment—but, of course, there are limits to adaptability.

The Necessary Levels of Essential Minerals Are Available from Foods

From this discussion you have seen that innumerable factors influence the bioavailability of minerals and that minerals probably never function independently in the body. Knowing this, we can now examine each mineral individually—a convenient but not particularly realistic way of describing the roles minerals play in the body.

Different minerals have different biochemical functions, which fall into the general categories of structural and regulatory uses:

1. They form part of tissue structure.
2. They help maintain water and acid–base balance.
3. They form components of important organic molecules, such as enzymes and hormones that regulate body processes.
4. They facilitate nerve impulse transmission and muscle contraction.

Table 13.2 summarizes mineral functions, requirements, typical intakes, sources, and possible consequences of excesses or inadequacies. As you read it, keep in mind that some very valuable information about minerals can't fit into a table. You can get that information from the following text sections.

Calcium and Phosphorus

Calcium and phosphorus deserve early attention both because they are the minerals in the body in the greatest amounts and because they have many functions.

Calcium and phosphorus are well known for their contributions to body structure. In fact, 99% of the calcium and 85% of the phosphorus in the human body are found in bones and teeth, where they are part of the compound **hydroxyapatite,** a combination of calcium, phosphorus, oxygen, and hydrogen. Other minerals add to the high concentration of **ash** (total mineral content) in bones and teeth, but their functions there are less clear.

hydroxyapatite—a compound consisting of calcium, phosphorus, oxygen, and hydrogen that is found in bones and teeth

ash—the total mineral content of a tissue

Although bones contain a large proportion of minerals, these structures are not like rocks, which are solid minerals. Bones are living tissues. Their cells produce and secrete collagen, a protein that forms the framework of connective tissue and bone. Calcium and phosphorus are incorporated into bone when they crystallize in and around this matrix (framework). Figure 13.3 shows a cross section of a bone; you can see that it is not a solid mass of minerals.

Bones in living animals are always being *remodeled;* for example, bones must be enlarged as a person grows. During this process, cells in the bone continually dissolve some of the minerals, which are then carried away in the blood. Simultaneously, calcium, phosphorus, and various other minerals are brought from the blood into bone, where they are deposited to form

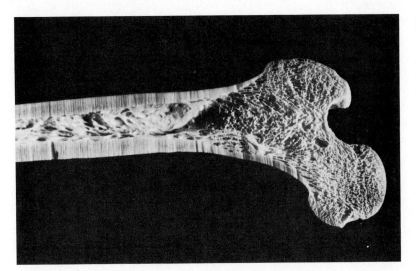

Figure 13.3 Cross section of **bone.** The lacy interior, called *trabecular bone,* shows how minerals are crystallized around a protein matrix (network). The compact bone at the exterior of the shaft is *cortical bone.*

part of its structure. When the amounts of minerals leaving and entering the bones are equal, a state of *homeostasis* or *dynamic equilibrium* exists. This is the desirable situation in fully grown, healthy adults.

Phosphorus is also present in cell membranes as part of phospholipids and in many other important body substances, such as DNA and RNA, certain coenzymes with a wide variety of functions, and adenosine triphosphate (ATP). In addition, it functions in acid–base balance. Calcium also performs additional critical functions: it is involved with other elements in nerve transmission and with vitamin K in blood clotting.

Bone Disorders   Because calcium is an important component of bone, it might seem logical that a dietary deficiency of calcium would affect the skeleton. But bone disease is not a simple topic.

Chapter 12 discussed two bone diseases, rickets and osteomalacia. These are skeletal conditions in which bone mineral salts are reduced in relation to the amount of matrix. This leads to softening of bones and to skeletal deformities. Even though these conditions involve calcium, they are not caused by low calcium intake; rather, inadequate vitamin D or physiological problems that impair calcium and phosphorus absorption and retention are likely to be the cause.

Osteoporosis is another sort of bone disorder. In this condition, both the protein matrix of bone and the mineral deposits are gradually lost, decreasing the total amount of bone and weakening the skeleton. This situation is four times more prevalent and severe in women than in men, and it becomes more common and rapid in women after menopause (Figure 13.4). Disability results if the weakened bones break, which is most likely to happen in the vertebrae, arms, and hips.

Every year in the United States, 2% of the women over 80 years of age break a hip. Less than a quarter of these women return to their previous level of functioning (Ford, 1989). At least 15–20 million people in the United States have osteoporosis; it contributes to 1.3 million bone fractures per year

osteoporosis—disease in which bone tissue is gradually lost, weakening the skeleton

Table 13.2 Key Information About Many Essential Minerals

Mineral	RDA for Healthy Adults Ages 19–50	Major Dietary Sources	Major Functions	Signs of Severe, Prolonged Deficiency	Signs of Extreme Excess
Major minerals					
Calcium	1200 mg for ages 19–24; 800 mg for 25 and older	Milk, cheese, dark green vegetables, legumes	Bone and tooth formation; blood clotting; nerve transmission	Stunted growth; perhaps less bone mass	Depressed absorption of some other minerals; perhaps kidney damage
Phosphorus	1200 mg for ages 19–24; 800 mg for 25 and older	Milk, cheese, meat, poultry, whole grains	Bone and tooth formation; acid–base balance; component of coenzymes	Weakness; demineralization of bone	Depressed absorption of some minerals
Magnesium	Females: 280 mg Males: 350 mg	Whole grains, green leafy vegetables	Component of enzymes	Neurological disturbances	Neurological disturbances
Sulfur	(Provided by sulfur amino acids)	Sulfur amino acids in dietary proteins	Component of cartilage, tendons, and proteins	(Related to protein deficiency)	Excess sulfur amino acid intake leads to poor growth; liver damage
Sodium	a	Salt, soy sauce, cured meats, pickles, canned soups, processed cheese	Body water balance; nerve function	Muscle cramps; reduced appetite	High blood pressure in genetically predisposed individuals
Potassium	a	Meats, milk, many fruits and vegetables, whole grains	Body water balance; nerve function	Muscular weakness; paralysis	Muscular weakness; cardiac arrest
Chloride	a	Same as for sodium	Plays a role in acid–base balance; formation of gastric juice	Muscle cramps; reduced appetite; poor growth	High blood pressure in genetically predisposed individuals
Trace minerals					
Iron	Females: 15 mg Males: 10 mg	Meats, eggs, legumes, whole grains, green leafy vegetables	Components of hemoglobin, myoglobin, and enzymes	Iron deficiency anemia, weakness, impaired immune function	Acute: shock, death; Chronic: liver damage, cardiac failure

Mineral	Dietary intake	Food sources	Functions	Deficiency	Toxicity
Iodine	0.15 mg	Marine fish and shellfish; dairy products; iodized salt, some breads	Component of thyroid hormones	Goiter (enlarged thyroid)	Iodide goiter
Fluoride	1.5–4.0 mg[b]	Drinking water, tea, seafood	Maintenance of tooth (and maybe bone) structure	Higher frequency of tooth decay	Acute: GI distress Chronic: mottling of teeth; skeletal deformation
Zinc	Females: 12 mg Males: 15 mg	Meats, seafood, whole grains	Component of enzymes	Growth failure; scaly dermatitis; reproductive failure; impaired immune function	Acute: nausea; vomiting; diarrhea; Chronic: adversely affects copper metabolism, anemia, and immune function
Selenium	Females: .055 mg Males: .070 mg	Seafood, meats, whole grains	Component of enzyme; functions in close association with vitamin E	Muscle pain; maybe heart muscle deterioration	Nausea and vomiting; hair and nail loss
Copper	1.5–3.0 mg[b]	Seafood, nuts, legumes, organ meats	Component of enzymes	Anemia; bone and cardiovascular changes	Nausea: liver damage
Cobalt	(Required as vitamin B-12)[a]	Animal products	Component of vitamin B-12	Not reported except as vitamin B-12 deficiency	With alcohol: heart failure
Chromium	0.05–0.2 mg[b]	Brewer's yeast, liver, seafood, meat, some vegetables	Involved in glucose and energy metabolism	Impaired glucose metabolism	Lung and kidney damage (occupational exposures only)
Manganese	2.0–5.0 mg[b]	Nuts, whole grains, vegetables and fruits, tea	Component of enzymes	Abnormal bone and cartilage	Central nervous system damage (occupational exposures)
Molybdenum	0.075–0.25 mg[b]	Legumes, cereals, some vegetables	Component of enzymes	Disorder in nitrogen excretion	Inhibition of enzymes; adversely affects copper metabolism

[a]No formal recommendation

[b]Estimated safe and adequate daily dietary intake

References: (1) Shils, M.E. 1988. Magnesium. In *Modern nutrition in health and disease*, eds. M.E. Shils and V.R. Young. Philadelphia: Lea & Febiger. (2) Fairbanks, V.F. and E. Beutler. Iron. (From same as [1].) (3) Solomons, N.W. Zinc and copper. (From same as [1].) (4) RDA Subcommittee. 1989. *Recommended dietary allowances*. Washington, DC: National Academy Press. (5) Underwood, E.J. 1977. *Trace elements in human and animal nutrition*. New York: Academic Press.

Figure 13.4 We normally lose bone starting in middle age. Women lose more bone and lose it faster, putting them at greater risk for osteoporosis. (*Source:* Anon. 1989. Links between nutrition and osteoporosis. Madison, WI: University of Wisconsin Extension.)

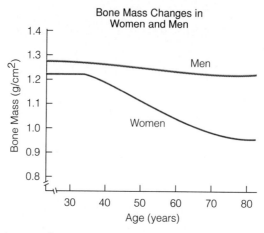

Bone Mass Changes in Women and Men

in people 45 years or older. It is estimated that the cumulative cost of osteoporosis is $7–10 billion annually (Surgeon General, 1988).

The causes of osteoporosis are not known for sure, although the data point to a number of risk factors. These include decreasing estrogen (female hormone) levels, advancing age, and too little or too much weight-bearing exercise. Although scientists have not found a consistent relationship between the incidence of osteoporosis and calcium intake, low calcium intake is a suspected risk factor as well. People who are thin and have a small body frame also are at greater risk. In addition, white women are at greater risk of developing osteoporosis than black women; this is at least partially because whites tend to have less bone mass, even though black women usually consume less calcium.

In recent years, many studies have attempted to clarify how calcium intake affects bone loss in women as they age. One group of researchers found that some women, especially after menopause, require an increase up to 1500 mg of calcium per day to achieve calcium balance (Heaney et al., 1982). In 1987, a group of Danish researchers reported that all types of bone do not change uniformly: in a two-year double-blind study with postmenopausal women, the researchers found that those who consumed 2000 mg of supplemental calcium daily lost **cortical bone** more slowly but lost **trabecular bone** at the same rate as women who took placebos. Women who used estrogen maintained a constant bone mass throughout the study (Riis et al., 1987). Yet another research group found that supplementation of the diet with calcium alone did not slow loss of trabecular bone in the spine; but if calcium and estrogen were taken together, less estrogen was necessary to reduce bone loss (Ettinger et al., 1987). In general, consumption of calcium supplements in excess of RDA level has not been proved to be an effective way to reduce bone loss.

Female marathon runners who have stopped menstruating or who menstruate only occasionally in association with strenuous training may have a higher incidence of osteoporosis. This may reflect tissue estrogen changes and/or poor calcium intake (Nelson et al., 1986).

A number of methods have been tried to halt the progress of existing osteoporosis. These include estrogen therapy; weight-bearing exercise regi-

cortical bone—the compact bone that surrounds the shaft of long bones

trabecular bone—bone tissue that forms a meshwork

mens; and the use of calcium, vitamin D, and fluoride supplements. Although some experiments show a certain degree of benefit from each of these methods, at this time scientists know of neither a sure cure nor a guaranteed preventive treatment for osteoporosis. Furthermore, they call for caution: excesses of each treatment can have negative consequences.

Many experts believe that the best protection against the adverse effects of bone loss is to maximize **peak bone mass** so that losses of bone with age weaken the structure more slowly. There are genetic limits to how much bone you can accumulate: scientists have found that adult daughters of women with osteoporosis have lower bone densities in their spines than other premenopausal women (Seeman et al., 1989).

peak bone mass—maximum amount of bone that can be achieved; occurs during the third decade of life

No matter what your genetic predisposition, you can take steps to maximize bone mass within your genetic potential. Many scientists believe that adequate intake of calcium during the teens and twenties may be more useful for reducing the risk of osteoporosis than suddenly becoming concerned about calcium later in life. Also, it is important to exercise regularly but not to extremes that induce cessation of menstruation. Weight-bearing activities such as walking or aerobics are better than those in which you are off your feet, such as swimming and biking. Finally, when you are nearing menopause, discuss estrogen replacement therapy with your physician to see whether it would be beneficial and appropriate in your case.

Deficiency Symptoms   Although calcium plays a role in blood clotting and nerve transmission, these functions are not affected when calcium intake is low because of regulatory mechanisms that maintain constant blood levels of calcium. Several hormones (one, a metabolite of vitamin D; another, parathyroid hormone) work together to increase the retention of calcium by the kidney and to withdraw calcium from bone. The vitamin D metabolite also increases calcium absorption in the gut. Accordingly, blood calcium levels are largely unaffected by dietary calcium intake. For this reason, it is not possible to use biochemical (blood or urine) tests to monitor the body's calcium status.

Several investigators have suggested that low calcium intakes may be related to a higher incidence of hypertension (Karanja and McCarron, 1986). Other investigators have suggested that high levels of calcium are protective against colon cancer (Wargovich, 1988). The relationships between calcium intake and hypertension and colon cancer have not been seen consistently and are subject to intensive research at this time. So although there is no doubt that calcium is essential, the consequences of taking in less than the RDA are not known for sure.

Recommended and Typical Intakes   Given the data available, it is not surprising that the RDA for calcium for adults has been the source of considerable controversy in recent years. A National Institutes of Health panel on osteoporosis suggested that women should consume 1000 to 1500 mg of calcium daily as a potential means of slowing the development of this disease (Consensus Conference, 1984).

The most recent RDA committee felt that higher intakes of calcium were apt to be beneficial in establishing maximal peak bone mass, which is attained during the third decade of life. Therefore, the RDAs for calcium and phosphorus are both 1200 mg (about ¼ teaspoon) daily for teens and adults through age 24. For men and women 25 and older, the RDA is 800 mg. Pregnant and lactating women should also consume 1200 mg per day of both calcium and phosphorus to supply resources for fetal growth and milk production.

Engrossed in the debate over optimal intakes of calcium, many people forget that most American women consume much less calcium than suggested in *any* of these recommendations (Figure 13.5). Women consumed an average of 570 mg of calcium daily in 1977 and 651 mg in 1985 (HNIS, 1985). On the other hand, the average calcium intake of men under 50 years of age in a national survey was 800 mg daily; this level was a reflection of their higher total energy intakes (Science and Education Administration, 1980).

Although many Americans consume less than recommended levels of calcium, most (especially men) consume adequate amounts of phosphorus. In fact, the average phosphorus intake of men in a national survey was 1400 mg daily (Science and Education Administration, 1980). The average intake of phosphorus by women is estimated to be about 1000 mg daily (HNIS, 1985). This finding suggests that young women are consuming less than the new RDA of 1200 mg. If you achieve the RDA goal for calcium from foods, you will get the RDA for phosphorus at the same time.

Sources Just as certain minerals are concentrated in specific tissues of your body, so are certain minerals concentrated in particular foods. Over half the calcium (55%) consumed by Americans is supplied by milk and milk products (Block et al., 1985). Table 13.3 shows what a rich source of calcium milk

Figure 13.5 How do American adults' calcium intakes compare with recommendations?

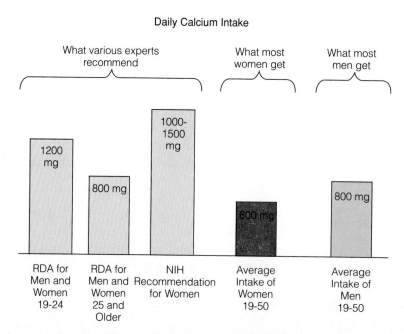

is. A cup of milk provides about 300 mg of calcium; to get an equivalent amount from other dairy products, you would have to consume $1\frac{1}{3}$ ounces of most hard cheeses (approximately $\frac{1}{3}$ cup, shredded), 2 cups of cottage cheese, $1\frac{1}{2}$ cups of ice cream, or 2 ounces of processed cheese food (approxi-

Table 13.3 Calcium and Phosphorus in Some Foods

The RDAs for calcium and phosphorus for adults through age 24 are 1200 mg/day; for people age 25 and older, the RDAs are 800 mg/day.

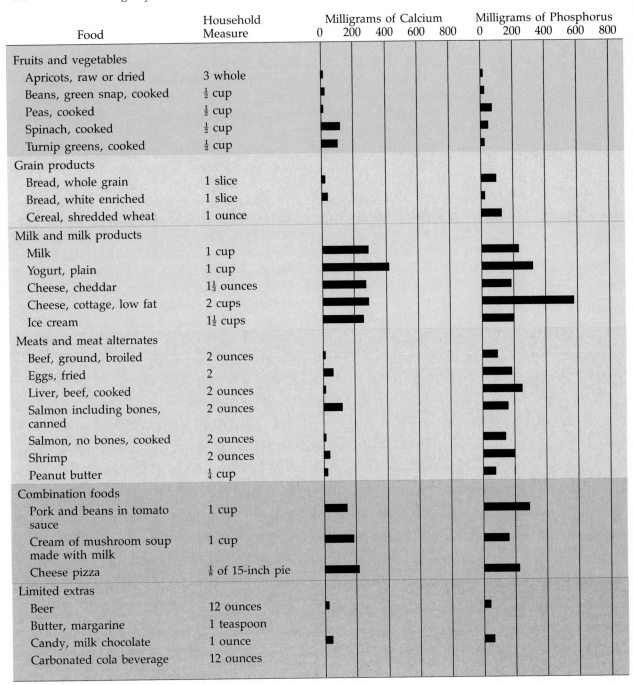

Food	Household Measure
Fruits and vegetables	
Apricots, raw or dried	3 whole
Beans, green snap, cooked	$\frac{1}{2}$ cup
Peas, cooked	$\frac{1}{2}$ cup
Spinach, cooked	$\frac{1}{2}$ cup
Turnip greens, cooked	$\frac{1}{2}$ cup
Grain products	
Bread, whole grain	1 slice
Bread, white enriched	1 slice
Cereal, shredded wheat	1 ounce
Milk and milk products	
Milk	1 cup
Yogurt, plain	1 cup
Cheese, cheddar	$1\frac{1}{3}$ ounces
Cheese, cottage, low fat	2 cups
Ice cream	$1\frac{1}{2}$ cups
Meats and meat alternates	
Beef, ground, broiled	2 ounces
Eggs, fried	2
Liver, beef, cooked	2 ounces
Salmon including bones, canned	2 ounces
Salmon, no bones, cooked	2 ounces
Shrimp	2 ounces
Peanut butter	$\frac{1}{4}$ cup
Combination foods	
Pork and beans in tomato sauce	1 cup
Cream of mushroom soup made with milk	1 cup
Cheese pizza	$\frac{1}{8}$ of 15-inch pie
Limited extras	
Beer	12 ounces
Butter, margarine	1 teaspoon
Candy, milk chocolate	1 ounce
Carbonated cola beverage	12 ounces

mately 3 wrapped slices). You might recognize these amounts as the serving sizes of dairy products in the Basic Food Guide, which were portioned that way to provide similar amounts of calcium. If you consume the three servings of milk or milk products per day recommended by the Basic Food Guide for teens and adults through age 24, you will ingest almost 900 mg of calcium, just 300 mg short of the RDA. The remainder is relatively easy to obtain from other foods.

Low calcium intakes are more likely among people who don't drink milk. If a person avoids milk because of lactose intolerance, lactase products can be used to make milk digestible (see Chapter 6). Ways to get calcium without drinking milk are to: (1) try different milk products, such as yogurt or cheese; (2) include milk and cheeses in sauces, casseroles, and desserts; and (3) consume vegetable products that are good sources of calcium (leafy vegetables, broccoli, legumes, and nuts). Be aware that some of the calcium from plant sources is apt to be unavailable because plant sources also contain phytate, fiber, and oxalates.

If for some reason you cannot tolerate foods that are high in calcium, you might benefit from a calcium supplement. Get professional advice about which kind to use, because the health risks and benefits of available products vary considerably. For example, bone meal (finely ground animal bones) contains all the typical bone minerals but may also contain lead that accumulated in the bones throughout the animal's lifetime (Miller, 1987).

Calcium supplements should be used in moderation. The idea is to consume adequate—not excessive—calcium. Overuse of some supplements could depress utilization of other minerals (Greger et al., 1987).

Many foods that are good sources of calcium are also good sources of phosphorus, as Table 13.3 shows; milk and other dairy products, fish with edible bones, legumes, and nuts are good examples. The reverse is not necessarily true; although meat, fish, poultry, and eggs are very rich sources of phosphorus, they usually contain little calcium.

Magnesium

Like calcium and phosphorus, magnesium has diverse functions. It, too, is a component of bone. It occurs in many enzymes as well, often catalyzing reactions in which phosphorus is involved. Along with calcium, it is necessary for the transmission of nerve impulses that influence the contraction and relaxation of muscles. It also helps stabilize DNA and RNA, the substances that direct cell division.

Recommended and Typical Intakes The recommended intakes for magnesium are 280 mg for women and 350 mg for men. Adults in the United States usually consume less: 226 mg per day is the average for women (HNIS, 1985) and 329 mg for men (HNIS, 1986). Despite these dietary shortfalls, Americans do not show overt symptoms of magnesium deficiency or evidence of biochemical impairment that can be directly related to magnesium status.

Several investigators have noted that in areas with "hard" drinking water, there is a lower incidence of hypertension. "Hard" water contains high concentrations of magnesium and calcium. However, data are inconsistent, making it impossible to determine the relationship of magnesium to high blood pressure (Surgeon General, 1988).

Sources The richest sources of dietary magnesium are nuts, legumes, seafood, and certain leafy green vegetables. Whole-grain products, meats, and milk contribute significant amounts of magnesium to the diets of Americans, as shown in Table 13.4.

Table 13.4 Magnesium in Some Foods

The RDA for magnesium is 280 mg/day for women; for men it is 350 mg/day.

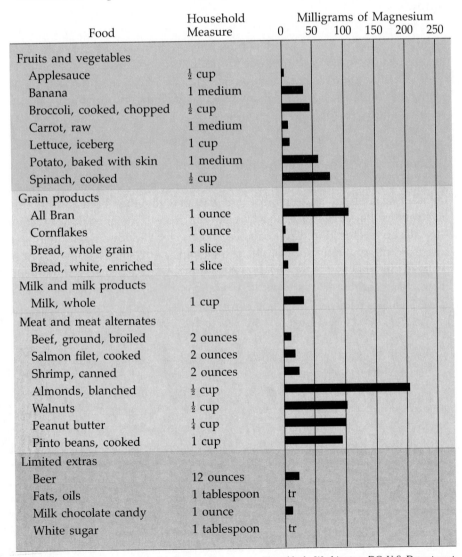

Food	Household Measure	Milligrams of Magnesium
Fruits and vegetables		
Applesauce	½ cup	
Banana	1 medium	
Broccoli, cooked, chopped	½ cup	
Carrot, raw	1 medium	
Lettuce, iceberg	1 cup	
Potato, baked with skin	1 medium	
Spinach, cooked	½ cup	
Grain products		
All Bran	1 ounce	
Cornflakes	1 ounce	
Bread, whole grain	1 slice	
Bread, white, enriched	1 slice	
Milk and milk products		
Milk, whole	1 cup	
Meat and meat alternates		
Beef, ground, broiled	2 ounces	
Salmon filet, cooked	2 ounces	
Shrimp, canned	2 ounces	
Almonds, blanched	½ cup	
Walnuts	½ cup	
Peanut butter	¼ cup	
Pinto beans, cooked	1 cup	
Limited extras		
Beer	12 ounces	
Fats, oils	1 tablespoon	tr
Milk chocolate candy	1 ounce	
White sugar	1 tablespoon	tr

Data sources: (1) HNIS. *Agriculture handbook 8 series on composition of foods.* Washington, DC: U.S. Department of Agriculture. (2) Leveille, G.A., M.E. Zabik, and K.J. Morgan. 1983. Nutrients in foods. Cambridge, MA: The Nutrition Guild.

Even though legumes, nuts, and products made from them are rich sources of magnesium, only 5% of the magnesium that the average Amerian consumes is from these sources. This demonstrates that a food is not a major source of magnesium for a given individual if it is not consumed in significant quantities. Grain products, which generally have less magnesium per serving, provide 21% of the average American intake; this amount is more than is contributed by any other group of foods (Science and Education Administration, 1980). Of the grain products, whole grains contain significantly more magnesium than refined grains do; therefore, an easy way to increase your magnesium intake is to consume a couple of servings of whole-grain products daily.

Sulfur

Sulfur is a component of two vitamins: thiamin and biotin. The majority of the sulfur in your body, though, is found in three amino acids: methionine, cystine, and cysteine. These amino acids are part of cellular proteins in both plants and animals. So, if a person's diet is adequate in protein, it will also be adequate in sulfur.

Potassium, Sodium, and Chloride

electrolytes—substances that carry an electrical charge when dissolved in water

Potassium, sodium, and chloride are grouped together because they are **electrolytes** that perform similar types of functions. One important function they all serve is to aid in water balance. In Chapter 4 we discussed the role of dissolved mineral ions and soluble proteins in controlling the movement of water from one region of the body to another. Recall that water moves through a membrane from the side with the lesser concentration of dissolved particles toward the side with the greater concentration until the concentrations are equalized. The electrolytes are the minerals most involved in water balance.

Potassium (K^+) is the electrolyte found in the highest concentration within body cells; magnesium, phosphates, and sulfates are also found there. Sodium (Na^+) and chloride (Cl^-) are found in highest concentration in extracellular fluids (outside cells) such as blood plasma. On each side of the membrane, the sum of the negatively charged ions is about equal to the sum of positively charged particles. Transmission of nerve impulses and muscle contraction depend on the rapid fluxes of these ions across membranes and back.

Chloride also functions in the body in a buffering system that compensates for excess acid or alkali.

Problems with Excess Although the body has mechanisms for dealing with considerable variation in levels of potassium, sodium, and chloride, it is possible to overwhelm the body's systems. The following Slice of Life about

Ryan, an infant who died from potassium intoxication, is a catastrophic example.

Ryan's case was an example of acute overdose of potassium, in which the excess was large and was ingested over a short period of time. Excesses of sodium and chloride are more apt to be chronic, which occurs when smaller excesses are ingested over a longer period of time.

Many scientists believe that chronic excess consumption of sodium may be related to the development of **essential hypertension,** or unexplained high blood pressure, which is a major risk factor for cardiovascular disease and stroke. Almost 58 million people in the United States have hypertension, including 39 million who are under the age of 65. The incidence of hypertension increases with age and is more prevalent in blacks (38%) than in whites (29%) (Surgeon General, 1988).

essential hypertension—high blood pressure of unexplained origin

The Surgeon General's 1988 Report notes: "While some people maintain normal blood pressure levels over a wide range of sodium intake, others appear to be 'salt sensitive' and display increased blood pressure in response to high sodium intakes." Since there is no quick, practical way to identify people who are sensitive to salt, and since no one would be harmed by moderate sodium restriction, many experts recommend moderate sodium restriction by everyone.

For many patients with high blood pressure, medications such as diuretics (which increase urinary sodium losses) are often used to help control

Slice of Life

The Colic "Cure" That Was a Killer

Ryan was a pleasant infant. He ate well and fell asleep soon after each feeding. One day, when he was 10 weeks old, he became quite irritable. After ruling out various other possibilities, his mother concluded he was having "colic" and sought advice from Adelle Davis's book *Let's Have Healthy Children.* The book suggests giving potassium supplements and reports that 653 colicky babies experienced "dramatic improvement" when given from 1000 to 3000 mg of potassium chloride by mouth.

Trusting the book, Ryan's mother offered him the recommended dosage of potassium from a bottle obtained at a health food store. According to the official report of the county medical examiner, Ryan received two doses of potassium chloride totaling 3000 mg along with breast milk on the first day. On the following morning, his symptoms recurred and he was given 1500 mg more. A few hours later, he became listless and stopped breathing. Despite resuscitation efforts and intensive hospital treatment, he died of potassium intoxication about 36 hours later. It was calculated that Ryan had received at least four times the dose needed for treatment *if he had been deficient in potassium,* which he was not.

Many people, unfortunately, hold the belief that "if a little is good, more is better." The above case report is a dramatic example that the idea is not true when it comes to nutrients. ▲

Reference: Marshall, C.W. 1983. *Vitamins and minerals: Help or harm?* Philadelphia: George F. Stickley Company.

Blood pressure can be affected by nutrition. If you have inherited the tendency to have high blood pressure, certain dietary factors may hasten or delay the onset of hypertension.

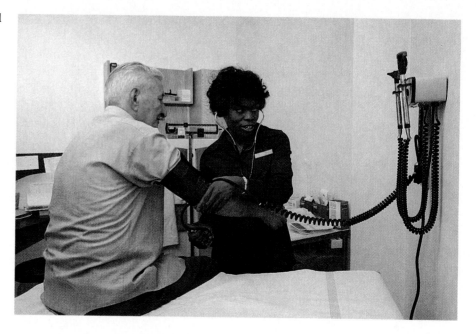

hypertension. Because these medications may have side effects, some physicians encourage hypertensive patients to restrict their sodium intakes because doing so may lessen the doses of medication needed to control the blood pressure. Some types of diuretics also cause loss of potassium, so patients need to be deliberate about replacing it.

It would be a mistake to assume that all research on hypertension centers on sodium metabolism. A number of investigators have suggested that excessive intakes of chloride; low intakes of potassium, calcium, and/or magnesium; obesity; and excess alcohol intake are related to hypertension (Surgeon General, 1988). Several investigators have noted interactions among these elements that may be helpful in explaining apparently conflicting data (Greger, 1989a). For example, ingestion of high levels of sodium chloride tends to increase urinary losses of calcium.

Requirements and Recommendations The Subcommittee on the RDAs did not establish recommendations for sodium, potassium, and chloride. However, the committee estimated that the average adult who does not sweat actively has a "minimum requirement" of 500 mg of sodium, 2000 mg of potassium, and 750 mg of chloride per day.

As you know from the discussion above, there is concern that Americans may get too much sodium rather than not enough. Although the 1989 RDA did not state an upper limit for sodium, it referred to the recommendation in the National Research Council's report *Diet and Health:* limit intake of sodium chloride to 6 grams per day or less, which is approximately 2400 mg of sodium at the upper end.

What about the electrolyte requirements of people such as athletes who sweat profusely? Sodium and chloride are the two primary electrolytes lost in sweat. (Potassium is lost to a much lesser degree.) But the solution of sodium and chloride that leaves the body as perspiration is only about one-third as concentrated as the solution of those same electrolytes in normal body fluids. Therefore, when you perspire, you lose relatively more water than electrolytes, and sodium and chloride become more concentrated within body fluids. For this reason, it is important to restore water losses but generally unnecessary to worry about sodium and chloride repletion. Exercise physiologist David Costill notes that distance runners studied in his laboratory who lost 6 to 9 pounds of sweat and drank nearly half a gallon of water per day retained normal plasma levels of sodium, chloride, and potassium (Costill, 1986) even when their food was unseasoned.

Some people take salt tablets in a well-intentioned effort to replace sodium and chloride. This is not recommended because it can make the overall situation worse: concentrated salt in the GI tract will result in water initially moving *from* surrounding tissues into the lumen, aggravating dehydration. Again, water must be restored first, and salt restored later if necessary. A different potential problem with taking salt tablets is that they may resist being dissolved and stick to the lining of the stomach where they can cause irritation.

Typical Intakes and Sources Foods produced by nature contain only modest amounts of sodium, with animal products having more than plant foods. Processing often adds much more sodium to a food than was there to begin with: pickles, salty snack foods, processed cheeses, and smoked meats and sausages often contain several hundred milligrams of sodium per serving. Experts believe that at least one-third of the sodium ingested in foods by most Americans was added during processing (Surgeon General, 1988). Much of this sodium is added in the form of sodium chloride—ordinary table salt. Table 13.5 enables you to compare the sodium contents of processed and unprocessed foods. Little data are available on the chloride content of food, but you can assume that salted foods will contain concentrated amounts of chloride as well as sodium.

Experts estimate that we add to food about one-third of the sodium we consume, but people vary a great deal in the amount of salt they add. These data cannot be obtained from diet recalls or records, because people cannot accurately remember how much salt they added. The method scientists use is to measure sodium and salt excretion in urine, since more than 90% of ingested sodium and chloride is excreted by healthy adults. On that basis, experts have estimated that men in Western cultures consume approximately 11 grams of salt daily. Because salt is 40% sodium and 60% chloride, that means that such men might consume more than 4 g of sodium and 6 g of chloride daily (Sanchez-Castillo et al., 1987). These intakes are a great deal above the minimum required levels, and some experts believe they are excessive (Surgeon General, 1988). Most adults could reduce their sodium intake considerably by restricting their addition of salt to food and reducing their intake of certain processed foods.

Water usually also contains some sodium. The level of sodium that occurs in the natural (hard) water supply varies considerably from one region to

Table 13.5 Sodium and Potassium in Some Foods

Food	Household Measure	Milligrams of Sodium (0–1500)	Milligrams of Potassium (0–1000)
Fruits and vegetables			
Apple	1 medium		
Banana	1 medium		
Beans, green, cooked without salt	½ cup		
Beans, green, canned with salt	½ cup		
Cucumber	1 large		
Dill pickle	1 large, 3¾ inches		
Orange juice	½ cup		
Peach, fresh	1 medium		
Peaches, canned, juice pack	½ cup		
Potato, baked	1 average		
Potato chips	1 ounce (14 chips)		
Grain products			
Biscuit, homemade	1 medium		
Bread, whole grain	1 slice		
Bread, enriched	1 slice		
Macaroni, cooked without salt	½ cup	tr	
Milk and milk products			
Milk	1 cup		
Cheese, cheddar	1⅓ ounces		
Cheese, processed	2 ounces		
Yogurt, plain	1 cup		
Meats and meat alternates			
Beef, ground, cooked without salt	2 ounces		
Corned beef, canned	2 ounces		
Frankfurter	2 ounces		
Salmon, fresh	2 ounces		
Salmon, canned with salt	2 ounces		
Walnuts, chopped	½ cup		
Peanut butter	¼ cup		
Combination foods			
Bean burrito	3 oz beans		
Cheese pizza	⅛ of 15-inch pie		
Cream of mushroom soup made with milk	1 cup		
Spaghetti, canned entree with meat	1 cup		
Limited extras			
Beer	12 ounces		
Butter	1 teaspoon		
Salt	1 teaspoon	▶ 2000	
Soy sauce	1 tablespoon		
Sugar	1 tablespoon	tr	tr

another. Home water softeners can add still more of this mineral to water, because the softening process substitutes sodium for the calcium and magnesium that made the water hard. Nonetheless, water is usually only a minor source of sodium; the average person will ingest less than 100 mg of sodium daily from water (based on amounts typically used in food preparation and as a beverage), assuming whatever water is used contains approximately 20 mg of sodium per quart (Safe Drinking Water Committee, 1980).

Foods and water are not the only sources of sodium. Many medications, including over-the-counter drugs, contain more than 200 mg of sodium per dose.

As Table 13.5 shows, potassium is widespread in the food supply; many fruits, vegetables, milk and yogurt, meats, legumes, and nuts are especially good sources. But potassium tends to be lost when foods are processed. Experts at FDA estimate that typical men and women consume about 2000 and 2900 mg of potassium daily (Pennington et al., 1989). These amounts are only slightly above estimated minimum requirements.

Iron

Now for a discussion of the trace minerals. The first is iron.

Iron, like many other minerals, is a component of many enzymes. It is also a part of the blood protein **hemoglobin** and the muscle protein **myoglobin,** both of which can bind (carry) oxygen. Although iron accounts for less than 1% of the weight of these proteins, it enables them to perform the essential ongoing tasks of moving oxygen and carbon dioxide to and from all body cells.

hemoglobin—the iron-containing protein in blood that carries oxygen to cells and carbon dioxide away

myoglobin—the iron-containing protein in a muscle cell

Anemia: A Possible Symptom of Iron Deficiency   When humans consume amounts of iron that are inadequate to meet their needs, they become anemic. Iron deficiency is not the only cause of anemia, however.

Anemia is a condition in which a person's blood hemoglobin level or the hematocrit (concentration of red blood cells) is lower than normal. When this condition occurs, body cells receive less oxygen, and carbon dioxide wastes are removed less efficiently. These compromised functions cause an individual to feel tired or "run down."

Anemia can result from a number of causes, such as loss of blood due to surgery, accidents, or disease, including duodenal or stomach ulcers or cancers; genetic conditions; and various vitamin or mineral deficiencies. The most common cause of anemia is iron deficiency. The age groups most apt to develop anemia are children aged 1 to 5, pregnant women and adolescents, and young adult women. In the U.S., people whose family incomes are below the poverty level are more apt to have low hemoglobin levels than members of more affluent families.

The incidence of anemia among children in the United States has declined steadily during the last 20 years, and only 2.9% of children ages 6 months to 5 years were anemic in 1985 (Dallman and Yip, 1989). This improvement

anemia—general term indicating that the concentration of blood hemoglobin or of red blood cells is lower than normal

reflects the effect of iron supplementation of formulas and cereals and major public health efforts, such as the Supplemental Food Program for Women, Infants, and Children (to be discussed in Chapter 16).

Recently, a number of physicians have noted anemia among women athletes. The anemia is associated with low body stores of iron (Deuster et al., 1986). Although the anemia may be related to decreased iron absorption or increased iron losses in some women, many of the athletes report low intakes of iron.

Other Symptoms of Iron Deficiency People with iron deficiency also have depressed levels of iron-containing enzymes. This results in decreased work efficiency and decreased ability to maintain body temperature.

Iron deficiency is also associated with depression of immune function (Dallman, 1987). Repletion with iron must be done carefully in severely malnourished children because bacteria also need iron for growth. If too much iron is given too soon, it may promote bacterial proliferation faster than immune function recovery, which causes uncontrolled infections if antibiotics are not available. This is a concern particularly in the developing countries.

Iron Toxicity Although nutritionists are more concerned about iron *deficiency*, iron *toxicity* can also occur. Every year, about a dozen young children die from acute iron toxicity caused from having taken a large number of their mothers' iron supplements.

Chronic iron toxicity can occur in people with a genetic predisposition, especially men because they do not experience physiological losses of iron in menstruation and childbirth. Even when they consume fairly typical levels of iron, these men can experience iron overload, which can cause liver damage and, sometimes, cardiac failure. Excess use of alcohol exacerbates the problem in susceptible individuals.

Recommended and Typical Intakes Iron is an exception to the general rule that RDA values are higher for adult males than for adult females. Males, on the average, have larger bodies and more lean body mass, so they require more nutrients. However, the adult male RDA for iron is 10 mg, and that for females is 15 mg. Women require more dietary iron because of losses of iron during menstruation and childbirth.

The RDA for iron is 12 mg for adolescent males and 15 mg for adolescent females. These high iron recommendations reflect physiological changes that occur during the teen years. For males, the extra iron is used primarily to form additional lean body mass; for females, it is used both for additional lean body mass and to replace iron lost in menstruation.

The recommended intake of iron during pregnancy is 30 mg daily because of the large amount of iron needed by growing fetal, placental, and maternal tissues. It is impossible to obtain this level through diet alone during pregnancy, and the 1989 RDA Subcommittee recommended daily supplemental iron for this group.

For the general population, iron intakes do not parallel recommendations. The average adult male under 65 years in USDA surveys consumed more than 15 mg daily (Science and Education Administration, 1980), but the average female consumed 11 mg daily (HNIS, 1985). That means most men had adequate intakes of iron, but the average woman consumed only 74% of the RDA.

Sources Foods contain very uneven quantities of iron. Table 13.6 lists the iron content of common foods. Meat, fish, and poultry are superior sources because the heme iron and unidentified meat factor they contain make the iron in those foods very bioavailable. Eggs, legumes, nuts, whole grains, enriched cereal products, and leafy vegetables can also contribute significant amounts of iron to the diet.

Several foods are questionable sources of iron. For example, certain dried fruits, such as raisins and apricots, contain significant amounts of iron only if eaten in large amounts. (The drying process doesn't add iron to these foods; it just concentrates the iron and all other substances that were in the fresh product by removing most of the water.)

Molasses contains more iron than refined sugar does, but since it is very energy-dense, it is not suitable as a regular source of iron for most people: you would get a lot of kcalories with a little iron.

Iodine

Iodine makes its principal contribution to human functions as a component of thyroid hormones, primarily T3 and thyroxin (T4). (T3 has three iodines attached; thyroxin has four.) These hormones stimulate oxygen consumption and basal metabolic rates in tissues by a variety of mechanisms (Stanbury, 1988). They also affect cell development and growth in fetuses and children.

The RDA for adults for iodine is only 150 μg (0.15 mg) daily. This is truly a trace amount.

Sources Traditionally, the best dietary sources of iodine were ocean fish, other seafoods, and crops grown on land near the ocean. To supplement the diets of Amerians who did not live near salt water, iodine was added to table salt. This made iodized salt the major source of iodine for many Americans, especially those living in the Midwest.

In the 1970s, milk and grain products became the major dietary sources of iodine. This occurred because dairy cows were being fed more iodine, iodine-containing compounds were being used as disinfectant washes on cows' udders, and iodine-containing dough conditioners and other additives were used in commercially baked products.

Table 13.6 Iron in Some Foods

The RDA for iron for women is 15 mg/day; for men it is 10 mg/day.

Food	Household Measure	Milligrams of iron
Fruits and vegetables		
Apricots, raw	3 medium	
Apricots, dried	6 large halves	
Beans, green snap, cooked	½ cup	
Broccoli, chopped, cooked	½ cup	
Corn, cooked	½ cup	
Lettuce, iceberg	1 cup	
Orange juice	½ cup	
Peas, green, cooked	½ cup	
Potatoes, mashed with milk	½ cup	
Raisins	¼ cup	
Spinach, chopped, cooked	½ cup	
Turnip greens, chopped, cooked	½ cup	
Grain products		
Bread, whole grain	1 slice	
Bread, white enriched	1 slice	
Cereal, bran flakes, iron-fortified	1 ounce	
Cereal oat flakes, iron-fortified	1 ounce	
Cereal, shredded wheat	1 ounce	
Spaghetti, enriched	½ cup	
Milk and milk products		
Milk	1 cup	
Cheese, cheddar	1⅓ ounces	
Meats and meat alternates		
Almonds	½ cup	
Beans, canned with tomato sauce and pork	1 cup	
Beef, ground, broiled	2 ounces	
Chicken breast, cooked	2 ounces	
Eggs, hard-boiled	2	
Liver, beef, cooked	2 ounces	
Peanut butter	¼ cup	
Shrimp, canned	2 ounces	
Tuna, canned	2 ounces	
Walnuts, chopped	½ cup	
Limited extras		
Beer	12 ounces	
Butter, margarine	1 teaspoon	tr
Carbonated beverage, cola type	12 ounces	
Honey	1 tablespoon	
Molasses, light	1 tablespoon	
Sugar, white	1 tablespoon	tr

Because of these new sources of iodine, during the 1970s adult Americans may have consumed levels of iodine more than five times the 150 μg suggested in the RDAs. The Food and Drug Administration has successfully encouraged the food industry to reduce the use of iodine-containing compounds in recent years; FDA officials recently estimated a young man's typical intake to be 470 μg (313% of the RDA) for iodine (Pennington et al., 1989). They suggested that this decline reflected a lower iodine content in breads and cereals as a result of decreased use of a red dye that contained iodine. Decreased use of iodine-containing disinfectants on dairy farms may also have contributed to the decline.

Deficiency and Toxicity Enlargement of the thyroid gland, or **goiter,** is the most obvious symptom of iodine deficiency (see Figure 13.6). When iodine is inadequate in the diet, the thyroid gland does not have enough of this mineral to produce a normal amount of thyroid hormones. In an attempt to produce more of them, the thyroid gland enlarges. However, even with a larger mass of thyroid tissue, the gland may be unable to produce enough additional thyroid hormones.

In the early part of the twentieth century, goiters were very common in inland areas in the United States, especially in the Midwest. After iodized salt was accepted as a public health measure designed to increase iodine to recommended levels, the incidence of goiters dropped markedly. However, they are still **endemic** in inland areas of South America, Africa, and Asia.

Dietary factors and drugs that prevent the normal incorporation of iodine into thyroxin can also promote the development of goiters. This effect is accentuated in people who consume low or marginal levels of iodine.

goiter—enlargement of the thyroid gland, resulting primarily from iodine deficiency

endemic—very common in a population

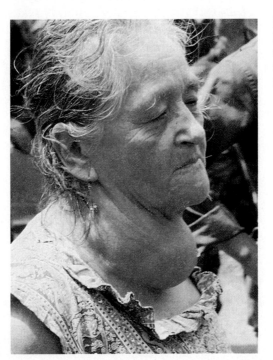

Figure 13.6 Goiter. Severe, long-term iodine deficiency results in enlargement of the thyroid gland, as you see in this woman.

cretinism—irreversible condition involving both mental and physical growth retardation; can occur in children of mothers who were severely iodine deficient during pregnancy

If iodine is deficient in the diets of pregnant women, there is the possibility of an additional penalty: the child may be born with **cretinism,** an irreversible condition characterized by both mental and physical growth retardation.

People who chronically ingest very high amounts of iodine may also develop goiter. This condition occurs among residents of certain areas of Japan who consume large amounts of iodine-rich seaweed (Stanbury, 1988).

Fluoride

Fluoride functions in teeth and bones by becoming part of the hydroxyapatite crystals and making them larger and less soluble. A certain minimal level of fluoride in the diet, therefore, increases resistance to dental caries.

The estimated adult safe and adequate intake range for fluoride is 1.5–4 mg daily. The major source of fluoride in most people's diets is water and (to a lesser extent) tea and the soft edible bones of fish. Topical application of fluoride by dentists, use of fluoride-containing toothpastes and powders, and ingestion of fluoride dentrifices are other sources of fluoride.

Fluoride is naturally present in the water supplies of some areas, but in regions with a temperate climate where less than 0.7 parts per million of fluoride is naturally found in water, public health agencies encourage that it be added to the level of 1 part per million. This level is equivalent to 1 ounce of fluoride in over 7750 gallons of water.

This small concentration of fluoride is associated with a reduced rate of dental caries (Sweeney and Shaw, 1988). Figure 13.7 shows the dramatic effect of adequate fluoride on the rates of decayed, missing, and filled teeth in children. Although fluoridation of water has had a very positive public health effect, the addition of fluoride to water remains controversial in some areas because of misinformation about its effects (Jones et al., 1989).

In 1990 officials at the Environmental Protection Agency indicated that they had preliminary data that suggested fluoride might be a weak carcinogen (Marshall, 1990). Their report has not yet been published, so there is no

Figure 13.7 The effect of fluoride on dental health. Here, you see the beneficial effect of adequate levels of fluoride intake. Children who did not ingest fluoride had two to three times more decayed, missing, and filled teeth than those who received at least 1 part per million of fluoride in their water supply. (From Sweeney and Shaw, 1988.)

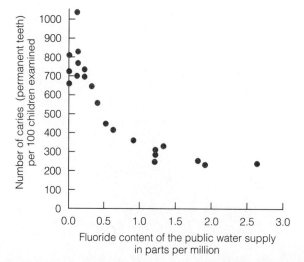

way to assess its validity. Experts are still recommending fluoridation of water.

The fact that small amounts of fluoride can lower the incidence of dental caries does not mean that *excess* fluoride is beneficial. People who habitually drink water that contains four or more times the recommended level may develop slight *mottling* (spotty discoloration) of their teeth. When the water supply contains eight times the recommended level, *fluorosis* may develop; this is a condition characterized by severe mottling of the teeth and eventual degenerative and crippling bone and joint disorders. Evidently, the safety range for fluoride is small, and addition of fluoride to water supplies must be done carefully.

Recently, physicians reported that treatment of osteoporotic women with large doses of "slow release" fluoride increased vertebral bone mass and decreased the frequency of vertebral fractures (Pak et al., 1989). They noted, however, that 16% of the patients had gastrointestinal or rheumatic complications. This therapy is experimental and the potential for toxicity is *great*; therefore, it should only be prescribed by physicians for postmenopausal women.

Zinc

Zinc makes its contribution to human health as a component of over 70 enzyme systems with a wide variety of functions. It is also necessary for adequate immune functions. If zinc is deficient in the diet, diverse symptoms occur, including loss of appetite, failure to grow, dermatitis, impaired healing of wounds, and decreased taste acuity.

Zinc Deficiency and Excess Zinc deficiency was first recognized in adults in villages in Iran and Egypt about 25 years ago. Investigators found adults who were unusually short and sexually immature; the abnormalities were corrected by zinc supplementation. It is not surprising, in retrospect, that the deficiency occurred: the local staple diet was low in zinc; the bioavailability of the small amount of zinc present was poor; and general infections and gut infestations resulted in high excretion of zinc.

Zinc deficiency is not limited to the Middle East. The symptoms of poor growth in children, poor wound healing in adults, scaly dermatitis, and impaired resistance to infections have also been seen in other parts of the world, including patients in North America. Some experts are particularly concerned about the zinc status of elderly people (Greger, 1989b), low-birth-weight infants, and infants with genetic defects (Hambidge et al., 1986). Figure 13.8 shows an infant with severe skin symptoms from zinc deficiency.

Because severe zinc deficiency was found to prevent sexual maturation and to impair sexual performance, some supplement promoters have suggested that normally healthy men can improve their sexual performance by taking zinc supplements. These claims are false: excessive zinc adds nothing

Figure 13.8 Zinc deficiency.
The skin of this infant shows the scaly dermatitis characteristic of severe zinc deficiency. (From Hambidge et al., 1978.)

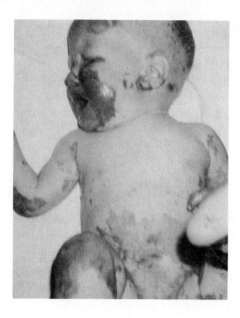

to performance beyond what is possible for the well-nourished individual.

On the other end of the spectrum, zinc toxicity can occur either as an **acute** or a **chronic** problem. Acute zinc toxicity with nausea and vomiting has been reported in some people who drank acidic beverages (such as lemonade) stored in galvanized (zinc-coated) containers. More frequently, chronic zinc toxicity has been reported among people who consumed high levels of zinc in supplements. The chronic ingestion of excess zinc depresses copper absorption and eventually *impairs* immune function and induces anemia (Fosmire, 1989).

acute—having a sudden onset and a short cause

chronic—persisting over a long period of time

Recommended Intakes and Sources The adult RDA for zinc is 15 mg for men and 12 mg for women. The average North American consumes less than 12 mg of zinc daily (Hambidge et al., 1986). Vegetarians, especially those who do not eat legumes frequently, and dieters with low energy intakes are likely to have low intakes of zinc.

Table 13.7 shows that the best dietary sources of zinc are seafood, red meats, nuts, and legumes. Other meat products, milk, and whole-grain products also contribute significant amounts to the diet. Of course, the bioavailability of zinc from some of these products—especially whole grains, legumes, and nuts—is lessened by the fiber and phytate they contain.

Selenium

Selenium is a trace mineral that came into the limelight in the 1980s. It is known to be interdependent with vitamin E, and in some instances a low level of one nutrient can be partly compensated for by the presence of the other.

Selenium is a component of an important enzyme called *glutathione peroxidase* that helps prevent damage to cell structures. A number of animal and epidemiological studies have shown that adequate selenium has a protective effect against certain cancers (Surgeon General, 1988), but the mechanism of this protective effect is not understood. Because it is known that excessive selenium intake can result in toxicity, the Surgeon General's Report states that "recommendations for increasing dietary intake are not warranted."

Selenium Deficiency and Excess The selenium content of grains varies according to the soil. Livestock that graze in regions with very low or high soil selenium levels suffer selenium deficiency and excess, respectively. But human diets, especially in the United States, are generally based on food-stuffs grown in a variety of areas; therefore, the overall selenium content of

Table 13.7 Zinc in Some Foods

The RDA for zinc is 15 mg for men; 12 mg for women per day.

Food	Household Measure	Milligrams of Zinc
Fruits and vegetables		
Apple	1 medium	tr
Banana	1 medium	▮
Corn, frozen, cooked	½ cup	▮
Peas, frozen, cooked	½ cup	▮
Grain products		
Bread, white	1 slice	▮
Bread, whole grain	1 slice	▮
Macaroni	½ cup	▮
Milk and milk products		
Milk, low fat	1 cup	▮
Meats and meat alternates		
Beef	2 ounces	▬▬
Chicken, dark meat	2 ounces	▮
Chicken, light meat	2 ounces	▮
Eggs	2	▮
Great northern beans, cooked	1 cup	▬
Walnuts	½ cup	▬
Peanut butter	¼ cup	▮
Shrimp, canned	2 ounces	▮
Fish, perch	2 ounces	▮
Combination foods		
Beef and vegetable stew	1 cup	▬▬
Lasagna, vegetarian	7.7 ounces	▮
Lasagna with meat	8.6 ounces	▬
Limited extras		
Fats, oils	1 tablespoon	tr
Gum drops, jelly beans	1 ounce	

Meat, fish, and poultry as sources of needed minerals. Iron and zinc are two minerals often found in short supply in the diets of Americans. Meat and fish are good sources of both. Furthermore, meat and fish furnish a form of iron that is absorbed better than that found in other foods.

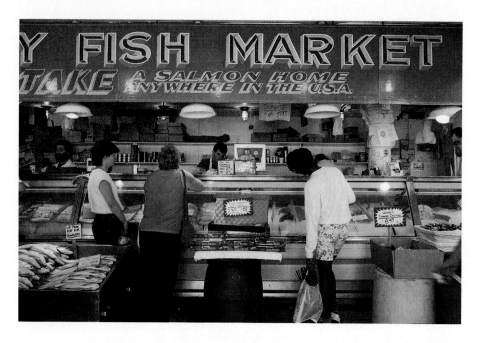

the diet is not much affected by the selenium content of the soils on which individual foods were grown.

There is one important exception. In a large area of western China, selenium intake is very low. There, a potentially fatal condition called *Keshan disease*, which is characterized by heart damage, is endemic in children and young women. In large studies in the 1970s, selenium supplements were given to thousands of children. The incidence of Keshan disease dropped to about 5% of the rate in controls. Despite this impressive response to raising selenium levels, the cause of Keshan disease is probably more complex than simple selenium deficiency. This belief is based on a number of observations; for one, in other locations with low selenium levels in foods, Keshan disease is not found (Levander, 1987).

Ironically, selenium *toxicity* has also been found in China; it has occurred naturally in some areas in which very high levels of selenium were found in local crops. In California, wildlife at the reservoir of a nature preserve suffered malformations due to very high levels of selenium in irrigation waters that drained into the reservoir. Toxicity has also occurred among people in the United States who consumed excess amounts of selenium supplements (Levander, 1988). Hair and nail loss were the most common symptoms that occurred with chronic ingestion of more than 1 mg of selenium daily.

Recommended Intakes and Sources   An RDA was set for selenium for the first time in 1989. For men, the recommended daily selenium intake is 70 μg (.07 mg); for women, it is 55 μg (.055 mg). These recommendations are based on extensive studies worldwide. Experts at FDA estimate that men and women in the United States typically consume 100 μg and 70 μg of selenium, respectively; therefore, American diets appear to be adequate in selenium.

Selenium is obtained primarily from grains, seafood, and meats. As mentioned above, the selenium content of grains is quite variable, depending on the selenium content of the soil on which they are grown. The bioavailability of different forms of selenium that occur in foods also varies.

Other Trace Minerals: Copper, Manganese, Cobalt, Chromium, Molybdenum, and Boron

These minerals have a variety of functions. Copper is a component of many enzymes and is important in the synthesis of collagen, normal cardiovascular function, and normal immune function. Since copper influences iron metabolism, copper deficiency can result in anemia.

Manganese and molybdenum, like many other minerals, are best known as components of enzymes with a variety of functions. Cobalt also is needed in the diet only insofar as it is a component of vitamin B-12. Other cobalt that may be present does not have any biological function.

Chromium aids in normal glucose metabolism, apparently by working with insulin.

Boron is essential for plants, but it has not been established as essential for animals. One group of researchers has observed that ingestion of additional boron increased circulating estrogen levels and reduced urinary calcium losses in postmenopausal women (Nielsen et al., 1987). It is too early to draw conclusions from these limited data.

Estimated Safe and Adequate Intakes and Typical Intakes   The 1989 RDA gives safe and adequate daily dietary ranges for these trace elements. The recommended range of intake for copper is 1.5–3 mg daily. The typical daily copper intake of most adult North Americans is believed to be 0.8–1.2 mg (Pennington et al., 1989). Experts are concerned, but recognized symptoms of copper deficiency are rarely seen.

The recommended range of intake for manganese is 2.0–5.0 mg per day. Typical intakes of adults in the United States are believed to be within the lower part of this range, approximately 2–3 mg/day (Pennington et al., 1989).

Recommended intakes for adults for chromium are 50 to 200 μg daily. Those for molybdenum are 75–250 μg daily. Reliable data on typical intakes are not available. As yet, there has been no recommendation made for boron intake.

Sources   For several reasons, it is not possible to give reliable data for the copper, manganese, chromium, and molybdenum content of foods. First, the analyses for chromium, molybdenum, and boron are difficult to perform, and those that have been done have resulted in only a limited amount of usable information. Second, the amounts of trace minerals in many foods are extremely variable, depending on the minerals' concentration in the soil, in the water, and/or in the fertilizer involved in food production. The amounts of certain trace minerals in root vegetables can vary by severalfold (Allaway, 1986); the trace mineral content of seafood is also affected by environmental conditions. For these reasons, no single value can be regarded as representative of any of these minerals in a particular food.

Despite analytical problems and natural variation, these trace minerals are thought to be widely distributed in foods as they come from nature; people who eat a wide variety of foods are likely to get what they need. Furthermore, since the foods available in any given part of North America have come from many different regions, the likelihood is greater that at least some good sources of these minerals will be present.

Because refinement processes generally remove much of the trace mineral content of foods, you will get more trace minerals from minimally processed items such as whole grains; but you will get very little from such foods as white flour, sugars, and fats.

Nonetheless, it is a mistake to think that food processing always decreases the trace mineral content of foods. Trace elements are sometimes added intentionally and unintentionally during processing. We'll talk more about the effects of processing on minerals in Chapter 14.

Mineral Intake Should Be Neither Too Low Nor Too High

We have mentioned that different mineral deficiencies have different results; for example, low iron intake can lead to a type of anemia, low iodine can result in goiter, and prolonged low calcium intake by children and young adults may result in a lower peak bone mass that increases the risk of osteoporosis. Does this mean that mineral deficiencies are rampant in developed countries?

Deficiencies

Generally speaking, deficiencies are more likely to occur if several precipitating factors are present at the same time. The following factors, usually in combination, are likely to cause mineral deficiencies:

1. The diet is limited in overall quantity, resulting in low intake of minerals and all other nutrients.
2. The diet is poorly selected for mineral content because of lack of knowledge, unavailability of certain foods, or poverty.
3. Bioavailability of minerals is low, for any of the many reasons discussed early in this chapter.
4. The individual cannot absorb, utilize, or maintain minerals normally because of inborn metabolic problems, disease conditions, or alcohol or other drug use.

5. Requirements for minerals are unusually high because of rapid growth or disease.

Given these factors, it's not hard to predict which categories of people will be most at risk of mineral deficiency. As an example, some elderly individuals may have limited total food intake owing to medical, social, or psychological problems that result in low intakes of zinc; they may selectively avoid meat, a good source of zinc, because they have trouble chewing it; they may suffer from a variety of conditions that cause zinc to be used inefficiently; and they may use a variety of medications that interfere with zinc utilization (Greger, 1989b).

Another group at risk for zinc deficiency is pregnant vegan women. A pregnant woman has a high requirement for minerals, but a vegan may be consuming a diet with low levels of zinc and other minerals or a diet with poor mineral bioavailability. Poverty, especially in developing countries, tends to exacerbate these problems; therefore, more individuals tend to be at risk in developing countries than in developed countries. Keep in mind that being "at risk" does not *guarantee* that a person will develop a deficiency but makes it statistically *more likely* to occur.

As with vitamin deficiencies, mild mineral deficiencies are not apt to produce distinct symptoms; rather, they may have certain common consequences, such as a decline in reproductive performance and compromised ability to deal with injury or infection.

Excesses

The old saying, "If a little is good, more is better" is not true for any nutrients, including minerals. It is definitely possible to ingest quantities that are too large. Ingesting unbalanced amounts of individual trace minerals is not only unscientific but also potentially dangerous. Finding the range between too little and too much is the key to good mineral nutrition.

Interference with Other Minerals   We have already mentioned one way in which mineral excess may be damaging: a large dietary intake of one mineral, such as zinc, can depress the absorption of another mineral, such as copper. And if the intake of copper is already low, the excess of zinc, although not toxic per se, will interfere with copper status.

Such imbalances rarely occur when people get their minerals in food, but they can occur fairly easily if people supplement their diets with individual minerals. Consumers should be very cautious about taking a mineral supplement to ensure their health; they may do more harm than good.

Toxicities   There are two general types of toxicities: acute and chronic. *Acute* toxicities occur when very large doses of a mineral are consumed; the effects are rapid and severe. We have already mentioned examples, such as when picnickers store acidic lemonade in galvanized (zinc-coated) containers or when a child consumes a bottle of Mother's iron supplements. Acute poisonings of this sort usually cause nausea, vomiting, and diarrhea; they can be fatal.

Most cases of mineral toxicity occur more gradually and are due to *chronic* exposure to lower-level excesses of the mineral. Three examples—iodine, fluoride, and iron—have already been discussed. Other minerals are also known for their toxicity; these include lead, cadmium, and mercury. Although many of the reported cases of such toxicities were due to industrial exposure, occasionally these minerals enter the food supply in sufficient quantities to be toxic. This topic will be discussed in Chapter 15.

A number of factors can affect the development of toxicity. In general, children are more sensitive than adults to toxic doses of minerals, particularly because of their smaller size. Also, there is considerable individual variation in sensitivity. Genetics also plays a role; as mentioned earlier, some people have a genetic predisposition to accumulate iron to abnormally high levels over time.

This chapter's Nutrition for Living section offers general suggestions for achieving adequate, but not excessive levels of minerals in your diet.

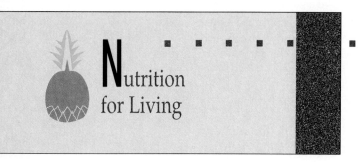

Nutrition for Living

There are several measures you can take to optimize your overall intake of minerals. Fortunately, these suggestions dovetail with many recommendations we have made previously for improving your diet in regard to other nutrients.

- Emphasize the Basic Food Guide foods in your diet. If you need more food than the minimum number of servings suggest, eat more foods from the basic groups rather than eating large amounts of limited extras.
- Vary your choices of food even within the basic food groups; this will increase your chances of getting the variety of trace minerals you need as well as the recommended amounts of major minerals.
- Choose foods that are less processed rather than the highly processed forms; minimally processed foods usually furnish more of the minerals you need (such as the trace minerals and potassium) and less of the mineral many of us should get less of (sodium).
- If you are a vegan, be especially careful to include good sources of calcium, zinc, and iron in your diet. This is important not only because plant foods are generally lower in these nutrients, but also because materials present in foods of plant origin may interfere with the bioavailability of the minerals.
- Don't resort to using mineral supplements to achieve recommended levels of intake; mineral supplements can interfere with metabolism of other minerals and are not recommended for most people.

There Are Several Ways to Evaluate Your Mineral Intake

Because we have discussed the difficulties in setting nutrition requirements and determining some mineral contents of foods, you might wonder if there is a way to evaluate your mineral intake with any reliability. Actually, we do have enough information to estimate the mineral adequacy of diets with some accuracy.

Methods You Have Already Used

You have been encouraged to use the Basic Food Guide (Assessment 2.2) as a technique for quickly evaluating overall diet quality and planning for adequate intakes. Although the guide is somewhat less useful for promoting adequate intakes of minerals than for most other nutrient groups, a diet that follows the recommendations of the Basic Food Guide is likely to contain at least one-half to two-thirds of the recommended levels of the essential minerals.

You have also had experience with using food composition tables to assess more specifically the level of nutrients in your diet. When you did Assessment 2.1, one of the things you determined was the status of your diet in regard to those minerals for which reliable data exist (information about these minerals is listed in Appendices E and F).

There is another way of looking at mineral intake that can be useful, especially for those minerals that are difficult for some people to consume in adequate amounts. This method involves determining nutrient density.

Calculation of Nutrient Density

Nutrient density is a term used to describe whether a food is a good source of a nutrient relative to the kcalories it contains. Usually, nutrient density is expressed as the quantity of a particular nutrient contained in 100 kcalories of the food. For example, a ground beef patty has a nutrient density for zinc of 2.1 mg per 100 kcalories; this was calculated from the food composition information that 245 kcalories of ground beef contains 5.1 mg of zinc.

Once you have determined the density of a given nutrient in a variety of foods, as shown in Assessment 13.1, you can readily make comparisons between the sources. If your diet is inadequate in a particular nutrient, knowing foods in which that nutrient is most dense can help you plan for a better intake. Assessment 13.1 guides you through an assessment of nutrient density.

Calculating Nutrient Density for a Selected Mineral

Because calcium, zinc, and iron are three minerals many people have trouble getting in the quantities suggested by the RDA, it makes sense to consider their density in various foods. The procedure is described below, and an example is given in Sample Assessment 13.1.

Assessment 13.1

1. Decide whether to evaluate your diet for its nutrient density of calcium, zinc, or iron. Check Assessment 2.1 (the first one you did) to see whether your intake of either of these was low; if so, use that nutrient.
2. Circle the name of the mineral you have chosen to assess in the third column heading of Assessment 13.1.
3. Copy your menu from Assessment 2.1 onto the sample assessment form for this chapter, and transfer to the appropriate columns the contents of the mineral in the foods you ate, the total, and your RDA for that mineral. In addition, copy the energy content of the foods.
4. Divide the mineral content of each food by the kcalorie value of the food; this will give you the nutrient density of the mineral per kcalorie of food. Since nutrient density is usually expressed in nutrient content per 100 kcalories of food, multiply your answer by 100, and enter the product in the nutrient density column.
5. Scan the nutrient densities of all foods in the column. Rank your top three sources next to their nutrient density values as (1), (2), and (3).
6. Now scan the column of absolute content for the mineral. Rank the top three next to their absolute values as (A), (B), and (C). These rankings will not automatically correspond with the nutrient density rankings, but they might.
7. Now that you've gathered the facts, go on to *Critical Thinking* 13.1 on page 464 to consider how you could use this information to improve the quality of your diet.

Food or Beverage	Approximate Measure	Absolute Calcium, Zinc, or Iron Content	Energy (Kcal)	Nutrient Density (mg/100 kcalories)
Egg bagel	1	20	180	11
Jelly	1 T.	2	49	4
Orange pop	12 oz.	15	170	9
McDonald's cheeseburger	2	398 (A)	620	64 (3)
French fries	regular	14	320	4
McDonald's cookies	small box	12	290	4
Cola drink	12 oz.	9	151	6
Pork chop—lean only	2½ oz.	3	172	2
Baked potato	1 avg.	8	145	6
Frozen peas, cooked	½ c.	19	63	30
Butter	2 t.	2	68	3
Iceberg lettuce	2 c.	22 (C)	14	157 (2)
French dressing	1 oz.	4	134	3
2% milk	½ c.	149 (B)	61	244 (1)
Graham crackers	2 squares	6	60	10
Total		683		
RDA		1200		

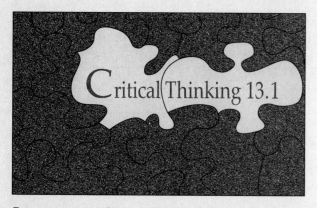

Critical Thinking 13.1

Improving Your Mineral Intake Using Nutrient Density Information

The situation

You analyzed your diet using food composition information in Assessment 2.1. In that assessment, you learned that your intake of one of the minerals most likely to be deficient in people's diets (calcium, zinc, or iron) was also inadequate in yours. Focusing on that mineral, you did Assessment 13.1 to learn about its density in the foods you ate that day.

Now you want to use this information to see how you could have improved your intake of that mineral on that particular day. You will use this information to help you in future food selection.

Is the information accurate and relevant?

■ If the day's intake you recorded is close to your average intake, the assessment will be relevant.
■ If your diet record and analysis and nutrient density calculations were carefully done, your findings should be accurate.

What else needs to be considered?

First, you need to decide how much of the mineral you need to add to your diet. Achieving the level of your RDA would be optimal, but your intake will vary somewhat from day to day. Since many experts regard 70% of the RDA as sufficient to meet many people's needs, taking in an amount that is 70–100% of the RDA each day would be a good goal.

As you consider how your diet might have been improved for the day you analyzed, keep in mind that you need to meet not only the scientific criteria, but also your own individual standards of acceptability. In other words, don't plan to eat in a way you know you won't.

As you plan dietary changes that will affect your intake of the mineral in question, keep the other nutrients in your diet in mind as well. As you think about adding (or increasing) some foods and excluding (or decreasing) others, don't jeopardize the adequacy of other important substances.

Also keep kcalories in mind. If your dietary changes would result in a net increase in kcalories and you don't want to gain weight, think of ways you could reduce the energy value of the diet while retaining nutritional value. Reducing the obvious fat in the diet is one effective way to do this.

What do you think?

What seems to you to be the best way to achieve an increase in the mineral in question?

■ Option 1 You could consume more of the food on your record that has the *highest nutrient density* for this mineral.
■ Option 2 You could consume more of the mineral source that was best on an *absolute basis*.
■ Option 3 You could look for other foods that are good sources of this mineral.
■ Option 4 You could consider a modest supplement of this mineral.

Do you see any other options? Given your own individual circumstances and preferences, which option do you prefer?

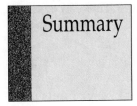

Summary

▶ Both vitamins and minerals are important micronutrients widespread in basic foods; the main difference between them is that vitamins are organic (carbon-containing) and **minerals** are inorganic, being simply individual chemical elements. Depending on the amounts present, essential minerals are categorized as either **macrominerals** or **trace minerals.** Some minerals present in the body are needed for growth, reproduction, and maintenance of health, and are considered essential. Minerals are not present in proportion to their importance; trace and major mineral deficiencies both can be damaging to health.

▶ Many factors can influence the **bioavailability** of minerals, making specific intake recommendations difficult to establish. For example, both vitamin C and the **unidentified meat factor** can increase the absorption of **nonheme iron** in the diet; and vitamin D is needed for optimal absorption of calcium and phosphorus. On the other hand, dietary fiber, **phytate, tannins,** and **oxalates** can depress the absorption of minerals, and minerals can compete with each other for absorption. Medications and physiological factors can also affect mineral absorption and excretion. Supplementing a diet with individual minerals may adversely alter the bioavailability of other minerals.

▶ Minerals function in four structural and regulatory ways: (1) they form part of tissue structure, (2) they help maintain water and acid–base balance, (3) they form components of enzymes and hormones, and (4) they facilitate the function of nerve and muscle cells. Tables 13.3–13.7 list food sources for essential minerals, and Table 13.2 summarizes key information about their RDAs, major functions, and signs of deficiency or excess.

▶ Mineral deficiencies are most likely to arise when the following combination of circumstances exists: (1) the overall diet is limited in quantity, (2) the diet is poorly selected for mineral content, (3) mineral bioavailability is low, and (4) mineral requirements are unusually high because of rapid growth or disease. All of these factors are less likely to occur simultaneously in the developed countries than in less developed parts of the world. The most common mineral deficiencies worldwide are for iron, iodine, and zinc.

▶ It is definitely possible to consume mineral overdoses; overdoses can both interfere with the absorption of other minerals and cause either acute or chronic toxicity symptoms, depending on the type and duration of exposure. The minerals necessary to health can be obtained in almost all cases by simply eating a balanced and varied diet; mineral supplements are not necessary for most people.

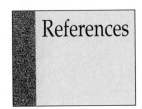

References

Allaway, W.H. 1986. Soil-plant-animal and human interrelationships in trace element nutrition. In *Trace elements in human and animal nutrition*, volume 2, ed. W. Mertz. Orlando, FL: Academic Press.

Block, G., C.M. Dresser, A.M. Hartman, and M.D. Carroll. 1985. Nutrient sources in the American diet: Quantitative data from the NHANES II Survey. I: Vitamins and minerals. *American Journal of Epidemiology* 122:13–26.

Consensus Conference. 1984. Osteoporosis. *Journal of the American Medical Association* 252:799–802.

Costill, D.L. 1986. *Inside running*. Indianapolis: Benchmark Press.

Dallman, P.R. 1987. Iron deficiency and the immune response. *American Journal of Clinical Nutrition* 46:329–334.

Dallman, P.R. and R. Yip. 1989. Changing characteristics of childhood anemia. *Journal of Pediatrics* 114:161–164.

Deuster, P.A., S.B. Kyle, P.B. Moser, R.A. Vigersky, A. Singh, and E.B. Shoomaker. 1986. Nutritional survey of highly trained women runners. *American Journal of Clinical Nutrition* 45:954–962.

Ettinger, B., H.K. Genant, and C.E. Cann. 1987. Postmenopausal bone loss is prevented by treatment with low-dosage estrogen with calcium. *Annals of Internal Medicine* 106:40–45.

Ford, A.B. 1989. Reducing the threat of hip fracture. *American Journal of Public Health* 79:269–270.

Fosmire, G.J. 1989. Possible hazards associated with zinc supplementation. *Nutrition Today* 24(no. 3):15–18.

Greger, J.L., C.E. Kryzkowski, R.R. Khazen, and C.L. Krashoc. 1987. Mineral utilization by rats fed various commercially available calcium supplements or milk. *Journal of Nutrition* 117:717–724.

Greger, J.L. 1989a. Effect of dietary protein and minerals on calcium and zinc utilization. *Critical Reviews of Food Science and Nutrition* 28:249–271.

———. 1989b. Potential for trace mineral deficiencies and toxicities in the elderly. In *Mineral homeostasis in the elderly*, ed. C.W. Bales. New York: Alan R. Liss, Inc.

Hambidge, K.M., C.E. Casey, and N.F. Krebs. 1986. Zinc. In *Trace elements in human and animal nutrition*, volume 2, ed. W. Mertz. Orlando, FL: Academic Press.

Heaney, R.P., J.C. Gallagher, C.C. Johnson, R. Neer, A.M. Parfitt, B. Chir, and G.D. Whedon. 1982. Calcium nutrition and bone health in the elderly. *American Journal of Clinical Nutrition* 36:986–1013.

HNIS (Human Nutrition Information Service). 1985. *Nationwide Food Consumption Survey, Continuing Survey of Food Intake by Individuals*. Rep 85-1. Hyattsville, MD: U.S. Department of Agriculture.

———. 1986. *Nationwide Food Consumption Survey, Continuing Survey of Food Intake by Individuals. Men 19–50 Years, 1 Day*. Report 85-3. Hyattsville, MD: USDA.

Johnson, M.A. and C.L. Murphy. 1988. Adverse effects of high dietary iron and ascorbic acid on copper status in copper-deficient and copper-adequate rats. *American Journal of Clinical Nutrition* 47:96–101.

Jones, R.B., D.N. Mormann, and T.B. Durtsche. 1989. Fluoridation referendum in LaCrosse, Wisconsin: Contributing factors to success. *American Journal of Public Health* 79:1405–1408.

Karanja, N. and D.A. McCarron. 1986. Calcium and hypertension. *Annual Reviews of Nutrition* 6:475–484.

Levander, O.A. 1987. A global view of human selenium nutrition. *Annual Reviews of Nutrition* 7:227–250.

Lonnerdal, B. 1987. Protein-mineral interactions. In *Nutrition 1987*. Washington, DC: Federation of American Societies of Experimental Biology.

Marshall, E. 1990. The fluoride debate: one more time. *Science* 247:276–277.

Merhav, H., Y. Amitai, H. Patti, and S. Godfrey. 1985. Tea drinking and microcytic anemia in infants. *American Journal of Clinical Nutrition* 41:1210–1213.

Miller, S.A. 1987. Lead in calcium supplements. *Journal of the American Medical Association* 257:1810.

Monsen, E.R. 1988. Iron nutrition and absorption: Dietary factors which impact iron bioavailability. *Journal of the American Dietetic Association* 88:786–790.

Munoz, L.M., B. Lonnerdal, C.L. Keen, and K.G. Dewey. 1988. Coffee consumption as a factor in iron deficiency anemia among pregnant women and their infants in Costa Rica. *American Journal of Clinical Nutrition* 48:645–651.

National Research Council. 1989. *Diet and health*. Washington, DC: National Academy Press.

Nelson, M.E., E.C. Fisher, P.D. Catsos, C.N. Meredith, R.N. Turksoy, and W.J. Evans. 1986. Diet and bone status in amenorrheic runners. *American Journal of Clinical Nutrition* 43:910–916.

Nielsen, F.H., C.D. Hunt, L.M. Mullen, and J.R. Hunt. 1987. Dietary boron effects mineral estrogen and testosterone metabolism in postmenopausal women. *FASEB Journal* 1:394–397.

Pak, C.Y., K. Sakhaee, J.E. Zerwelch, C. Parcel, R. Peterson, and K. Johnson. 1989. Safe and effective treatment of osteoporosis with intermittent slow release sodium fluoride: Augmentation of vertebral bone mass and inhibition of fractures. *Journal of Clinical Endo-*

crinology and Metabolism 68:150–159.

Pennington, J.A., B.E. Young, and D.B. Wilson. 1989. Nutritional elements in U.S. diets: Results from the Total Diet Study, 1982–1986. *Journal of the American Dietetic Association* 89:659–664.

Raper, N.R., J.C. Rosenthal, C.E. Woteki. 1984. Estimates of available iron in diets of individuals 1 year and older in the Nationwide Food Consumption Survey. *Journal of the American Dietetic Association* 84:783–787.

RDA Subcommittee. 1989. *Recommended dietary allowances.* Washington, DC: National Academy Press.

Riis, B., K. Thomsen, and C. Christiansen. 1987. Does calcium supplementation prevent post-menopausal bone loss? *New England Journal of Medicine* 316:173–177.

Safe Drinking Water Committee. 1980. *Drinking water and health,* volume 3. Washington, DC: National Academy of Sciences.

Sanchez-Castillo, C.P., W.J. Branch, and W.P. James. 1987. A test of the validity of the lithium-marker technique for monitoring dietary sources of salt in men. *Clinical Science* 72:87–94.

Sanchez-Castillo, C.P., S. Warrender, T.P. Whitehead, and W.P. James. 1987. An assessment of the sources of dietary salt in a British population. *Clinical Science* 72:95–102.

Science and Education Administration. 1980. *Food and nutrient intakes of individuals in 1 day in the United States, Spring, 1977.* Nationwide food consumption survey 1977–78; preliminary report No. 2. Washington, DC: U.S. Department of Agriculture.

Seeman, E., J.L. Hopper, L.A. Bach, M.E. Cooper, E. Parkinson, J. McKay, and G. Jerums. 1989. Reduced bone mass in daughters of women with osteoporosis. *New England Journal of Medicine* 320:554–558.

Solomons, N.W. 1988. Physiological interaction of minerals. In *Nutrient interactions,* eds. C.E. Bodwell and J.W. Erdman. New York: Marcel Dekker.

Stanbury, J.B. 1988. Iodine. In *Modern nutrition in health and disease,* eds. M.E. Shils and V.R. Young. Philadelphia: Lea & Febiger.

Surgeon General. 1988. *Surgeon General's report on nutrition and health.* Washington, DC: U.S. Department of Health and Human Services.

Sweeney, E.A. and J.A. Shaw. 1988. Nutrition in relation to dental medicine. In *Modern nutrition in health and disease,* eds. M.E. Shils and V.R. Young. Philadelphia: Lea & Febiger.

Wargovich, M.J. 1988. Calcium and colon cancer. *Journal of the American College of Nutrition* 7:295–300.

Weaver, C.M., B.R. Martin, J.S. Ebner, and C.A. Krueger. 1987. Oxalic acid decreases calcium absorption in rats. *Journal of Nutrition* 117:1903–1906.

FOOD SAFETY: A CONCERN OF THE 90s

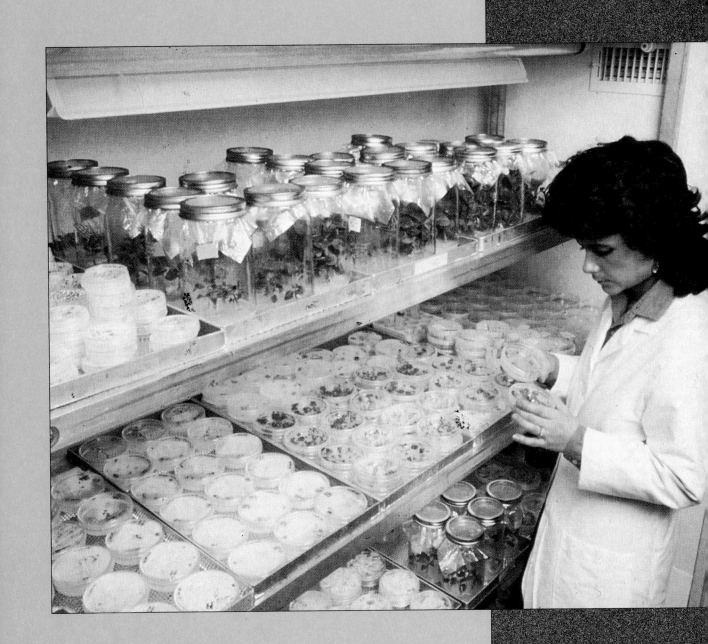